Advances and Technical Standards in Neurosurgery

Volume 51

This series, which has earned a reputation over the years and is considered a classic in the neurosurgical field, is now relaunched under the editorship of Professor Di Rocco, which relies on the collaboration of a renewed editorial board.

Both volumes focused on recent advances in neurosurgery and on technical standards, and monographs devoted to more specific subjects in the neurosurgical field will implement it. Written by key opinion leaders, the series volumes will be useful for young neurosurgeons in their postgraduate training but also for more experienced clinicians.

Nobuhito Morota • Paul Steinbok
Editors

Dorsal Rhizotomy: Neurosurgery for Childhood Spasticity

Vol. 51

Springer

Editors
Nobuhito Morota
Department of Neurosurgery
Kitasato University Hospital
Minami-Ku, Sagamihara, Japan

Paul Steinbok
Division of Neurosurgery, Department of Surgery
British Columbia Children's Hospital and University of British Columbia
Vancouver, BC, Canada

ISSN 0095-4829 ISSN 1869-9189 (electronic)
Advances and Technical Standards in Neurosurgery
ISBN 978-3-031-86440-7 ISBN 978-3-031-86441-4 (eBook)
https://doi.org/10.1007/978-3-031-86441-4

This Springer imprint is published by the registered company Springer Nature Switzerland AG
The registered company address is: Gewerbestrasse 11, 6330 Cham, Switzerland

This book is primarily dedicated to the disabled children who, despite experiencing spasticity, live actively lives in the face of their challenges.

This book is also dedicated to the parents and family members, who provide support and closely accompany their disabled children or sibling. Observing their deep affection for their children underscored our recognition of the limitations in our ability to effectively manage spasticity and enhance the daily happiness of these individuals. Their encouragement and heartfelt words served as the most potent and motivating force, propelling us to relentlessly pursue improved surgical interventions for spasticity.

Finally, this book is devoted to our dedicated team, "Rhizotomy for spasticity," comprising multidisciplinary medical professionals. Without their collaborative effort, the execution of rhizotomy surgery would be unattainable.

Preface to the Series

Advances and Technical Standards in Neurosurgery (ATSN) represents the successful achievement of the wish of Jean Brihaye, Bernard Pertuised, Fritz Loew, and Hugo Krayenbuhl to provide the European neurosurgeons in training with a high-level publication to accompany the teaching provided by the European postgraduate course. The project was conceived during the joint meeting of the German and Italian Neurosurgical Societies in Taormina in 1972, and the first volume was published in 1974. The English language was chosen to facilitate the international exchange of information and the circulation of scientific progress. Since then, the ATSN has hosted chapters by eminent European neurosurgeons and has become one of the most renowned educational tools on the continent for both young and experienced neurosurgeons. The successive editorial boards have maintained the ATSN's high scientific quality and ensured a good balance between contributions dealing with advances in neurosciences over the years and detailed descriptions of surgical techniques as well as analyses of clinical experiences. Additional appeal has been added by freedom granted by the editor and publisher in the length, style, and organization of the published papers.

The current series aims to preserve the original spirit of the publication and its high-level didactic function but intends to present itself not only as a historic European publication but also as a truly international forum for most advanced clinical research and modern operating standards.

Hannover, Germany

Concezio Di Rocco

Preface

Given the recent surge in interest in dorsal rhizotomy, this book aims to disseminate the latest information on dorsal rhizotomy for children with disabling, intractable spasticity caused by various pathologies. Several textbooks focusing on the treatment of spasticity, including dorsal rhizotomy, have been published previously. However, this is the first book dedicated exclusively to dorsal rhizotomy, serving as a practical guide and comprehensive source of information.

The book addresses recent surgical and intraoperative neurophysiological advancements, catering to pediatric neurosurgeons experienced in dorsal rhizotomy surgery. Furthermore, it aims to introduce dorsal rhizotomy to pediatric neurosurgeons worldwide, especially those in developing low- and middle-income countries, expanding the potential reach of the surgery to countless spastic children in need.

The book is structured into five sections:

1. The first section describes the history and neuroanatomical background of dorsal rhizotomy and spasticity.
2. The second section discusses selection and preoperative evaluation of surgical candidates.
3. The third section covers various surgical and intraoperative neurophysiological procedures used during the surgery. This section is critical for readers who are interested in learning the surgical procedure of the dorsal rhizotomy.
4. The fourth section emphasizes the importance and role of postoperative rehabilitation, functional evaluation, and long-term follow-up after the surgery, and discusses surgical outcomes.
5. The fifth section explores future perspectives of dorsal rhizotomy and offers guidance on initiating a rhizotomy program.

We hope this book contributes to the well-being of disabled children and families and enhances the practice and understanding of spasticity management for interdisciplinary dorsal rhizotomy teams.

Both editors sincerely thank Madona Samuel and Donatella Rizza for their invaluable cooperation, professional contributions, and efforts in editing this book. Special and heartfelt acknowledgment is extended to Professor Concezio Di Rocco for his unwavering support. Without his guidance and encouragement, this book would not have been initiated nor brought to fruition.

Minami-Ku, Sagamihara, Japan — Nobuhito Morota
Vancouver, BC, Canada — Paul Steinbok

Contents

Chapter 1
Introduction

Nobuhito Morota and Paul Steinbok

Over four decades have passed since the resurgence of dorsal rhizotomy for relief of spasticity, initiated by work of the Italian neurosurgeon Fasano [1]. He introduced the concept of intraoperative neurophysiology using 50 Hz electrical stimulation to discern dorsal roots/rootlets involved in the spastic process (abnormal) and therefore to be cut from the normal ones to be preserved [2]. Peacock, a pediatric neurosurgeon in South Africa, subsequently modified Fasano's procedure by shifting the surgical field from the conus medullaris to the cauda equina [3]. His modification made the procedure easier, safer, and facilitated precise spinal level identification and differentiation of the dorsal from the ventral root. As a result, it ignited the spread of the procedure in the world. Both Fasano and Peacock stand as founders of modern dorsal rhizotomy for spasticity. A variety of modified surgical procedures and intraoperative neurophysiological procedures to be applied during dorsal rhizotomy have been reported since then. A PubMed search for "rhizotomy and spasticity" indicates an initial surge in publication in 1990, following Peacock's contribution (Fig. 1.1). Then, came a second surge in 2019, the reason for which is not clear. This perhaps reflects the increased acceptance and more detailed outcome analysis of the rhizotomy procedure for treatment of spasticity, together with expanding the indication other than spastic cerebral palsy.

Looking back at the history of rhizotomy, Abbe, a neurosurgeon in the New York City, performed the first rhizotomy as a treatment of intractable pain in the late nineteenth century [4]. The German neurosurgeon and neurologist Foerster

N. Morota (✉)
Department of Neurosurgery, Kitasato University Hospital, Minami-Ku, Sagamihara, Japan

P. Steinbok
Division of Neurosurgery, Department of Surgery, British Columbia Children's Hospital and University of British Columbia, Vancouver, BC, Canada
e-mail: psteinbok@cw.bc.ca

N. Morota, P. Steinbok (eds.), *Dorsal Rhizotomy: Neurosurgery for Childhood Spasticity*, Advances and Technical Standards in Neurosurgery 51,
https://doi.org/10.1007/978-3-031-86441-4_1

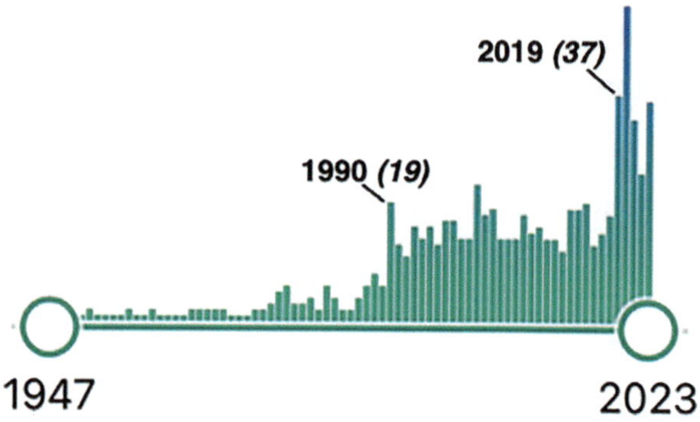

Fig. 1.1 The PubMed search for "rhizotomy and spasticity". It reveals an initial surge in publication in 1990, followed by the second surge in 2019

introduced dorsal rhizotomy for spasticity reduction in 1908. In his publication of 1913, he advocated the need for postoperative long-term rehabilitation and recommended preservation of the L4 posterior root for truncal support [5]. The procedure was known as "Foerster's operation" until World War II, establishing Foerster as the father of dorsal rhizotomy for spasticity. We still have a lot to learn from those pioneers of dorsal rhizotomy.

Many congenital or acquired central nervous system disorders lead to exaggerated spasticity, causing motor disability and great burden for caregivers. Cerebral palsy, resulting from various pathological conditions during embryonic and neonatal period, is the most common cause of spasticity, affecting approximately 0.2% of live births worldwide. There is not a big difference between the countries regardless of the geographic location or economic development. Among children with cerebral palsy, about 60% suffer spastic para-/tetraparesis. Dorsal rhizotomy, when appropriately and safely carried out, holds the potential for substantial positive impact on children, families, and society.

References

1. Fasano VA, Urciuoli R, Broggi G, Barolat-Romana G, Benech F, Ivaldi A, Sguazzi A. New aspects in the surgical treatment of cerebral palsy. Acta Neurochir Suppl (Wien). 1977;24:53–7.
2. Fasano VA, Barolat-Romana G, Zeme S, Sguazzi A. Electrophysiological assessment of spinal circuits by direct dorsal root stimulation. Neurosurgery. 1979;4:146–51.
3. Peacock WJ, Arens LJ. Selective posterior rhizotomy for the relief of spasticity in cerebral palsy. S Afr Med J. 1982;62:119–24.
4. Abbe R. Intradural section of the spinal nerves for neuralgia. Boston Med Surg J. 1896;135:329–44.
5. Foerster O. On the indications and results of the excision of posterior spinal nerve roots in man. Surg Gynecol Obstet. 1913;16:463–74.

Part I
Background of Dorsal Rhizotomy

Chapter 2
History of Dorsal Rhizotomy for Spasticity

Nobuhito Morota

Dorsal rhizotomy is a surgical procedure aimed at reducing spasticity by severing dorsal roots or rootlets [1, 2]. The evolution of this technique has been complex and marked by significant challenges over time (Figs. 2.1 and 2.2) [1, 3, 4]. The history of dorsal rhizotomy extends beyond the surgical procedure itself; it also encompasses the development of intraoperative neurophysiology for functional evaluation and preservation (Fig. 2.3). This chapter discusses the past, present, and future of dorsal rhizotomy for spasticity.

N. Morota (✉)
Department of Neurosurgery, Kitasato University Hospital, Minami-Ku, Sagamihara, Japan

N. Morota, P. Steinbok (eds.), *Dorsal Rhizotomy: Neurosurgery for Childhood Spasticity*, Advances and Technical Standards in Neurosurgery 51,
https://doi.org/10.1007/978-3-031-86441-4_2

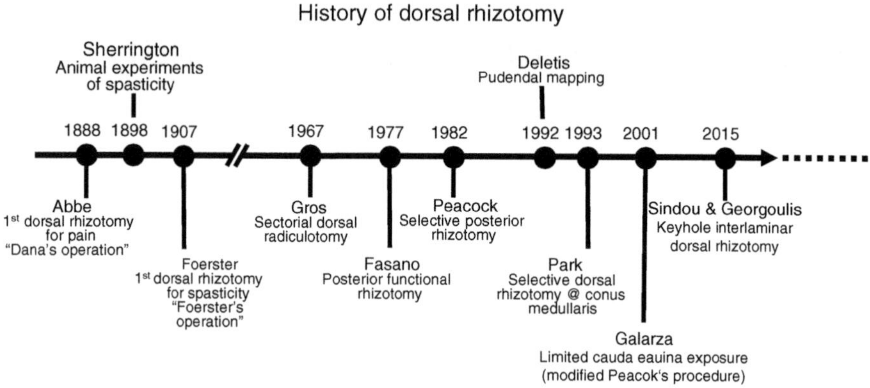

Fig. 2.1 History of dorsal rhizotomy: major events on the history of dorsal rhizotomy are chronologically shown

Fig. 2.2 Chronological change of the surgical site: change of the surgical site by pioneers are demonstrated

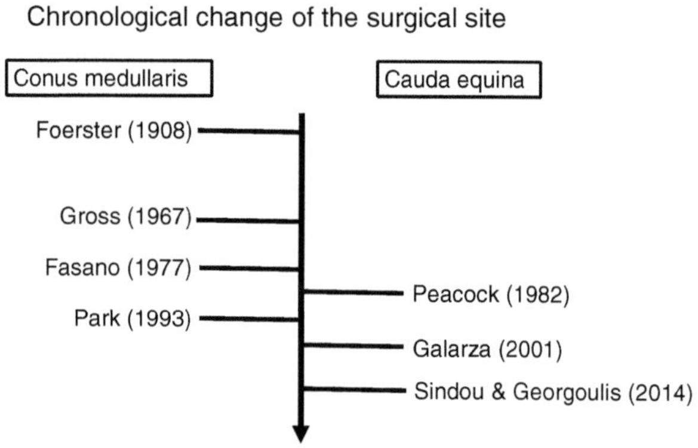

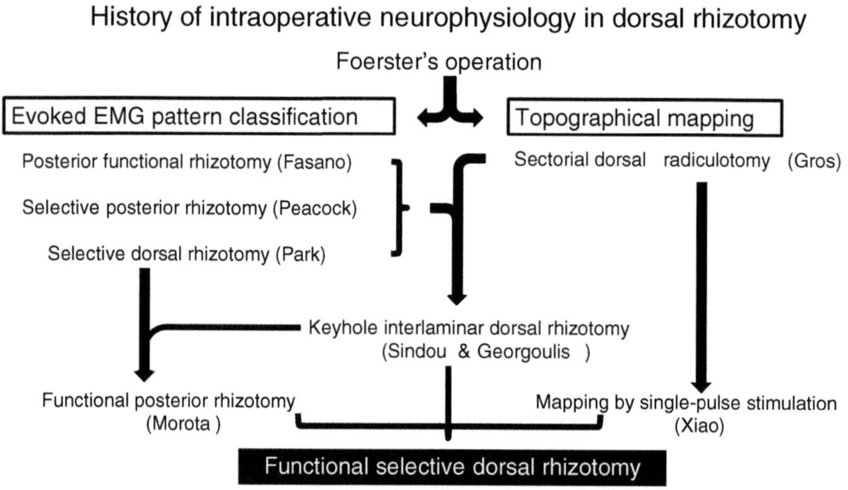

Fig. 2.3 History of intraoperative neurophysiology in dorsal rhizotomy: evolution and modification of intraoperative neurophysiological procedures are shown with the term of dorsal rhizotomy

2.1 Dawn and Decline (1880s ~ 1950s)

The history of dorsal rhizotomy dates back to 1888, more than a century ago. The late nineteenth century is the time of the infancy of modern neurosurgery, which coincided with advances in neuroscience and neurophysiology.

Dorsal rhizotomy was initially introduced as a treatment for intractable pain. The first successful dorsal rhizotomy was performed on December 31, 1888, by Robert Abbe, a neurosurgeon at New York Hospital, following the suggestion of neurologist Charles L. Dana [5]. The patient, a 44-year-old man, suffered from severe intractable neuralgia of the right brachial plexus, even after amputation of the arm. Abbe performed a total dorsal root sectioning from C6 to C7 on the right side following a C4–C7 laminectomy, but no pain relief was achieved. The patient returned to the operating room 48 h later for additional sectioning of the C8 dorsal root, which resulted in the disappearance of the phantom pain. Notably, Abbe mentioned "faradic battery … moderate current was used," suggesting that intraoperative neurophysiology was employed from the onset of dorsal rhizotomy.

Following this initial success, Abbe expanded his cases and published a three-case report in 1896 [5]. Later, in 1911, he published a report of six cases, which included four cases of pain and two of spasticity [6]. In this later report, he credited the German neurosurgeon and neurologist Otfrid Foerster for introducing dorsal rhizotomy as a treatment for spasticity. Although Abbe referred to the procedure as "Dana's operation" out of respect for the neurologist, it was commonly known as "Foerster's operation" at the time, as Foerster was the first to apply the procedure to reduce spasticity in 1907 [7]. Foerster's work was based on the findings of Sir Charles Sherrington, who demonstrated that dorsal root sectioning could reduce muscle tone in affected limbs [8]. Foerster himself arrived at this conclusion after observing a patient with tabes dorsalis and hemiplegia who did not develop spasticity on the paralyzed side.

Foerster's astute observations continue to influence current practice [7, 9]. He noted that surgical results for athetosis were generally poor, with some cases even experiencing increased spasticity. He stressed the importance of postoperative rehabilitation, stating that long and careful exercise treatment was necessary to regain locomotion gradually. His insights included the recommendation to preserve the fourth lumbar root, as it is crucial for standing and walking, and his observation that complete dorsal rhizotomy at two adjacent spinal levels would not result in sensory deficits. Finally, Foerster strongly advocated the use of intraoperative electrical stimulation (intraoperative neurophysiology) due to individual differences in dorsal nerve innervation. The author expresses deep admiration for Foerster's observations made over a century ago.

Dorsal rhizotomy emerged as a neurosurgical procedure for reducing spasticity, with its popularity peaking in the early twentieth century. However, the procedure involved the sectioning of multiple dorsal roots, leading to complications such as sensory disturbances, ulceration, and hypotonia, which gradually diminished its popularity after World War I [1, 3, 4].

2.2 Revival (1960s ~ 1970s)

During the decline of dorsal rhizotomy, the pioneering work of Abbe and Foerster was narrowly continued by French neurosurgeons after World War II. Claude Gros and his team modified Foerster's technique by preserving 1/5 of the rootlets instead of cutting the entire root [3, 10, 11]. They also developed a method to identify the topographical innervation map to target spastic muscles more precisely. This allowed them to differentiate between disabling spasticity and useful spasticity, selectively cutting dorsal roots to the responsible muscle groups. The procedure became known as "sectorial posterior radiculotomy (rhizotomy)" [11]. It is important to note that their goal was to create a more functional dorsal rhizotomy by selecting dorsal roots to be cut based on both clinical and neurophysiological findings.

In the late 1970s, Victor A. Fasano, an Italian neurosurgeon, played a pivotal role in the resurgence of dorsal rhizotomy for spasticity [12]. He was a pioneer in reintroducing and advancing the procedure. Fasano incorporated modern intraoperative neurophysiology into dorsal rhizotomy, using it not only for topographical mapping but also for assessing the abnormality of roots/rootlets through electromyography (EMG) patterns [12, 13]. His work was partially based on the study of the H-reflex recovery curve [14]. He developed a method to determine which dorsal roots/rootlets to section based on EMG patterns following repetitive electrical stimulation. Fasano posited that the loss of normal inhibitory reflexes due to central nervous system damage played a major role in spasticity. The loss of inhibitory function could be identified by observing muscle contraction outside the myotome of the stimulated spinal segment or sustained muscle contraction during repetitive electrical stimulation. Dorsal roots/rootlets exhibiting uninhibited abnormal EMG patterns were selected for sectioning. His approach introduced a new dimension to the use of intraoperative neurophysiology in dorsal rhizotomy, utilizing EMG as a guide to identify "abnormal" roots/rootlets. In essence, the quality of the muscle response demonstrated on EMG was used to determine which roots/rootlets to section. Fasano performed the surgery at the level of the conus medullaris (Th12–L1 laminectomy), coining the procedure termed "posterior functional rhizotomy."

The efforts of Gros, Fasano, and others to selectively target roots/rootlets responsible for harmful spasticity while preserving the neural integrity of motor and sensory functions led to the revival and resurgence of dorsal rhizotomy in the following decades.

2.3 Establishment (1980s ~ 2000s)

In the 1980s, pediatric neurosurgeon Warwick Peacock from South Africa played a pivotal role in the global dissemination of dorsal rhizotomy for spasticity [15, 16]. He shifted the surgical field from the conus medullaris to the cauda equina. His modification, which involved the exposure of the entire cauda equina, allowed for more precise localization of the spinal level of the dorsal root, thereby enhancing the safety of the rhizotomy procedure. Peacock also applied intraoperative neurophysiology based on Fasano's EMG pattern classification to determine which rootlets should be sectioned [16]. As Peacock moved to North America, the procedure gained popularity and became an accepted neurosurgical approach for managing childhood spasticity.

In the early 1990s, Park from St. Louis further modified the procedure by shifting the surgical field back to the conus medullaris, performing a single-level laminectomy (laminotomy), and introducing microsurgical techniques [17, 18]. His team modified Fasano's EMG pattern classification by incorporating a grading system to assess the abnormality of roots/rootlets [19]. After functional evaluation with tetanic electrical stimulation, roots were ranked according to their degree of abnormality, with higher-graded roots being sectioned. Various modifications of Park's procedure have since been developed [20].

Peacock's original procedure was also refined. Galarza introduced a limited exposure of the conus medullaris for children with mild spasticity [21]. Unlike the standard Peacock procedure, which exposed L2 to S2, the limited approach involved opening only the lower half, from L4 to S1. Sindou and Georgoulis combined Gros's and Peacock's concepts to develop a new surgical technique called "keyhole interlaminar dorsal rhizotomy," detailed in Chap. 12 [22, 23].

Advancements were also made in intraoperative neurophysiology. Deletis developed a technique known as "pudendal mapping," which localized the sacral distribution of the dorsal action potential of the pudendal afferent nerve [24]. By preserving the pudendal potential, this technique helped prevent postoperative urological complications [25, 26].

Dorsal rhizotomy was firmly established as an effective neurosurgical treatment for spasticity in the late 1990s, following three consecutive randomized controlled studies that demonstrated its efficacy in reducing childhood spasticity [27–30]. The procedure was shown to improve lower leg spasticity, increase lower leg range of motion (ROM), and enhance Gross Motor Function Measure (GMFM) scores with a high degree of certainty. It also moderately improved locomotive function, with the surgical effects lasting for more than 5 years. Additionally, the procedure was found to have a remote effect in reducing spasticity in the upper extremities and trunk [31]. The evidence from these studies significantly contributed to the widespread adoption of dorsal rhizotomy worldwide.

2.4 Development (2010s~)

In the past decade, dorsal rhizotomy has experienced a new wave of development. The procedure has gained traction in more countries and continents as a treatment for childhood spasticity. As described in Chap. 1, we are currently witnessing a second surge in dorsal rhizotomy, characterized by technical modifications of surgical procedures, research into surgical indications and outcomes, and analysis of locomotive function, among other areas. Many of these topics are discussed in this book.

On the other hand, the role of intraoperative neurophysiology in dorsal rhizotomy has remained a subject of ongoing debate [32–35]. In most medical centers that perform dorsal rhizotomy, the cutting rate of the roots/rootlets is predetermined—typically between 40% and 60%—based on the degree of spasticity and clinical experience. This approach, often referred to as "experience-based medicine," is currently the mainstream method for selecting dorsal roots/rootlets for sectioning [36]. However, it differs from the approach originally adopted by Fasano.

Sindou and his team utilized intraoperative neurophysiology for both topographical mapping and physiological testing, balancing these techniques to inform decisions about dorsal root sectioning [37]. However, the quantity of dorsal root sectioning (cutting rate) was still predetermined according to the spinal root level and its innervating muscles (see Chap. 12). Xiao introduced a novel protocol for root selection, focusing on topographical mapping of muscle innervation through single-pulse stimulation of the dorsal root [38]. If the stimulated dorsal root innervated a muscle responsible for harmful spasticity, it was sectioned according to a predetermined rate (25–50%) (see Chap. 11).

Morota took a more classical approach, making full use of intraoperative physiological testing. In his cauda equina approach, whether by the standard or limited Peacock procedure, topographical mapping was not essential [39]. Neurophysiological testing included both 10 Hz tetanic stimulation and pudendal mapping. Root/rootlet sectioning was determined based on Fasano's EMG pattern classification, with the overall cutting rate estimated preoperatively using a formula based on the preoperative GMFM-88 score. Reduction in spasticity following rootlet sectioning was confirmed using the F-wave (see Chap. 14). Morota named the procedure "functional posterior rhizotomy" in honor of Fasano's pioneering work.

2.5 Future

It is logical to anticipate that the cutting rate should correlate with the severity of spasticity—lower rates for children with mild spasticity and higher rates for those with severe spasticity. The cutting rate should be individualized for each patient. The future of dorsal rhizotomy lies in this principle: to refine the procedure by minimizing the extent of root/rootlet sectioning while still achieving optimal surgical outcomes. This approach represents a truly functionally less invasive surgery.

It is worth noting that in the series by Xiao and Morota, the minimum overall cutting rate of roots/rootlets was less than 20% [38, 40]. Such an outcome could be achieved through meticulous and innovative application of intraoperative neurophysiology. We select children with spasticity for dorsal rhizotomy, we select roots/rootles to be cut for reducing spasticity. The role of intraoperative neurophysiology will become increasingly integral to making the surgery more functional and precise.

Given the functional nature of this surgery, it might be more appropriate to refer to it as "functional selective dorsal rhizotomy" in the future. Over the coming decades, it is expected that dorsal rhizotomy will continue to gain global recognition as a safe and effective functional neurosurgical procedure for reducing spasticity.

References

1. Abbott R, Forem SL, Johann M. Selective posterior rhizotomy for the treatment of spasticity: a review. Childs Nerv Syst. 1989;5:337–46.
2. Steinbok P. Selective dorsal rhizotomy for spastic cerebral palsy: a review. Childs Nerv Syst. 2007;23:981–90.
3. Sindou M, Georgoulis G, Mertens P. History of neurosurgical treatment for spasticity. In: Neurosurgery for spasticity. Wien: Springer; 2014.
4. Cespedes J, Vidarte OAE, Uparela MJ, Osorio-Fonseca E, Alvernia JE. History and evolution of surgical treatment for spasticity: a journey from neurotomy to selective dorsal rhizotomy. Neurosurg Focus. 2024;56(6):E2.
5. Abbe R. Intradural section of the spinal nerves for neuralgia. Boston Med Surg J. 1896;135:329–44.
6. Abbe R. Resection of posterior roots of spinal nerves to relieve pain, pain reflex athetosis and spastic paralysis-Dana's operation. Med Rec. 1911;79:377–81.
7. Foerster O. On the indication s and results of the excision of posterior spinal nerve roots in men. Surg Gynecol Obstet. 1913;16:463–4.
8. Sherrington CS. Decerebrate rigidity, and reflex coordination of movements. J Physiol. 1898;22(4):319–32.
9. Tan T-C. Otfrid Foerster (1873–1941). J Neurol. 2003;250:513–4.
10. Privat JM, Benezech J, Frerebeau P, Gros C. Sectorial posterior rhizotomy, a new technique of surgical treatment for spasticity. Acta Neurochir. 1976;35:181–95.
11. Gros C. Spasticity. Clinical classification and surgical treatment. In: Krayenbuhl H, editor. Advances and technical standards in neurosurgery 6. Wien/New York: Springer; 1979. p. 55–97.
12. Fasano VA, Barolat-Romana G, Zeme S, Sguazzi A. Electrophysiological assessment of spinal circuits by direct dorsal root stimulation. Neurosurgery. 1979;4:146–51.
13. Fasano VA, Broggi G, Zeme S. Intraoperative electrical stimulation for functional posterior rhizotomy. Scand J Rehab Med Suppl. 1988;17:149–54.
14. Futagi Y, Abe J. H-reflex study in normal children and patients with cerebral palsy. Brain Dev. 1985;7:414–20.
15. Peacock WJ, Arens LJ. Selective posterior rhizotomy for the relief of spasticity in cerebral palsy. S Afr Med J. 1982;62:119–24.
16. Peacock WJ, Arens LJ, Berman B. Cerebral palsy spasticity. Selective posterior rhizotomy. Pediatr Neurosci. 1987;13:61–6.
17. Park TS, Gaffney PE, Kaufman BA, Molleston MC. Selective lumbosacral dorsal rhizotomy immediately caudal to the conus medullaris for cerebral palsy spasticity. Neurosurgery. 1993;33:929–34.
18. Park TS, Johnston JM. Surgical techniques of selective dorsal rhizotomy for spastic cerebral palsy. Technical note. Neurosurg Focus. 2006;21:e7.

19. Phillips LH II, Park TS. Electrophysiologic studies of selective posterior rhizotomy patients. In: Park TS, editor. Neurosurgery: state of the art reviews 4. Management of spasticity in cerebral palsy and spinal cord injury. Philadelphia: Hanley & Belfus; 1989. p. 459–69.
20. Warsi NM, Tailor J, Coulter IC, Shakil H, Workewych A, Haldenby R, Breibart S, Strantzas S, Vandenberk M, Dewan MC, Ibrahim GM. Selective dorsal rhizotomy: an illustrated review of operative techniques. J Neurosurg Pediatr. 2020;25:540–7.
21. Galarza M, Fowler EG, Chipps L, Padden TM, Lazareff JA. Functional assessment of children with cerebral palsy following limited (L4-S1) selective posterior rhizotomy – a preliminary report. Acta Neurochir. 2001;143:865–72.
22. Sindou M, Georgoulis G, Mertens P. Dorsal rhizotomy for children with cerebral palsy. In: Neurosurgery for spasticity. Wien: Springer; 2014.
23. Sindou M, Georgoulis G. Keyhole interlaminar dorsal rhizotomy for spastic diplegia in cerebral palsy. Acta Neurochir. 2015;157:1187–96.
24. Deletis V, Vodusek D, Abbott R, Epstein F, Turndorff H. Intraoperative monitoring of the dorsal roots: minimizing the risk of iatrogenic micturition disorders. Neursurgery. 1992;30:72–5.
25. Ogiwara H, Morota N. Pudendal afferents mapping in posterior sacral rhizotomies. Neurosurgery. 2014;74:171–5.
26. Morota N. Pudendal mapping of S1 rootlets in a functional posterior rhizotomy: when an S1 posterior root shows a high pudendal dorsal action potential—a technical note. Childs Nerv Syst. 2020;36:1971–5.
27. Steinbok P, Reiner AM, Beauchamp R, Armstrong RW, Cochrane DD. A randomized clinical trial to compare selective posterior rhizotomy plus physiotherapy with physiotherapy alone in children with spastic diplegic cerebral palsy. Dev Med Child Neurol. 1997;39:178–84.
28. McLaughlin JF, Bjornson KF, Astley SJ, Graubert C, Hays TS, Roberts TS, Price R, Temkin N. Selective dorsal rhizotomy: efficacy and safety in an investigator-masked randomized clinical trial. Dev Med Child Neurol. 1998;40:220–32.
29. Wright FV, Sheil EMH, Drake JM, Wedge JH, Naumann S. Evaluation of selective dorsal rhizotomy for the reduction of spasticity in cerebral palsy: a randomized controlled trial. Dev Med Child Neurol. 1998;40:239–47.
30. McLaughlin J, Bjorson K, Temkin N, Steinbok P, Wright V, Reiner A, Roberts T, Drake J, O'Donnell M, Rosenbaum P, Barber J, Farrel A. Selective dorsal rhizotomy: meta-analysis of three randomized controlled trials. Dev Med Child Neurol. 2002;44:17–25.
31. Steinbok P. Outcomes after selective dorsal rhizotomy for spastic cerebral palsy. Childs Nerv Syst. 2001;17:1–18.
32. Steinbok P, Tidemann AJ, Miller S, Mortenson P, Bowen-Roberts T. Electrophysiologically guided versus non-electrophysiologically guided selective dorsal rhizotomy for spastic cerebral palsy: a comparison of outcomes. Childs Nerv Syst. 2009;25:1091–6.
33. De Vloo P, Huttunen TJ, Forte D, Jankovic I, Lee A, Hair M, Cawker S, Chugh D, Carr L, Crowe BHA, Pitt M, Aquillina K. Intraoperative electrophysiology during single-level selective dorsal rhizotomy: technique, stimulation threshold, and response data in a series of 145 patients. J Neurosurg Pediatr. 2020;25:597–606.
34. Wolter S, Spies C, Martin JH, Schultz M, Sarpong-Bengelsdorf A, Unger J, Thomale UW, Michael T, Murphy JF, Haberi H. Frequency distribution in intraoperative stimulation-evoked EMG responses during selective dorsal rhizotomy in children with cerebral palsy—part 1: clinical setting and neurophysiological procedure. Childs Nerv Syst. 2020;36:1945–54.
35. Joud A, Sindou M, Stella I, Wiedemann A, Klein O. Dorsal rhizotomy in cerebral palsy: how root sectioning is influenced by intraoperative neuromonitoring? Neurochirurgie. 2022;68:e16–21.
36. Morota N. What we have gained and what have remained controversial in the field of rhizotomy for spasticity since 2007. Childs Nerv Syst. 2020;36:1887–94.
37. Georgoulis G, Brînzeu A, Sindou M. Dorsal rhizotomy for children with spastic diplegia of cerebral palsy origin: usefulness of intraoperative monitoring. J Neurosurg Pediatr. 2018;22:89–101.

38. Xiao B, Constantini S, Browd SR, Zhan Q, Jiang W, Mei R. The role of intra-operative neuroelectrophysiological monitoring in single-level approach selective dorsal rhizotomy. Childs Nerv Syst. 2020;36:1925–33.
39. Morota N, Ihara S, Ogiwara H. Neurosurgical management of childhood spasticity: functional posterior rhizotomy and intrathecal baclofen infusion therapy. Neurol Med Chir (Tokyo). 2015;55:624–39.
40. Morota N. Clinically practical formula for preoperatively estimating the cutting rate of the spinal nerve root in a functional posterior rhizotomy. Childs Nerv Syst. 2019;35:665–72.

Chapter 3
Neurophysiological and Neuroanatomical Background of Spasticity: Surgical Implication for Dorsal Rhizotomy in Cerebral Palsy

Marc Sindou, Anthony Joud, and George Georgoulis

3.1 Introduction

Hypertonia is a frequent clinical condition in children affected with cerebral palsy (CP) that may be caused by several mechanisms, among which spasticity is predominant.

The physiological definition of spasticity, given by Lance in 1980, remains the most widely accepted: "Spasticity is a motor disorder characterized by a velocity-dependent increase in tonic stretch reflexes with exaggerated tendon jerk, resulting from hyperexcitability of the stretch reflex, as one of the components of the upper motor neuron syndrome" [1].

Whereas Lance referred to the pathophysiological mechanisms, Sanger et al. stayed closer to the clinical phenomena and defined spasticity as "hypertonia in which one or both of the following signs are present: (I) resistance to externally imposed movement that increases with increasing speed of stretch and varies with the direction of joint movement, and/or (II) resistance to externally imposed movement rises rapidly above a threshold speed or joint angle" [2].

M. Sindou (✉)
University of Lyon, Lyon, France

Groupe ELSAN, Clinique Bretéché, Nantes, France
e-mail: marc.sindou@orange.fr

A. Joud
Department of Pediatric Neurosurgery Centre Hospitalo-Universitaire de Nancy, Nancy, France
e-mail: a.joud@chru-nancy.fr

G. Georgoulis
Department of Neurosurgery, General Hospital of Athens "G. Gennimatas", Athens, Greece

N. Morota, P. Steinbok (eds.), *Dorsal Rhizotomy: Neurosurgery for Childhood Spasticity*, Advances and Technical Standards in Neurosurgery 51,
https://doi.org/10.1007/978-3-031-86441-4_3

In 2005, the SPASM consortium (established to develop Standardized Measures of Spasticity) introduced a new definition of spasticity using a motor control approach: “Disordered sensorimotor control, resulting from an upper motor neuron lesion, presenting as intermittent or sustained involuntary activation of muscles” [3, 4]. This definition includes the entire range of signs and symptoms that are collectively described as excess features and not exclusively the hyperactive stretch reflex [5].

All these various definitions are mutually compatible.

Spasticity may be either useful, by compensating for a decrease in motor strength; or harmful, by limiting both passive and active motion and at the extreme leading to irreducible contractures and deformities; or as in most cases, harmful and useful in the same patient. In CP patients, spasticity is frequently associated with dystonia, which is a sustained hypertonic state induced by attempts at voluntary motion. The proper aim of dorsal rhizotomy (DR) is to reduce the excess of the spastic component.

3.2 Mechanisms of Hypertonia in Cerebral Palsy

The initial background for understanding the pathophysiology of spasticity was the pioneering work of Sherrington [6]. The experiments were on decerebrate animals and demonstrated that spasticity was associated with hyperexcitability of the stretch (= myotatic) reflex related to the loss of inhibitory influences from descending supraspinal structures. Actually, Sherrington’s experimental model interrupted not only the corticospinal tract but also, and mainly, the (inhibitory) reticulospinal tract and likely also the vestibulospinal tract (Fig. 3.1). Therefore, *spasticity would result not only from gamma loop’s hyperexcitability but also from lack of inhibition of the IA afferent fibers at the level of their spinal cord interneurons*, which have GABA as their main synaptic neurotransmitter [7].

Further studies of the underlying mechanisms of spasticity have shown that *neurobiological responses of the central nervous system to damages* entail reorganization of synapses and the creation of new connectivity for the reestablishment of residual functions in partially impaired structures. Spasticity, which—by definition—opposes to muscle stretching and lengthening, has two important consequences. First, the muscles tend to remain in a shortened position, which in turn results in soft tissue changes and contracture. The second consequence is that movements are restricted. Both—hypertonia and lack of mobilization—create a vicious circle leading to severe locomotor disability (Fig. 3.2).

Hypertonia has at the same time a neural component due to spasticity and a biomechanical component linked to *soft tissue changes*. This biomechanical hypertonia is not velocity dependent; it limits movements even at a slow velocity. As pointed out by Barnes, the biomechanical component will not respond to antispastic agents; the only therapeutic possibility is physiotherapy [8].

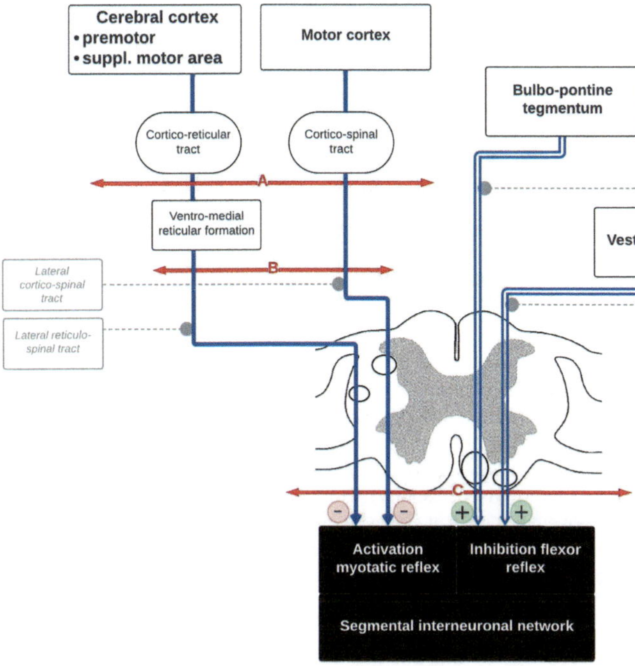

Fig. 3.1 Schematic representation of the "supraspinal descending systems" exerting (inhibitory and excitatory) control on segmental muscular tone. Sites of the various anatomical/pathological lesions and corresponding mechanisms that lead to spastic disorders: (*A*) lesion affecting the corticospinal tract and the cortico-reticular tract, which are facilitating structures of the main inhibitory system, namely, the reticulospinal tract; (*B*) lower brainstem lesion affecting the corticospinal fibers and the lateral reticulospinal tract; and (*C*) spinal cord (complete) lesion affecting the corticospinal fibers together with the lateral reticulospinal fibers and (also) the excitatory pathways—namely, the medial reticulospinal tract and the vestibulospinal tract—which exert activation influence onto the segmental inhibition of the spinal flexor reflexes. Minus symbol indicates inhibitory pathways and plus symbol excitatory pathways

Practically, it reveals often difficult to determine the relative responsibility of each of the components because of the frequent association of neural and biomechanical hypertonia and therefore decide the appropriate treatment.

Muscle overactivity, linked to disruption of the central nervous system (CNS) command, becomes superimposed to paresis and soft tissue contracture as a third factor of impairment in those paretic/spastic patients. Pathogenesis involves adaptive sprouting in the CNS, as well as reciprocal potentiation between spastic overactivity and contracture, and evolves in parallel with the paresis–underuse–paresis cycle. None of the three factors, paresis, contracture, and muscle overactivity, is symmetrically distributed between agonists and antagonists, which creates torque imbalance in joints then deformities.

Training in the less overactive muscle groups together with concomitant stretch, and if necessary focal weakening agents in their more overactive and shortened

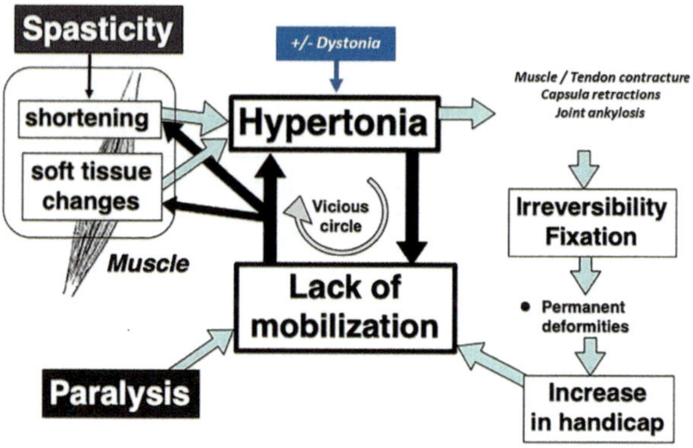

Fig. 3.2 The vicious circle of hypertonia and lack of mobilization. Spasticity, which by definition opposes to muscle stretching, has two important consequences. First, the muscles tend to remain in a shortened position, so that movements are restricted. Second, hypertonia and lack of mobilization result in soft tissue changes (loss of viscoelasticity). This biomechanical component, which is not velocity dependent, limits movements even at slow velocity that will not respond to antispastic agents. Risk of irreversibility induced by this vicious circle is a plea to actively reduce hypertonia/spasticity before disorders become fixed

antagonists, should be carried out to disrupt the vicious circle of contracture and paresis [9].

Furthermore, *spasticity is frequently associated with dystonia*, which is a stereotype pattern of contorted and sustained hypertonic state induced by attempts at voluntary motion. When examined, the limb resists to passive mobilization. Like spasticity, dystonia is very susceptible to anxiety and emotional factors. Spasticity and dystonia have to be distinguished in clinical practice. They are two symptoms with a completely different pathophysiology, dystonia being linked to basal ganglia impairment. Dorsal rhizotomy will not significantly influence the dystonic component.

Hypertonia and dystonia may be also affected by the coexistence of choreoathetoid "parasite" movements that will not be influenced by the treatment of hypertonia and spasticity.

Coming back to the role of spasticity in locomotor disability, its participation is more complex than the content of its strict definition. As proposed by Sheean, the term "spastic motor overactivity" would be more appropriate [7]. The proposed term includes spasticity (as defined by Lance), spastic co-contractions (which refers to the simultaneous contraction of agonist and antagonist muscles), and spastic dystonia. The substrate of co-contraction is impairment of reciprocal inhibition in the spinal cord, co-contraction being activated and/or deactivated at cortical level [10], as well as by other afferents [11].

As regard to spastic dystonia, its motor drive is not a spinal reflex; it is efferent mediated rather than afferent mediated. This has essential therapeutic implications.

Spastic dystonia should not be expected to respond well to antispastic treatments, whether pharmacological or by dorsal rhizotomy, which aim to reduce reflex activity. Spastic dystonia should better respond to treatments that modify motor nerve and/or motor activity, such as dantrolene, botulinum toxin injections, motor blocks, or peripheral neurotomies.

The most frequent cause of spasticity and hypertonia in childhood is by far cerebral palsy (CP), a term that was established by Osler in 1889 [12], almost three decades after the first clinical description given by Little in 1861 [13]. The presently adopted description of CP, proposed by Ingram in 1955 [14], is used to designate nonprogressive disorders of the motor and related functions that result from an insult to the brain, the insult having occurred in the prenatal, perinatal, or approximately 2-year postnatal period or due to excessive prematurity. There are different clinical patterns of hypertonia within the frame of CP disorders; they are described in detail in most pediatric neurological handbooks [15].

Children with CP do not have contractures and skeleton deformities at birth; those are acquired during childhood. *Spasticity and reduced activity lead to a lack of muscle lengthening, contractures, and then fixed deformities.* According to Graham and Selber, limb pathology can be considered in three stages [16].

- In stage 1 (younger age), spasticity is dynamic and reversible. This is the phase when spasticity management, gait training, and use of orthoses is most useful.
- In stage 2, contractures become fixed.
- In stage 3, irreducible deformities appear in long bones (leading especially to medial femoral torsion and/or lateral tibial torsion) and also in joints (producing hip subluxation and subtalar collapse in the hindfoot).

Based on this evolution, clinical management should anticipate irreducible contractures and fixed deformities.

3.3 Anatomical Bases of Tone and Spasticity

Spasticity has many clinical expressions, with a varied distribution among different muscle groups and by different responses to physiological stimuli that may be proprioceptive, exteroceptive, or interoceptive.

The spinal motoneuron is under permanent influence of peripheral afferent fibers, interneurons, and descending projections from supraspinal structures, not only the corticospinal tract but also the (predominantly inhibitory) reticulospinal tract. Basically, by definition, spasticity corresponds to the exaggeration of the monosynaptic reflex, but not exclusively.

The following anatomical brief of the main structures and pathways implicated in the regulation of tone will help to understand the mechanisms, as well as the diversity, of the clinical spastic states observed in the affected patients.

3.3.1 The Spinal Reflexes Involved in the Genesis of Spasticity

Basically, spasticity corresponds to exaggeration of the monosynaptic reflex elicited by *the IA afferent fibers*, which originate from the primary muscle spindle endings, to the corresponding alpha motoneurons (Fig. 3.3a). The monosynaptic myotatic reflex can be easily explored by recording the H-reflex and spasticity quantified with the Hmax/Mmax ratio (Fig. 3.3b). However, several other important spinal reflexes do play a role in spasticity after anatomical damages. Among them, the presynaptic inhibition (explored by vibratory inhibition of the H-reflex) is reduced; the ones responsible for reciprocal inhibition, for IB nonreciprocal inhibition, and for the recurrent Renshaw inhibition (all explored by H-reflex conditioning) are similarly reduced.

Beside the role of the IA fibers, the implication of *the afferents of group II*, originating from the secondary muscle spindle endings (and that can be explored by study of the long latency reflexes), is crucial [17]. Their role has even been considered more powerful than the role of the IA fibers in spastic patients. Fibers II are activated, like fibers IA, by muscle stretching, although they are less sensitive to the velocity of the stretching.

Nowadays, the most accepted basis of the stretch reflex hyperexcitability—which underlies the clinical signs of enhanced tendon reflexes, clonus, reflex

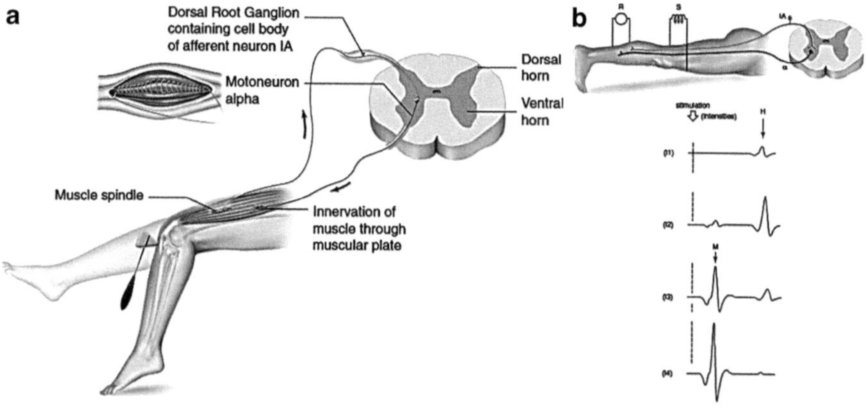

Fig. 3.3 (**a**) The myotatic reflex is a muscle contraction in response to its stretching (for instance, when the patellar tendon is tapped with a reflex hammer). This reflex provides automatic regulation of the muscle length. When a muscle is lengthened, its spindle, which is its sensory receptor, is stretched, increasing its nerve activity. The afferent volley in the IA fiber excites the alpha motoneuron, causing the muscle to contract, thus resisting the stretching. (**b**) The H-reflex explores the monosynaptic pathways between the afferent IA fiber and the alpha motoneuron. The method consists in stimulation (*S*) of the tibial nerve at the popliteal fossa and recording (*R*) of the motor response of the soleus muscle. Increasing the stimulation intensities results in the occurrence of the H-reflex (*i1*, *i2*). When stimulation intensities continue to increase, the H-reflex disappears, by collision with the recruitment of motor fibers that is manifested by an increasing amplitude of direct motor response (*M*) (*i3*, *i4*)

diffusion, and spasticity itself—is *abnormal processing of the proprioceptive information* within the spinal cord [18]. This reflexologic mechanisms would prevail over the one of an increased fusimotor activity via the gamma motoneuron system [19].

Similar abnormal processing that motoneurons themselves had become hyperexcitable, ready to overreact in response to afferent input, would also operate for the exaggerated cutaneous/nociceptive reflexes that are frequently associated with severe spasticity (namely, flexor withdrawal spasms, more rarely extensor reflexes) [7].

These spinal cord mechanisms, which involve interneurons that are under strong supraspinal control, are complex and still remain incompletely elucidated.

3.3.2 The Organization of the Spinal Cord

Knowledge was established from a large number of anatomical and physiological works, conducted in animal experiments and human studies, and synthetically collected in basic anatomical books [20–24].

3.3.2.1 The Alpha Motoneurons

The alpha motoneurons are located in the ventral horn. Those innervating the same muscle group are associated in a motoneuronal group, itself organized in longitudinal motor columns that can extend over 2–4 metameric levels.

3.3.2.2 The Primary Afferents

All the Rexed laminae receive primary afferents directly, except lamina VIII, which is an area of intercommissural exchange. The fibers of large diameter project onto laminae III, IV, V, VI, and IX, and the fibers of small diameter project onto the superficial laminae I and II and the deeper laminae V and X. Some proprioceptive IA fibers project directly onto the lamina IX motor neurons to trigger the monosynaptic reflex. However, the majority of these proprioceptive afferents ends onto *lamina VI*, at the base of the dorsal horn, which constitutes a real "proprioceptive layer" where the primary afferent fibers connect with the interneurons that are the origin of the ascending pathways.

In the entry zone of the dorsal rootlets, anatomical and physiological studies in humans revealed the existence of a spatial organization of the primary afferents according to their size and their destination in the spinal cord [25] and therefore to their functions. Thus, the fine fibers (Aδ and C), primarily nociceptive, regroup at the ventrolateral region of the dorsal root entry zone; they then cross through the tract of Lissauer (in its medial part) to reach the uppermost layers of the dorsal horn.

The large fibers (Aβ), which are located dorsomedially in the dorsal root entry zone, reach the dorsal column and destinate to the brainstem lemniscal pathways.

Briefly, the *neurotransmitters* released by the afferents are on one side excitatory amino acids, mainly the glutamate and aspartate, and on the other side, inhibitory amino acids, mainly the gamma-aminobutyric acid (GABA) and glycine. They all play a determining role in the neuromodulation of tone.

3.3.2.3 The System of Spinal Interneurons

The interneurons of the spinal cord, named propriospinal interneurons, have their cell bodies located in all laminae of the gray matter. However, the interneurons located in laminae VII and VIII particularly control the intersegmental spinal reflexes. The axons of short interneurons travel to the dorso- and ventrolateral tracts on 4–8 adjacent metameres to project predominantly onto the motoneurons of the flexor muscles in the lateral part of lamina IX. The intermediate interneurons send their axons via the ventrolateral tract onto lamina IX of even larger adjacent metameres, particularly on the columns of the motoneurons of the extensor muscles. The long interneurons make connections with the quasi-totality of the spinal cord segments. All of these interneurons are targets of converging information from peripheral origin but also from the suprasegmental descending pathways. After processing this information, the interneurons send a modulatory resulting command, inhibitory or facilitatory, on the pool of motoneurons.

The neurotransmitters are crucial in the control of tone (Fig. 3.4). The inhibitory interneurons have glycine as their predominant neurotransmitter. Most of other interneurons are GABAergic and enkephalinergic. Renshaw cells are mainly glycinergic and in some cases GABAergic; they are activated by the recurrent motoneuron fibers using acetylcholine. They in turn have an inhibitory (hyperpolarizing) action on the same alpha or gamma motoneurons. These Renshaw interneurons are themselves modulated by afferent fibers and descending pathways of supraspinal origin. Another population of GABAergic interneurons acts through a presynaptic, axono-axonal inhibition of afferent fibers. Receptors may be either GABA-A (coupled to a transmembrane Cl^- channel benzodiazepine agonist) or GABA-B (K^+ channel baclofen agonist). The activated GABA-A and GABA-B receptors lead to membrane hyperpolarization and thus reduce motoneuron excitability. These inhibitory interneurons can be activated either by primary afferents or by descending monoaminergic pathways. They activate receptors of type alpha-2 (for noradrenergic pathways) and type 5-HT1 (for serotonergic pathways). The enkephalinergic interneurons are located in large number in the superficial laminae of the dorsal horn and exert an inhibitory effect specifically on nociceptive transmission via opioid receptors mu, delta, and kappa.

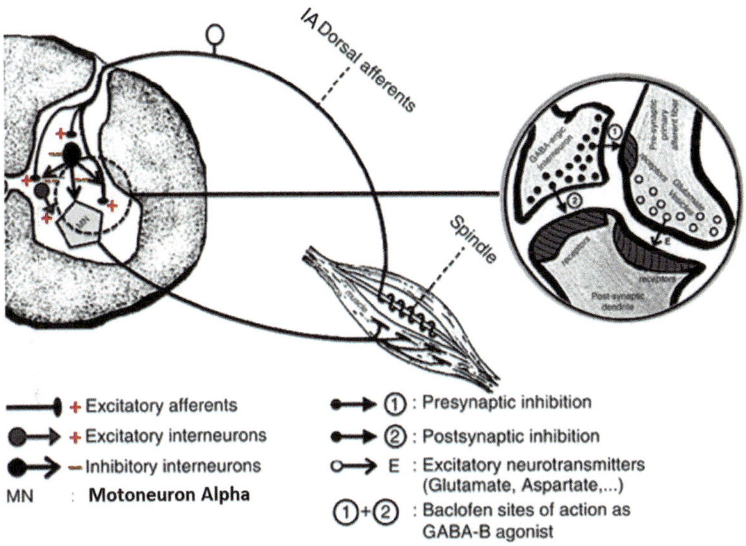

Fig. 3.4 The dorsal horn and ventral horn synapses, with excitatory and inhibitory neurotransmitters. The figure also shows baclofen sites of action. Baclofen is a lipophilic **GABA-B receptor agonist** that affects type B receptor. Baclofen is a transmembrane protein that controls calcium and potassium channels. By activation of the GABA-B receptors, which decreases the influx of calcium into the presynaptic terminals of the afferent fibers, baclofen reduces the release of the excitatory transmitters and thereby produces a decrease in monosynaptic and polysynaptic spinal reflexes. Baclofen also affects the postsynaptic membrane by increasing potassium influx and thus raises the membrane potential and inhibits neuronal firing. Intrathecal baclofen given to a spastic patient markedly decreases muscle tone and spasticity. The reason that baclofen is so effective in reducing spasticity is that the same changes in the spinal cord that produce spasticity enhance the sensitivity to baclofen

3.3.2.4 The Ascending Pathways

The spinocerebellar tracts are essentially secondary neurons that consist of axons from the Clarke and Betcherew nuclei of lamina VI and also of laminae IV–IX. These ascending tracts travel within the lateral column, and they are differentiated into a ventral bundle of proprioceptive contralateral fibers carrying information from the limbs (fasciculus of Gowers) and a dorsal bundle of ipsilateral fibers carrying information from the trunk (fasciculus of Flechsig).

The ventral column harbors *the spino-reticular tract* that originates from the deep layers of laminae VII, VIII, and X with ipsi- and contralateral projections principally to the ponto-bulbar reticular formation. This tract plays a role not only in the nociception but also in the field of the motor control, through the reticular formation [26].

3.3.3 *The Supraspinal Descending Pathways*

3.3.3.1 The Corticospinal System

Its fibers originate from large areas of the frontoparietal cortex (e.g., Brodmann areas 4, 3a, 3b, 1, 2, 5, SII, supplementary motor area). They constitute the axons of neurons located in layer V of the cerebral cortex (i.e., the internal pyramid layer of those cortical areas).

The majority of the corticospinal fibers decussates in the medullary pyramids and descends in the medial part of the dorsolateral column. They project onto the alpha motoneurons in the ventral horn. A minority of fibers remains ipsilateral and descends in the ventral column before crossing the midline at the level of their metameric projection onto the motoneurons. Most of these corticospinal fibers end in the ventral horn, but some end also on laminae IV–IX spreading over the dorsal horn and intermediate zone [27, 28]. This system has been unequivocally shown to *code for individual fine movements of the fingers*. The fibers of parietal origin project preferentially on the dorsal horn (laminae IV–VI), while the fibers from the motor cortex project preferentially on the interneurons of the intermediate zone and on the ventral horn.

3.3.3.2 The Descending Lateral Brainstem System

This system includes *the rubrospinal and the reticulospinal pathways* coming from the lateral pontine and medullary reticular formation (the gigantocellular nucleus). These pathways are regrouped in the dorsolateral column and project contralaterally to lamina I and the lateral part of laminae V, VI, VII, and IX. This system subserves the possibility of performing independent flexion or extension movements of the elbow and hand.

3.3.3.3 The Descending Medial Brainstem System

Its fibers have wide spread origins, mainly *from the reticular formation*, to which fibers from the vestibular and also the cerebellar nuclei and tectum are associated. Then, fibers travel in both the ventrolateral and ventral columns, bilaterally or ipsilaterally, and project onto laminae VI, VII, VIII, and IX. The main function of this system is the maintenance of the erect position, body and neck/head orientation, body–limb interaction, and synergistic global movement of a limb.

3.3.4 *Importance of the Reticular Formation*

Most patients affected with excessive spasticity, particularly children with cerebral palsy, are hampered by additional manifestations linked to *over-reactivity* that strongly aggravates their disability. These manifestations consist, among others, of startle responses to even minor physical or psychological irritations, parasite motor reactions, and incongruous movements to any close or remote stimuli. The whole central nervous system is involved in those manifestations not only via the propriospinal interneuron network but also, and to a significant extent, through the reticular formation (RF) and its widespread connections.

The RF is composed of widely spaced neurons loosely arranged into nuclear groups throughout the entire brainstem tegmentum. The huge dendritic trees and the highly branched afferent and efferent network of axons that separate the RF perikarya cause its "reticular" appearance in microscopic sections. The RF extends continuously throughout the entire length of the tegmentum. It fills all of the space not occupied by cranial nerve nuclei, supplementary sensory and motor nuclei, and long and short tracts. The bulbo-medullary junction is generally regarded as its caudal limit. From the anatomic point of view, the rostral limit of the RF is at the midbrain–diencephalon junction, but functionally, it represents a continuum between spinal cord and diencephalic and cerebral connections.

The RF receives impulses from and sends impulses to all of the central nervous system; thus, it influences all mental, motor, and sensory functions. Physiologically, RF neurons are characterized by recruitment, divergence, and after-discharge. The RF is particularly sensitive to general anesthetics and certain psychoactive drugs that have much less effect on the lemniscal and other specific afferent sensory systems.

3.3.4.1 The Reticular Formation Afferents

The RF receives collaterals from most ascending or descending pathways through the brainstem, regardless of the location of a pathway's origin in the spinal cord or in the brain and of the pathway's function, visceral or somatic, motor or sensory.

3.3.4.2 The Specific Efferent Reticular Formation Pathways

The RF efferent pathways are the reticulobulbar and the reticulospinal tracts with their specific neurotransmitter pathways.

The *reticulobulbar tracts* run to all cranial nerve nuclei.

The *reticulospinal tracts* run within the ventrolateral columns of the spinal cord and end into laminae VII, VIII, and IX at all cord levels, where they overlap extensively with the termination fields of the vestibular nuclei. These pathways act on the axial muscles, particularly those of the neck, to mediate postural reflexes and muscle tone. Their field of termination overlaps also with the terminals of the corticospinal and rubrospinal tracts. Whereas a minority of reticulospinal axons ends on the ventral motoneurons, most end on internuncial neurons of laminae VII–IX.

3.3.5 In conclusion and brief

Spasticity corresponds to the exaggeration of the myotatic reflex and more generally to an hyperexcitability of the motoneurons. This hyperexcitability results from a loss of inhibitory control from the supraspinal descending pathways, not only the corticospinal tract but also and even more the brainstem descending inhibitory pathways, principally the inhibitory reticular formation. Also important, spinal plasticity after pathological process plays a crucial role in hyperexcitability. Two mechanisms may occur: (I) axonal growth (collateral sprouting) from intact nerve fibers in the direction of synaptic sites vacated by the degeneration of lesioned nerve fibers [29] and (II), to a lesser extent, a phenomenon of hypersensitivity of neuronal receptors, compensating for the loss of presynaptic afferents.

3.4 Surgical Implications for Dorsal Rhizotomy

3.4.1 *Considering the neurophysiological mechanisms of spasticity in CP children,* the criteria to be optimal candidate for dorsal rhizotomy (DR) *are the following*

- Hypertonia: disabling.
- Spasticity: predominant over dystonia.
- Abnormal movements: absent.
- Tendino-muscular contractures, capsular retractions, and bone/joint deformities: absent or at least minimal.
- Muscle power especially in antigravity muscular groups: good.
- Voluntary motility hidden behind hypertonia: still present.
- I.Q.: good.
- Cooperation of child and family: active.

3.4.2 The Appropriate Time for the Neurosurgical Treatment Is Still Controversial

Theoretically, time is when an excess of hypertonia has been recognized to be harmful and before contractures and deformities appear.

In fact, the optimal time is difficult to determine; too early would impact the developmental maturation of the central nervous system and capacities of further locomotion skills; too late would entail the risk of irreducible contractures and deformities. For our team, the decision should be based not only on the age itself but also—and primarily—*on functional status deterioration*. This can be objectively quantified and followed on the classic scoring scales, especially the Gross Motor Function Measure (GMFM) score (Fig. 3.5).

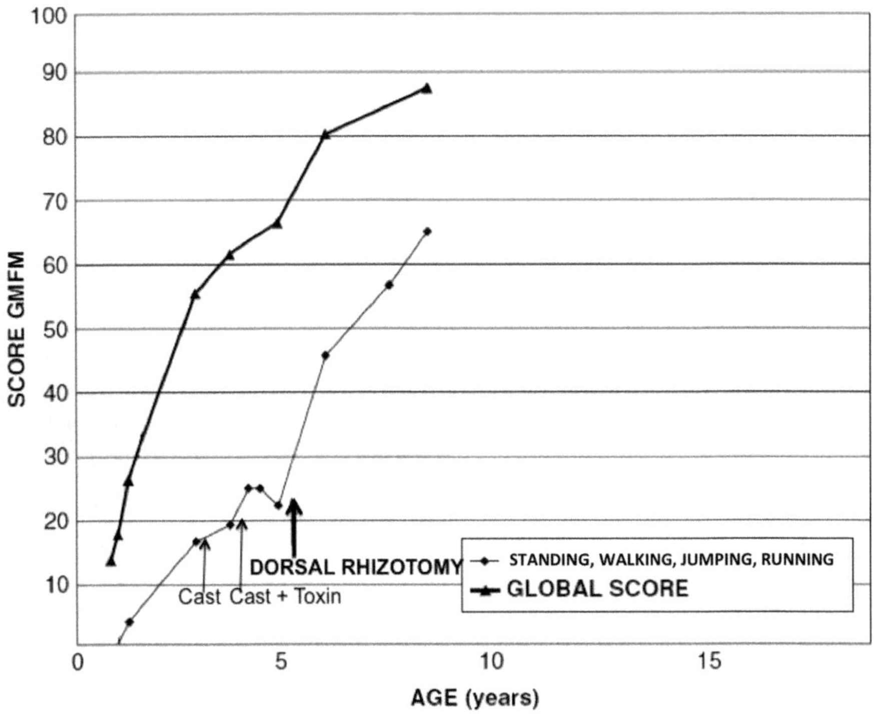

Fig. 3.5 Time course (in years) of dimensions on the Gross Motor Function Measure. Diplegic child with cerebral palsy: global score and targeted score on standing/walking/running/jumping. Note that dorsal rhizotomy (DR) was indicated after cast and cast + botulinum toxin injections failed. Also note that the score improved significantly after DR was performed

3.4.3 There Are Many Different Ways That Have Been Developed to Perform DR

The most important types are illustrated in Fig. 3.6 [30–32].

Some teams use extended approaches, others limited openings. Some teams target every dorsal root as a whole, others target rootlet by rootlet individually. Some teams perform detailed mapping and detailed testing of roots, others more rudimentary monitoring. All these methods have been recently reviewed in an excellent article by Enslin et al. [32].

The question of the *proportion of roots/rootlets to be cut* still remains a debate. There is an empirical consensus that an average of 60% ± 10% should be cut, depending on the preoperative status of the child. Morota in a recent paper proposed the following formula established on the GMFM-88 system: $y = 100 - x$ (where y

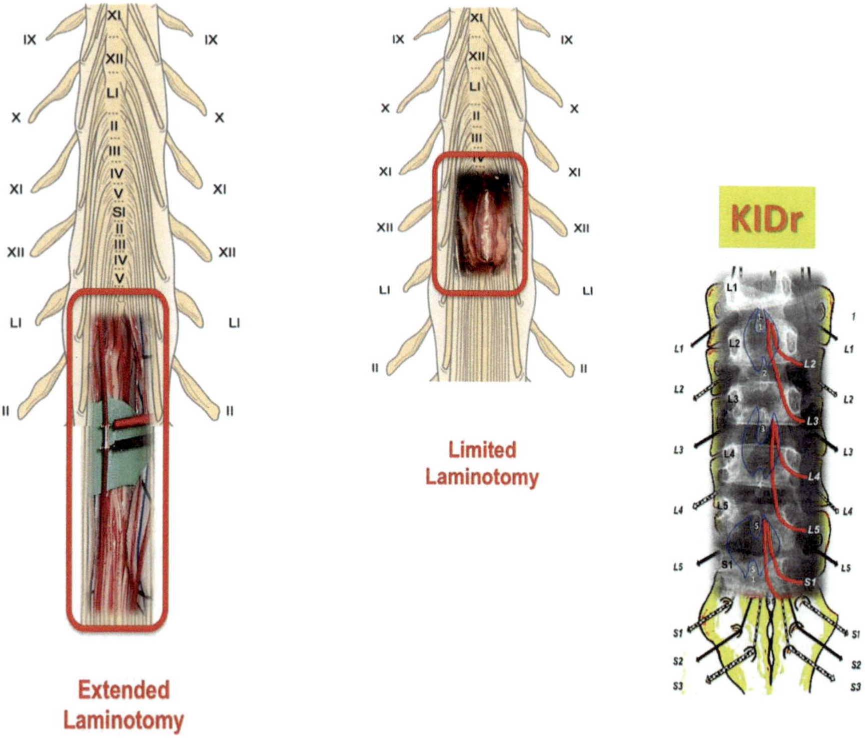

Fig. 3.6 Main variants for dorsal rhizotomy. *Left*: extended laminotomy from L1 to S1 to expose all roots of the entire cauda equina. *Middle*: limited laminotomy at caudal part of the conus medullaris (from Th11 to L1). Through such approach, L2 and L3 (ventral and dorsal) roots can be identified at their respective dural sheaths, while the dorsal rootlets from L4 to all sacral segments are identified at their entry into the dorsolateral sulcus of the conus medullaris. *Right*: Keyhole Interlaminar Dorsal rhizotomy (KIDr) through enlarged interlaminar spaces to target all lumbosacral (ventral and dorsal, individually) from L2 to S2, intradurally at their respective dural sheaths

is the estimate cutting rate and x the preoperative GMFM score) [33]. Whatever the method used, DR should be a tailored operation adapted to every particular child that must be decided by a multidisciplinary pediatric team and adjusted by a rigorous intraoperative neurophysiological monitoring [15]. Because most reports, as well as our recent study on the functional anatomy of the lumbar–sacral roots [34], show important interindividual variability and some asymmetry of myotome innervation, intraoperative guidance by a strict intraoperative neuromonitoring seems to us of practical interest. Therefore, we currently perform at each radicular level, from L2 to S2, on both sides, stimulation of every ventral root *for anatomical mapping* (Fig. 3.7, **upper row**) and stimulation of every dorsal root *for physiological testing*

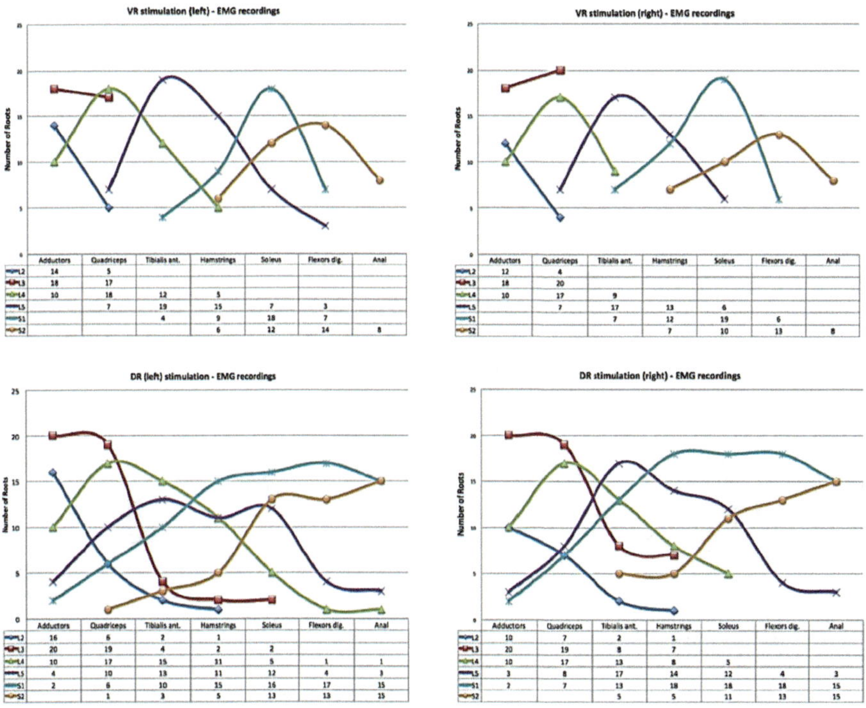

VR stimulation (left) - EMG recordings

	Adductors	Quadriceps	Tibialis ant.	Hamstrings	Soleus	Flexors dig.	Anal
L2	14	5					
L3	18	17					
L4	10	18	12	5			
L5		7	19	15	7	3	
S1			4	9	18	7	
S2				6	12	14	8

VR stimulation (right) - EMG recordings

	Adductors	Quadriceps	Tibialis ant.	Hamstrings	Soleus	Flexors dig.	Anal
L2	12	4					
L3	18	20					
L4	10	17	9				
L5		7	17	13	6		
S1			7	12	19	6	
S2				7	10	13	8

DR (left) stimulation - EMG recordings

	Adductors	Quadriceps	Tibialis ant.	Hamstrings	Soleus	Flexors dig.	Anal
L2	16	6	2	1			
L3	20	19	4	2	2		
L4	10	17	15	11	5	1	1
L5	4	10	13	11	12	4	3
S1	2	6	10	15	16	17	15
S2		1	3	5	13	13	15

DR stimulation (right) - EMG recordings

	Adductors	Quadriceps	Tibialis ant.	Hamstrings	Soleus	Flexors dig.	Anal
L2	10	7	2	1			
L3	20	19	8	7			
L4	10	17	13	8	5		
L5	3	8	17	14	12	4	3
S1	2	7	13	18	18	18	15
S2			5	5	11	13	15

Fig. 3.7 Distribution of muscle responses to stimulation: of ventral roots (myotome) (upper row) and dorsal roots (according to excitability degree) (lower row). Figure shows strong overlapping between root territories, in spite of intensity of stimulation of root just above threshold (in a personal 20 patients' series). Distribution of muscular responses to *stimulation of each ventral root (VR)*, as assessed by electromyography (EMG) recordings to L2–S2 VR stimulation. Columns show the number of patients in whom each muscle contracted after stimulation of each of the six VRs. Each column corresponds to one of the muscles (eight for VR stimulation, including psoas that was examined only by physiotherapist). Data from left and right sides are illustrated separately to compare symmetry. Distribution of muscular responses to *stimulation of each dorsal root (DR)*, as assessed by electromyography (EMG) recordings to L2–S2 DR stimulation. Columns show the number of patients in which each muscle contracted after stimulation of each of the six DRs. Each curve corresponds to one of the muscles (seven for DR stimulation). Data from left and right side are illustrated separately to compare symmetry

of the excitability of the segmental circuitry (Fig. 3.7, **lower row**) [35, 36]. This led to frequently modify the initial program of the sectioning quantification, as much as in three-fourths of our surgically treated children [37].

Although intraoperative recordings have been widely used and described by a majority of teams [38–43], only a few systematic studies have compared reflexive excitability between the various segmental levels of the conus medullaris [44–45]. The use in a personal study of similar stimulation parameters for all the exposed dorsal roots to be targeted confirmed significant differences in the degree of reflexive excitability among the various L2–S2 lumbosacral segments tested and also the existence of important interindividual variability among patients [36], as illustrated in (Figs. 3.7 and 3.8). The degrees of excitability in L2 and L3 were found to be lower than expected, especially for L2. The degrees of excitability in L4 and L5 were both substantially elevated, so that it was considered that those roots had to be targeted despite the (known) danger of weakening antigravity function and pelvic stability. The excitability in S1 was found to be high, as expected. For the S2 root, because the degree of excitability was substantially high, its partial sectioning was deemed justified provided taking into account the potential risk on the genitourinary

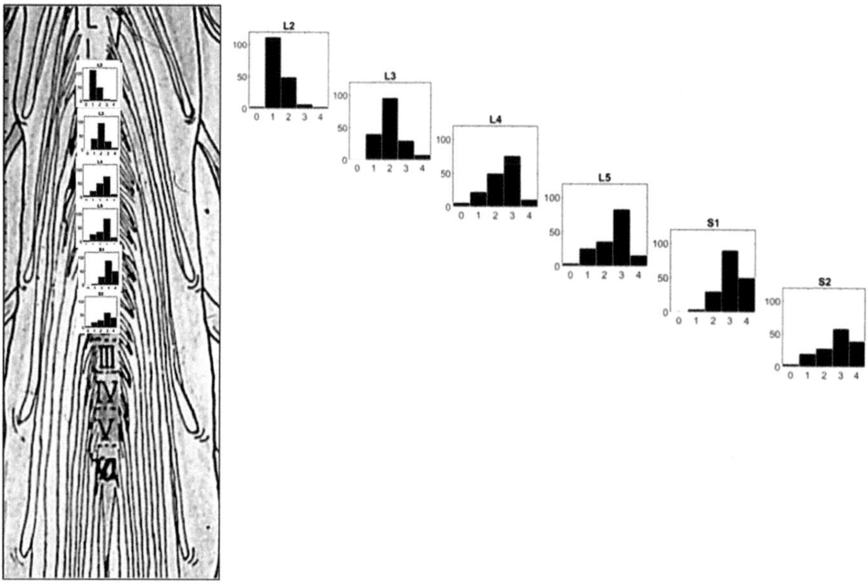

Fig. 3.8 Grades of reflexive excitability according to spinal cord metameric levels. Figure presents grades of reflexive excitability—according to the scale 0–4 described by Fasano—of each of the L2 to S2 radiculo-medullary segments, in a personal series of 46 children spastic CP children who underwent the Keyhole Interlaminar Dorsal rhizotomy (KIDr) procedure used by the authors. All explored levels (assessed by clinical observation of the physical therapist and EMG recordings, from both sides) manifested increased excitability, with higher grades in lower segments. These neurophysiological findings have practical implications for multidisciplinary surgical preplanning and operative procedure. Bar graphs on conus medullaris (L2 through S2) show the number of "cases" for each grade of excitability according to the grading scale 0–4 described by Fasano

function. Accuracy and safety implicate intraoperative mapping and monitoring of the lower limb muscle groups and of the anal/bladder sphincters [46–49].

3.4.4 Is There Anatomical/Physiological Justification to Consider Dorsal Rootlets Individually and Independently?

This is still a to-day controversial subject.

- *In the one-single-level laminectomy/laminoplasty approach at the conus*, only the L2/L3 roots can be anatomically identified, the L4–S2 roots being not exposed at their dural sleeve entry. Further, those dorsal roots cannot be anatomically individualized ones from the others. Identification of levels can be performed only electrophysiologically. Given the significant overlap in muscle innervation, the surgeon relies on the muscle displaying the largest EMG response [44]. Following identification, the roots are arbitrarily divided into a number of rootlets of similar thickness, in general four components on average. Then, excitability of each dissected element "considered rootlet or group of rootlets" is tested individually. First, a threshold intensity, defined as the current needed to elicit a noticeable response (a compound muscle action potential), is determined by increasing the current intensity incrementally (from 0.1 mA to a seldom reached maximum of 10 mA) until a potential is evoked. Then, using the previously identified threshold intensity, a 1-s, 50-Hz train stimulation is delivered at the same spot in the rootlet, following which the elicited response is classified according to the five-level grading score of Fasano [45]. Such limited approach, which has the advantage of a minimal spine opening, is intrinsically approximative in terms of identification of topographic radicular level. Further, testing excitability at the level of the rootlet structure, which needs to divide each dorsal root into three to seven rootlets (median four rootlets), entails the risk of traumatizing or at least striking the manipulated rootlets and therefore modifying excitability.
- For the teams which follow Peacock's method of using an *extended laminotomy approach from L1–S1* [50, 51], identification of roots, as well as of all their constituting rootlets, can by principle be accurately performed. The procedure was estimated reliable by most of the adepts of the method, as particularly well-documented by Mittal et al. [52]. However, it might be that the wide exposure in this technical modality do not provide sufficient delicacy to respect the physiology of the neurophysiological events. Stimulation of the dorsal roots/rootlets is generally accomplished after their extensive dissection and elevation from the pool of cerebrospinal fluid, which may provoke some harmful stretching and modify electrophysiology.
- In most reports, whatever the extent of the chosen laminotomies and cauda equina exposures, *the strength of the stimulus* was mentioned "adjusted to pro-

vide a maximal dorsal root potential, whilst taking care to keep the stimulus intensity low enough to prevent the spread of current to adjacent roots" [52]. However, because intensity generally varied as highly as 5–15 mA, stimulation might well manifest some parasite diffusion, especially when dealing with individual rootlets' testing.

- De Vloo et al., in a recent article on their own results and that visited literature, concluded that "the responses to stimulation appeared to be relatively stable between patients, … and that there were limited inter- and intra-subject variabilities" [44]. However, their estimations remain in conflict with those from two studies that reported substantial variability upon retesting the stimulation threshold and responses [53, 54].
- Up to now, as claimed by Cohen and Webster, *stimulation rootlet by rootlet* (or group of rootlets by group of rootlets) has not proven any superiority (or no inferiority either) compared to individual global stimulation of the entire dorsal roots [55]. In their article, the authors concluded: "Arbitrary subdivision of dorsal roots at surgery may lead to widely varying numbers of IA spindle afferents traveling within each dorsal rootlet". This alone could explain significant variation in responses. In addition, the use of repetitive short-duration stimuli delivered at supramaximal threshold probably also leads to response variability.
- Since our work on the anatomical/histological structure of the dorsal root entry zone (DREZ), published in the *Journal of Comparative Neurology* [25], to our knowledge, no study was conducted on the comparative organization of the various afferent fibers in between the constituting rootlets of the dorsal roots (Fig. 3.9). In our study, no significant difference in histology was found among the rootlets letting know that some of them would be preferentially devoted to a myotatic or any form of tonigenic function. However, one study using electron microcopy, by Fukuhara et al., found an association between grades of stimulation response and histopathological characteristics of the rootlets, with axonal degeneration and dysmyelination apparent only in rootlets with an abnormal response to stimulation [56].

3.4.5 Mechanisms of Postoperative Hypotonia Are Complex

Reduction of tone after DR is primarily linked to the (planned) cutting of the dorsal roots, the aim of which is to interrupt not only the afferent IA fibers, which are responsible for the (monosynaptic) myotatic reflex, but also all types of tonigenic (polysynaptic) fibers, which converge onto the segmental interneurons and exert their excitatory input to the ventral horn motor neurons [7, 57, 58].

Noteworthy, in a large number of patients, DRs are followed in the early postoperative period by hypotonia that may be excessive, which may worry the patient and the caregivers. In fact, after approximately 6 ± 3 months, in most cases, the tone reaches an appropriate level and so for a long-term therapeutic effect. Likely, part of the decrease in tone observed immediately after the surgery can be related to the

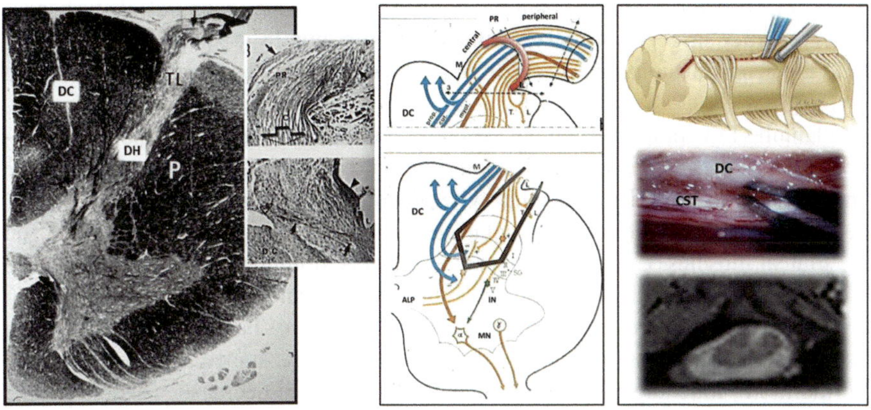

Fig. 3.9 The dorsal rootlet entity and the dorsal root entry zone (DREZ). *Left:* transverse hemisection of the spinal cord (at the lower cervical level) with myelin stained with luxol fast blue and fuchsin, showing the myelinated rootlet afferents that reach the dorsal column (DC) and the ventral horn through the dorsal horn (DH). *P* pyramidal tract, *TL* tract of Lissauer. Small arrow indicates the pial ring of the dorsal rootlet (diameter: 1 mm). Histological insert and schematic representation of DREZ: each rootlet can be divided, owing to the transition of its glial support, into a peripheral and a central segment. The transition between the two segments is at the pial ring (PR), which is located approximately 1 mm outside the penetration of the rootlet into the dorsolateral sulcus. Peripherally, the fibers are mixed together. As they approach the pial ring, the fine fibers (considered nociceptive) are located toward the rootlet surfaces (small arrows). In the central segment, they group in the ventrolateral portion of the DREZ and enter the dorsal horn through the tract of Lissauer (TL). The large myotatic fibers (myot) are situated in the middle of the DREZ to reach the ventral horn, whereas the large myelinated sensory fibers (proprioceptive and cutaneous epicritic) are located dorsomedially to reach the dorsal column (DC). On the schematic drawing, note the monosynaptic excitatory arc reflex of the myotatic fibers on the ventral horn alpha motoneurons (MN), the inhibitory influence of the recurrent collaterals of the large fibers to the dorsal column on dorsal horn cells and interneurons (IN), the fine fiber excitatory input onto the dorsal horn cells and the interneurons, the origin of the spino-reticulo-thalamic anterolateral pathways (ALP), and the projections of the interneurons onto the motoneurons (MN). The Microsurgical DREZoTomy (MDT) target (arrowhead), which aims to interrupt most of the fine tonigenic and the myotatic fibers, enters the medial (excitatory) portion of the tract of Lissauer and penetrates deeply in I–VI Rexed laminae of the dorsal horn. Sg, substantia gelatinosa. *Right (from top to bottom):* drawing of the MDT procedure; operative view of the MDT lesioning, performed inside the DREZ and the DH, after opening of the dorsolateral sulcus and working on high magnification of the operative microscope between the dorsal column (DC) and the corticospinal tract (CST); and MRI postoperative aspect of the MDT lesion

surgical manipulations, especially in the modalities that use rootlets' individual dissection and stimulation.

Progressive, late return of tone may have several (other) sources: refunctioning of some of the surgically traumatized fibers, synaptic rearrangement of the remaining dorsal root fibers, and their functional reorganization to reestablish their output to ventral horn through neural plasticity. These hypotheses are corroborated by clinical and neurophysiological observations. Hyperesthesia and paresthesias, which may be present immediately after surgery, slowly disappear in most cases.

The somatosensory-evoked potential study shows that the (eventual) disturbances observed after surgery normalize within the next 6 months [59]. This is concordant with the neurophysiological knowledge on the segmental organization of the spinal cord [60].

Planning DR should take into account not to decrease too much tone in the antigravity muscles and in the muscles contributing to pelvis stability, especially in the children able to walk. Briefly, antigravity predominantly (although not exclusively) depends on the quadricipital muscular group and stability of pelvis principally on the gluteal muscles. Considering metameric levels, dominant responsible roots are L3/L4 and L5, respectively. Also of paramount importance is not to produce excessive hypotonia in the triceps surae muscles; as a matter of fact, creating a talus foot would result in the impossibility to trigger walk with its stance and swing phases. Furthermore, touching S2—which would be justified to decrease spasticity in the hamstrings—entails the risk of detrusor and sphincter hypotonia, with its harmful consequences. For these reasons, and because—on another hand—there is an important interindividual variety among patients, intraoperative neuromonitoring/mapping seems to us mandatory in the decision process of identifying roots (and the amount of their fibers) to be cut.

3.4.6 Mechanisms of Distant Effects

Importantly, effects of dorsal rhizotomy (D.Rh.) should include the so-called distant effects. Those have been recognized as soon as the 1970s. It was pointed out that lumbosacral rhizotomy alleviates not only spasticity but also—frequently—dystonia in the upper limbs [61, 62]. This suprasegmental phenomenon was named by Gros: "distant effects" [61]. Also, parasite functional disturbances in the neck and cephalic extremity, as well as emotional over-reactivity, can be favorably influenced after D.Rh. [15].

Hypotheses on mechanisms are plural.

1. The predominant one is input decreased onto the reticular formation and input particularly conveyed by the ascending spinoreticular tract, structure described in the anatomical bases section of this article.
2. Distant effects of D.Rh. can also be linked to decreased input within two longitudinal systems coordinating reflex activity of the spinal cord and medulla oblongata, known to be activated through dorsal root stimulation at any level [63, 64].

    2.1 The first system consists of spinal afferent volleys that ascend the spinal cord and reach the medulla oblongata where they relay. Some of the impulses then reenter the spinal cord to reach spinal motor outflows; they correspond to spino-bulbo-spinal reflexes. The other impulses continue to ascend the brainstem to influence cranial motor outflows; they correspond to spino-

bulbo-cranial reflexes. Interaction between systems takes place predominantly within the midline bulbar reticular formation [65].
2.2 The second system corresponds to the propriospinal reflexes, which—differently—do not depend on bulbar relay but are self-sufficient within the spinal cord. Those reflexes, elicited by electrical stimulation of the dorsal roots, can be observed and recorded in spinalized animals [66].
2.3 These propriospinal reflexes are sustained by interneurons that have their cell bodies located in all laminae of the gray matter, with fibers, diffusely projecting, abundantly crossing from one side of the spinal cord to the other, and projecting to all motor nuclei. Propriospinal reflexes can be initiated from muscular as well as cutaneous afferents and cause discharges in both flexor and extensor motor neurons.

Both systems are implicated in interlimb, trunk, and head coordination mechanisms. D.Rh., by reducing input in those systems, not only diminishes spasticity in lower limbs and reduces abnormal postures but also improves gait, alleviates pain, eases comfort, and facilitates nursing from caregivers.

Also, D.Rh. by its effect on both systems, which have intimate central connections with the regulation centers of the autonomic nervous system, may favorably influence harmful dysautonomic/vegetative manifestations.

According to our experience, such distant effects can be particularly interesting in quadriplegic children by dramatically diminishing the parasite movements and improving the postural maintain in the upper limbs, neck, and trunk. Also handicapping emotional over-reactivity can be significantly reduced [15].

Therefore, we recommend lumbosacral D.Rh. not only for diplegic but also quadriplegic children for making positioning more comfortable, cares easier, pain more bearable, and emotional over-reactivity lesser.

3.5 Conclusions

Indications for dorsal rhizotomy in cerebral palsy should be based on the particular neurophysiological mechanisms of hypertonia, after recognition of the importance of the spastic component in the disorder. The procedure should be designed in accordance with the known functional anatomy of the radicular myotome innervation. Surgery should be decided and tailored through a multidisciplinary team [67]. The procedure should be guided by a strict intraoperative neuromonitoring, with ventral root stimulation for anatomical mapping and dorsal root stimulation for quantification of roots/rootlets to be cut [36]. The next period should be devoted to launch in-depth studies, principally neurophysiologic confronted to anatomy, with the aim to further improve efficacy, selectivity, and innocuity of the neurosurgical treatment of the disabling hypertonia affecting CP children.

Acknowledgments To Ms. Adelaide Croizé-Pourcelet for contribution to iconography.

References

1. Lance JW. Spasticity: disordered motor control. Chicago: Year Book Medical Publishers; 1980. p. 485–95.
2. Sanger TD, Delgado MR, Gaebler-Spira D, Hallett M, Mink JW. Classification and definition of disorders causing hypertonia in childhood. Pediatrics. 2003;111:e89–97.
3. Burridge JH, Wood DE, Hermens HJ, et al. Theoretical and methodological considerations in the measurement of spasticity. Disabil Rehabil. 2005;27:69–80.
4. Pandyan AD, Gregoric M, Barnes MP, et al. Spasticity: clinical perceptions, neurological realities and meaningful measurement. Disabil Rehabil. 2005;27:2–6.
5. Van den Noort JC, Bar-On L, Aertbeliën E, Bonikowski M, Braendvik SM, Broström EW, et al. European consensus on the concepts and measurement of the pathophysiological neuromuscular responses to passive muscle stretch. Eur J Neurol. 2017;24(7):981–e38.
6. Sherrington CS. Decerebrate rigidity and reflex coordination of movements. J Physiol. 1898;22(4):319–32.
7. Sheean G. Neurophysiology of spasticity. In: Barnes MP, Johnson GR, editors. Upper motor neuron syndrome and spasticity. Cambridge: Cambridge University Press; 2008. p. 9–63.
8. Barnes MP, Johnson GR. An overview of the clinical management of spasticity. In: Barnes MP, Johnson GR, editors. Upper motor neurone syndrome and spasticity. 2nd ed. Cambridge: Cambridge University Press; 2008. p. 1–8.
9. Gracies JM. Pathophysiology of spastic paresis. II: emergence of muscle overactivity. Muscle Nerve. 2005;31:552–71.
10. Humphrey DR, Reed DJ. Separate cortical systems for control of joint movement and joint stiffness reciprocal reactivation and coactivation of antagonist muscles. In: Desmedt JE, editor. Motor control mechanisms in health and disease. New-York: Raven Press; 1983. p. 347–72.
11. Delwaide PJ, Olivier E. Pathophysiological aspects of spasticity in man. In: Beneeke R, Conrad B, Marsden CD, editors. Motor disturbance I. London: Academic Press; 1987. p. 153–68.
12. Osler W. The cerebral palsies of children: a clinical study from the infirmary for nervous diseases. Philadelphia: Blakiston; 1889.
13. Little WJ. On the influence of abnormal parturition, difficult labours, premature birth and asphyxia neonatorum on the mental and physical condition of the child, especially in relation to deformities. Trans Obstet Soc Lond. 1861;3:293–344.
14. Ingram TT. A study of cerebral palsy in childhood population of Edinburgh. Arch Dis Child. 1955;30:85–98.
15. Sindou M, Georgoulis G, Mertens P. Neurosurgery for spasticity: a practical guide for treating children and adults. Wien: Springer; 2014.
16. Graham HK, Selber P. Musculoskeletal aspects of cerebral palsy. J Bone Joint Surg (Br). 2003;85(2):157–66.
17. Simonetta-Moreau M, Marque P, Marchand-Pauvert V, Pierrot-Deseilligny E. The pattern of excitation of human lower limb motoneurones by probable group II muscle afferents. J Physiol. 1999;517(Pt 1):287–300.
18. Burke D, Gandevia SC, McKeon B. The afferent volleys responsible for spinal proprioceptive reflexes in man. J Physiol. 1983;339:535–52.
19. Burke D. Critical examination of the case for or against fusimotor involvement in disorders of muscle tone. Adv Neurol. 1983;39:133–50.
20. Kuypers HGJM. A new look at the organization of the motor system. In: Kuypers HGJM, Martin GF, editors. Progress in brain research [Internet]. Elsevier; 1982 [cité 4 avr 2021]. p. 381–403. Disponible sur: https://www.sciencedirect.com/science/article/pii/S0079612308641382
21. Pierrot-Deseilligny E. Electrophysiological assessment of the spinal mechanisms underlying spasticity. Electroencephalogr Clin Neurophysiol. 1990;41:264–73.
22. Nieuwenhuys R, Voogd J, C van Huijzen. The human central nervous system: a synopsis and atlas [Internet]. 3rd ed. Berlin/Heidelberg: Springer; 1988 [cité 4 avr 2021]. Disponible sur: https://www.springer.com/gp/book/9783662103432

23. Jeanmonod D. Neuroanatomical bases of spasticity. In: Sindou MP, Abbott IR, Keravel Y, editors. Neurosurgery for spasticity: a multidisciplinary approach [Internet]. Vienna: Springer; 1991 [cité 4 avr 2021]. p. 3–14. Disponible sur: https://doi.org/10.1007/978-3-7091-6708-3_1.
24. Mertens P. Bases anatomiques de la motricité appliquée à l'étude de la spasticité [Internet]. In: EM-Consulte. Masson: Elsevier; [cité 4 avr 2021]. Disponible sur: https://www.em-consulte.com/article/118641/fgures/bases-anatomiques-de-la-motricite-appliquees-a-l-e
25. Sindou M, Quoex C, Baleydier C. Fiber organization at the posterior spinal cord-rootlet junction in man. J Comp Neurol. 1974;153:15–26.
26. Willis WD. Ascending somatosensory systems. In: Yaksh TL, editor. Spinal afferent processing [Internet]. Boston: Springer; 1986 [cité 4 avr 2021]. p. 243–74. Disponible sur. https://doi.org/10.1007/978-1-4684-4994-5_11.
27. Kuypers HGJM. Anatomy of the descending pathways. In: Brooks VB, editor. Handbook of physiology, section 1, nervous system. Baltimore: Williams and Wilkins; 1981. p. 597–666.
28. Walberg F. Paths descending from the brain stem. An overview. In: Sjölund B, Björklund A, editors. Brainstem control of spinal mechanisms. Amsterdam: Elsevier; 1982. p. 1–27.
29. McCouch GP, Austin GM, Liu CN, Liu CY. Sprouting as a cause of spasticity. J Neurophysiol. 1958;21(3):205–16.
30. Warsi NM, Tailor J, Coulter IC, Shakil H, Workewych A, Haldenby R, Breitbart S, Strantzas S, Vandenberk M, Dewan MC, Ibrahim GM. Selective dorsal rhizotomy: an illustrated review of operative techniques. J Neurosurg Pediatr. 2020;7:1–8.
31. Abbott R. The selective dorsal rhizotomy technique for spasticity in 2020: a review. Childs Nerv Syst. 2020;36(9):1895–905.
32. Enslin JMN, Langerak NG, Fieggen AG. The evolution of selective dorsal rhizotomy for the management of spasticity. Neurotherapeutics. 2019;16(1):3–8.
33. Morota N. Clinically practical formula for preoperatively estimating the cutting rate of the spinal nerve root in a functional posterior rhizotomy. Childs Nerv Syst. 2019;35(4):665–72.
34. Georgoulis G, Sindou M. Muscle responses to radicular stimulation during lumbo-sacral dorsal rhizotomy for spastic diplegia: insights to myotome innervation. Clin Neurophysiol. 2020;131:1075–86.
35. Sindou M, Georgoulis G. Keyhole interlaminar dorsal rhizotomy for spastic diplegia in cerebral palsy. Acta Neurochir. 2015;157(7):1187–96. https://doi.org/10.1007/s00701-015-2453-1.
36. Sindou M, Georgoulis G, Joud A, Neromyliotis E, Dinopoulos A. Excitability of the radiculo-medullary circuitry in spastic cerebral palsy: an intraoperative neurophysiological study in children undergoing selective dorsal rhizotomy. Dev Med Child Neurol. 2022;00:1–8. https://doi.org/10.1111/dmcn.15315.
37. Georgoulis G, Brinzeu A, Sindou M. Dorsal rhizotomy for children with spastic diplegia of cerebral palsy origin: usefulness of intraoperative monitoring. J Neurosurg Pediatr. 2018;22(1):1–13.
38. Park TS, Gaffney PE, Kaufman BA, Molleston MC. Selective lumbosacral dorsal rhizotomy immediately caudal to the conus medullaris for cerebral palsy spasticity. Neurosurgery. 1993;33:929–34.
39. Turner RP. Neurophysiologic intraoperative monitoring during selective dorsal rhizotomy. J Clin Neurophysiol. 2009;26:82–4.
40. Hays RM, McLaughlin JF, Bjornson KF, Stephens K, Roberts TS, Price R. Electrophysiological monitoring during selective dorsal rhizotomy, and spasticity and GMFM performance. Dev Med Child Neurol. 1998;40(4):233–8.
41. Logigian EL, Shefner JM, Goumnerova L, Scott RM, Soriano SG, Madsen J. The critical importance of stimulus intensity in intraoperative monitoring for partial dorsal rhizotomy. Muscle Nerve. 1996;19(4):415–22.
42. Newberg NL, Gooch JL, Walker ML. Intraoperative monitoring in selective dorsal rhizotomy. Pediatr Neurosurg. 1991–1992;17(3):124–7.

43. Steinbok P, Kestle JR. Variation between centers in electrophysiologic techniques used in lumbosacral selective dorsal rhizotomy for spastic cerebral palsy. Pediatr Neurosurg. 1996;25(5):233–9.
44. De Vloo P, Huttunen TJ, Forte D, Jankovic I, Lee A, Hair M, Cawker S, Chugh D, Carr L, Crowe BHA, Pitt M, Aquilina K. Intraoperative electrophysiology during single-level selective dorsal rhizotomy: technique, stimulation threshold, and response data in a series of 145 patients. J Neurosurg Pediatr. 2020;25:597–606.
45. Wolter S, Spies C, Martin JH, Schulz M, Sarpong-Bengelsdorf A, Unger J, Thomale UW, Michael T, Murphy JF, Haberl H. Frequency distribution in intraoperative stimulation-evoked EMG responses during selective dorsal rhizotomy in children with cerebral palsy-part 1: clinical setting and neurophysiological procedure. Childs Nerv Syst. 2020;36(9):1945–54.
46. Lang FF, Deletis V, Cohen HW, Velasquez L, Abbott R. Inclusion of the S2 dorsal rootlets in functional posterior rhizotomy for spasticity in children with cerebral palsy. Neurosurgery. 1994;34(5):847–53. discussion 853.
47. Sindou M, Joud A, Georgoulis G. Usefulness of external anal sphincter EMG recording for intraoperative neuromonitoring of the sacral roots—a prospective study in dorsal rhizotomy. Acta Neurochir. 2021;163(2):479–87.
48. Sindou M, Brinzeu A, Georgoulis G. Chapter 35: Neurosurgical lesioning procedures for spasticity and focal dystonia. In: Deletis V, Shils J, Sala E, Seidel K, editors. Neurophysiology in neurosurgery. A modern approach. 2nd ed. London: Academic Press; 2020. p. 499–513.
49. Deletis V, Vodusek DB, Abbott R, Epstein FJ, Turndorf H. Intraoperative monitoring of the dorsal sacral roots: minimizing the risk of iatrogenic micturition disorders. Neurosurgery. 1992;30:72–5.
50. Peacock WJ, Arens LJ. Selective posterior rhizotomy for the relief of spasticity in cerebral palsy. S Afr Med J. 1982;62:119–24.
51. Abbott R, Johann-Murphy M, Shiminski-Maher T, Quartermain D, Forem SL, Gold JT, Epstein FJ. Selective dorsal rhizotomy: outcome and complications in treating spastic cerebral palsy. Neurosurgery. 1993;33(5):851–7. discussion 857.
52. Mittal S, Farmer JP, Poulin C, Silver K. Reliability of intraoperative electrophysiological monitoring in selective posterior rhizotomy. J Neurosurg. 2001;95:67–75.
53. Warf BC, Nelson KR. The electromyographic responses to dorsal rootlet stimulation during partial dorsal rhizotomy are inconsistent. Pediatr Neurosurg. 1996;25:13–9.
54. Weiss IP, Schiff SJ. Reflex variability in selective dorsal rhizotomy. J Neurosurg. 1993;79:346–53.
55. Cohen AR, Webster HC. How selective is selective posterior rhizotomy? Surg Neurol. 1991;35:267–72.
56. Fukuhara T, Nakatsu D, Namba Y, Ichiro Y. Histological evidence of intraoperative monitoring efficacy in selective dorsal rhizotomy. Childs Nerv Syst. 2011;27:1453–8. https://doi.org/10.1007/s00381-011-1462-5.
57. Pierrot-Deseilligny E, Mazieres L. Spinal mechanism underlying spasticity. In: Delwaide PJ, Young RR, editors. Clinical neurophysiology in spasticity. Amsterdam: Elsevier; 1985.
58. Pierrot-Deseilligny E, Morin C, Bergego C, Tankov N. Pattern of group I fibre projections from ankle flexor and extensor muscles in man. Exp Brain Res. 1981;42(3–4):337–50.
59. Parise M, Sindou M, Mertens P, Maugière F. Somatosensory evoked potentials following functional posterior rhizotomy in spastic children. Stereotact Funct Neurosurg. 1997;69:268–73.
60. Jeanmonod D, Sindou M, Mauguiere F. The human cervical and lumbo-sacral evoked electrospinogram. Data from intraoperative spinal cord surface recordings. Electroencephalogr Clin Neurophysiol. 1991;80(6):477–89.
61. Gros C. Spasticity: clinical classification and surgical treatment. Adv Tech Stand Neurosurg. 1979;6:55–97.
62. Sindou M, Abbott R, Keravel Y. Neurosurgery for spasticity: a multidisciplinary approach. Wien: Springer; 1991.

63. Shimamura M, Livingston RB. Longitudinal conduction systems serving spinal and brainstem coordination. J Neurophysiol. 1963;26:258–72. https://doi.org/10.1152/jn.1963.26.2.258. PMID: 13988518
64. Shimamura M, Akert K. Peripheral nervous relations of propriospinal and spino-bulbo-spinal reflex systems. Jpn J Physiol. 1965;15:638–47.
65. Shimamura M. Longitudinal coordination between spinal and cranial reflex systems. Exp Neurol. 1963;8:505–21.
66. Shimamura M. Spino-bulbo-spinal and propriospinal reflexes in various vertebrates. Brain Res. 1973;64:141–65. https://doi.org/10.1016/0006-8993(73)90175-3. PMID: 4781342
67. Sindou M, Duraffourg M, Georgoulis M. Neurosurgery for spasticity: a practical guide for treating children and adults. 2nd ed. Wien: Springer; 2022.

Part II
Patient Selection and Functional Evaluation

Chapter 4
Role of Dorsal Rhizotomy in the Comprehensive Management of Childhood Spasticity

Nobuhito Morota

Abbreviations

BTX	Botulinum toxin
GMFCS	Gross Motor Function Classification System
GMFM	Gross Motor Function Measurement
ITB	Intrathecal baclofen infusion
LMIC	Low- to middle-income country
QOL	Quality of life

4.1 Introduction

A variety of pathologies, which affect the central nervous system (CNS), lead to motor dysfunction such as mono-, para-, and tetra-paresis/palsy. These pathological findings, collectively referred as "negative phenomena," are primarily characterized by muscle weakness. Conversely, spasticity is characterized by muscle hyperactivity and hypertonia, representing a category of "positive phenomena" in the spectrum of CNS-related impairments [1].

Spasticity is a common finding in children who have suffered CNS damage. Concurrent with exaggerated motor tone, spasticity often serves as a detrimental factor affecting the motor function. Over the long term, spasticity leads to joint contracture and deformity, exacerbating the decline of motor function and diminishing the overall quality of life (QOL) in daily activities. Severe spasticity can induce pain and suffering in seriously disabled children and increase the burden of

N. Morota (✉)
Department of Neurosurgery, Kitasato University Hospital, Minami-Ku, Sagamihara, Japan

N. Morota, P. Steinbok (eds.), *Dorsal Rhizotomy: Neurosurgery for Childhood Spasticity*, Advances and Technical Standards in Neurosurgery 51,
https://doi.org/10.1007/978-3-031-86441-4_4

caregivers, further intensifying the impact on QOL for both children and caregivers. This underscores the critical importance of spasticity management to enhance both motor function and QOL in disabled children experiencing spasticity.

Various interventions, including oral medications, neurorehabilitation, and surgical procedures, have been used in the management of childhood spasticity [2]. The intricacies of addressing spasticity in disabled children necessitate a holistic and integrated approach, where a comprehensive multidisciplinary team plays a critical role [3].

Dorsal rhizotomy stands as a neurosurgical intervention designed to manage spasticity by selectively and functionally severing root/rootlets during the surgical procedure [4–10]. This chapter provides an in-depth exploration of the role of dorsal rhizotomy in the comprehensive management of childhood spasticity, elucidating its position within the broader context of concurrent therapeutic modalities.

4.2 Treatment Modalities for Childhood Spasticity

The medical management of spasticity encompasses two distinct treatment modalities: basic management and active management [11–14]. The basic management involves noninvasive interventions such as antispastic medications and neurorehabilitation through physio- and occupational therapies. These modalities are administered on a long-term basis to control spasticity and enhance or maintain motor function. In contrast, active management entails invasive treatments aimed at reducing spasticity and improving motor function. Notable procedures in the field of active management include dorsal rhizotomy, orthopedic surgery, intrathecal baclofen infusion (ITB), and local injection of botulinum toxin (BTX) [2, 15, 16]. It is crucial to note that dorsal rhizotomy, ITB, and BTX are specifically applied to alleviate spasticity, whereas orthopedic surgery is indicated for joint complications secondary to spasticity.

There are advantages and limitations inherent in each active management procedure employed for the reduction of spasticity. Table 4.1 provides a comprehensive overview of the characteristics associated with these treatments. Dorsal

Table 4.1 Factors influencing the selection of spasticity treatment

	FPR	ITB	Botox
Pathology	Mainly spastic cerebral palsy	Any spasticity	Any spasticity
W. dystonia	+	+++	+ ~ ++
Extent of spasticity	General (L/E > U/E)	General (L/E > U/E)	Focal
Degree	Mild ~ severe	Severe	Mild ~ moderate
Age	2.5 y.o. and over to adolescent	3 y.o. and over (BW. > 15Kg)	No age limitation (Insurance coverage over 2 y.o. in Japan)

rhizotomy, primarily indicated for spastic cerebral palsy, demonstrates versatility by extending its application to spasticity stemming from diverse pathologies [17, 18]. While effective for any degree of spasticity, preference is given to cases with mild to moderate spasticity, corresponding to Gross Motor Function Classification System (GMFCS) levels 1–3 [19, 20]. Surgical indications remain a subject of global debate, with the youngest age recommended at 2.5–3 years old [4, 8, 17, 21]. Dorsal rhizotomy may extend to young adults without joint complications, although its efficacy is a matter of controversy. ITB, recognized for its efficacy across varied spasticity backgrounds, proves effective at any spasticity level through catheter tip adjustments. Commonly applied for moderate to severe spasticity (GMFCS levels 3–5), ITB may have a role in the management of associated dystonia [22, 23]. Surgical indications lean more toward body weight than age, with a preference for a body weight exceeding 15 kg, although acceptability at over 10 kg is acknowledged. The reported youngest and smallest patient was 11 months old with the body weight of 6.4 kg [24]. In contrast to dorsal rhizotomy and ITB, BTX is usually used for focal spasticity management, but its supplemental use extends to generalized spasticity. Without age restrictions, even infants can receive BTX treatment.

4.3 A Strategic Approach to Spasticity Management in Childhood

The management of childhood spasticity is strategically organized into three distinct modalities. The foundational approach involves basic management utilizing oral antispastic medication and neurorehabilitation, followed by active management aimed at reducing spasticity through interventions such as dorsal rhizotomy, ITB, and BTX. Additionally, there is a focus on active management for functional improvement and/or preservation through orthopedic surgery.

Given that most functional deterioration and joint complications are derived from spasticity, it is reasonable that management of spasticity comes first as a selection of treatment from the neurosurgeon's viewpoint. The adoption of a "spasticity first" policy is considered the initial step in the comprehensive management of spasticity, as illustrated in Fig. 4.1. This strategic framework provides a systematic approach to guide clinicians in optimizing the treatment trajectory for childhood spasticity.

In cases where basic management proves insufficient in controlling spasticity, active management comes to the forefront, as the first step. The choice of treatment is determined by a thorough consideration of multiple factors, as discussed in subsequent sections. Importantly, the reduction of spasticity is not limited to a single treatment modality; rather, combinations such as dorsal rhizotomy or ITB with BTX may be employed. For instance, generalized severe hypertonia can be reduced through dorsal rhizotomy or ITB, and subsequently, BTX may be indicated if focal

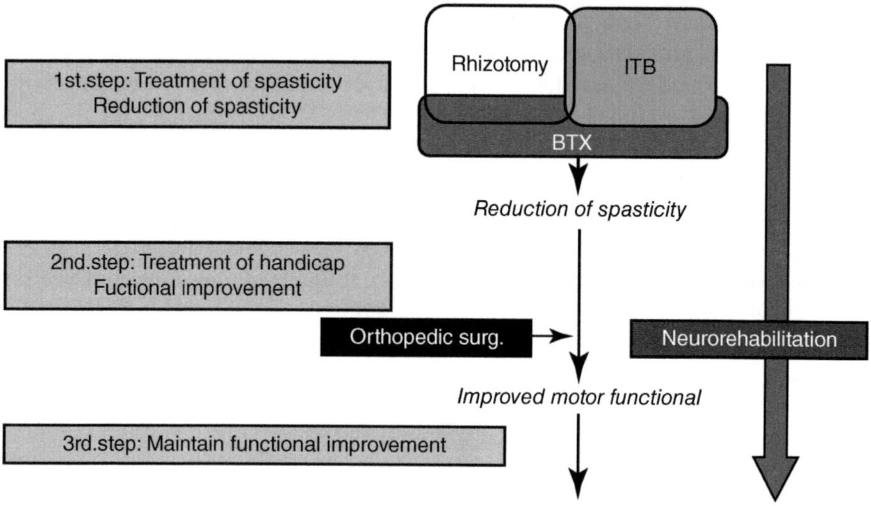

Fig. 4.1 Treatment strategy for childhood spasticity. The "spasticity first" policy represents the initial step in the comprehensive management of childhood spasticity. A comprehensive multidisciplinary team approach is essential for the successful treatment of spasticity in childhood

residual spasticity persists. The adoption of combination therapies is not uncommon, particularly in cases of severe spasticity, underscoring the flexibility and individualized nature of treatment planning.

The second step of the management of spasticity focuses the functional improvement. This phase is initiated following the successful reduction of spasticity in the first step. Neurorehabilitation takes precedence as the primary treatment during this phase; however, in cases where persistent joint or tendon complications contribute as underlining causes of impaired motor function, orthopedic surgery becomes a warranted intervention.

As the basic management, the long-term requirement of oral antispasticity medications will be necessary for children with severe spasticity. On the other hand, for cases with mild to moderate spasticity, the dosage of medication may be judiciously reduced or interrupted if satisfactory spasticity control is achieved. The imperative of neurorehabilitation extends throughout the lifespan, serving not only to enhance motor function but also to sustain the gains achieved. Over the course of spasticity treatment, the integral role of a comprehensive multidisciplinary team within a specialized spasticity clinic becomes paramount in determining the optimal treatment direction [3]. A crucial initial step involves collaborative discussions to ascertain the most suitable treatment modalities for each child at every stage, ensuring an integrated and personalized approach to spasticity management.

4.4 Comparative Assessment of Childhood Spasticity Treatments

Determining the position of dorsal rhizotomy within the spectrum of treatment modalities for childhood spasticity necessitates a comprehensive evaluation. Flett's classification, based on the severity of spasticity and the sustainability of treatment effects, serves as a benchmark [25]. According to this classification, dorsal rhizotomy is recommended for diffuse generalized hypertonia, offering an enduring and nonreversible effect. In comparison, ITB is indicated for a similar degree of hypertonia, but its effects are transient and reversible. Figure 4.2 illustrates a representative categorization of treatments for childhood spasticity, deviating from the original Flett classification by allowing each treatment to be applicable across varying degrees of spasticity. Dorsal rhizotomy can be considered for hemiparetic spasticity with favorable outcomes. BTX injection becomes a viable option for residual spasticity persisting after dorsal rhizotomy or ITB treatment.

The age of the patient is a factor in determining suitable spasticity interventions [10, 26, 27] (Fig. 4.3). Dorsal rhizotomy typically finds indication in toddlers through low to high teens, with a preference for candidates aged approximately 3–10 years [21, 28]. For infants, ITB becomes a viable option if the infusion pump can be implanted in the abdominal wall. Since both ITB and BTX treatments are reversible, they are intended for continued use throughout the patient's lifespan.

Another factor to be considered in the selection of treatment modalities for childhood spasticity is the extent of joint contraction and/or deformity [20] (Fig. 4.4). The tailored management of childhood spasticity based on the severity of musculoskeletal involvement is important. Dorsal rhizotomy, along with ITB and BTX, constitutes interventions aimed at reducing spasticity. Mild joint contraction can often be ameliorated, leading to improved range of movement following spasticity

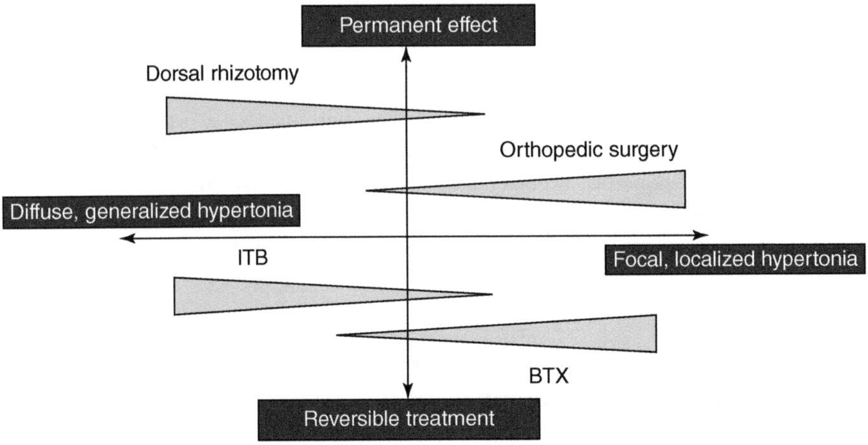

Fig. 4.2 Selection of childhood spasticity treatment. Dorsal rhizotomy is recommended for diffuse generalized hypertonia, providing a lasting and nonreversible effect. It can also be applied to localized hypertonia. (Modified from Reference 25)

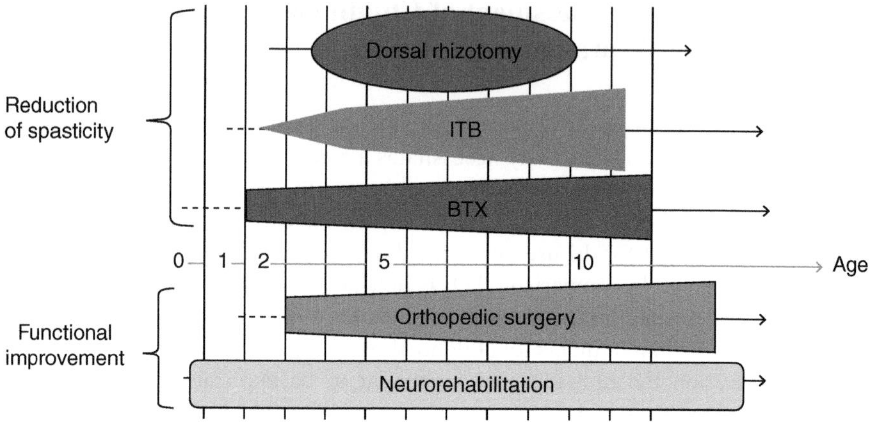

Fig. 4.3 Influence of age on the selection of treatment modality for childhood spasticity. Patient's age is an important factor in treatment selection. Dorsal rhizotomy is typically indicated in toddlers through the low to high teens

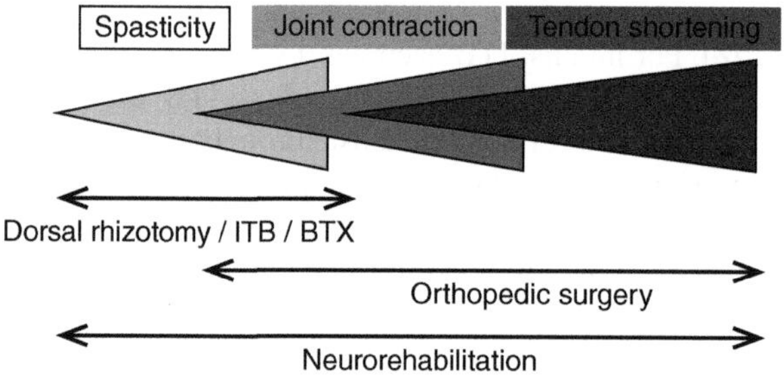

Fig. 4.4 Influence of joint complications on the selection of treatment modality for childhood spasticity. The extent of joint contraction and/or deformity affects the choice of treatment modality. Orthopedic surgery takes precedence if the joint complication is in an advanced stage

reduction. However, more advanced joint contractions or tendon shortening may remain despite the alleviation of hypertonia. In such instances, orthopedic surgery becomes an indicated intervention subsequent to spasticity reduction. In young children, timing of orthopedic surgery needs to be carefully judged. Observation for a few years after the reduction of spasticity is recommended. For older children and adolescents, orthopedic surgery may be considered as the primary treatment choice.

4.5 Dorsal Rhizotomy's Role in Comprehensive Spasticity Management

What is the role of dorsal rhizotomy? Dorsal rhizotomy is a surgical procedure to reduce spasticity. The role of dorsal rhizotomy in the comprehensive management of spasticity stems from its capability to reduce spasticity by a single surgical procedure. The surgical goals vary based on the preoperative condition, aiming for improved motor function in children with mild to moderate spasticity, while seeking relief from tonic pain associated with spasticity and alleviating the caregiving burden for severely disabled children.

Dorsal rhizotomy stands out among spasticity-reducing modalities as it offers a sustainable and long-term surgical effect (Table 4.1). This implies that a solitary intervention suffices to achieve spasticity reduction. Extensive literature has documented the efficacy of dorsal rhizotomy in managing spasticity related to cerebral palsy. Furthermore, its effectiveness across diverse pathologies is thoroughly reviewed in the Chap. 7 and other publications [17, 18]. In comparison with ITB and BTX treatments, dorsal rhizotomy appears to be cost-effective due to the absence of the need for lifelong refilling or repeated injection [29]. This cost-effectiveness holds particular significance for those low- to middle-income countries (LMICs), offering a valuable way to disseminate spasticity treatment to a broader population.

Dorsal rhizotomy has been recognized for its effectiveness in reducing generalized diffuse spasticity (Fig. 4.2). While it is acknowledged that dorsal rhizotomy improves spasticity in the body trunk and upper extremities, it is crucial to dispel the prejudice that it is exclusively indicated for diffuse spasticity. As previously highlighted, dorsal rhizotomy is effective and beneficial for cases of unilateral spasticity or instances where spasticity is localized at the ankle joint. To convey a more accurate representation, it is pertinent to emphasize that the efficacy of dorsal rhizotomy spans the entire spectrum of spasticity severity, encompassing any degree from mild to severe (Table 4.1).

The multifaceted role of dorsal rhizotomy can be delineated in four key points. First, it is indicated for spasticity across the entire spectrum. Cutting rate of dorsal roots/rootlets increases proportionally with advanced degree of spasticity. Generally, this cutting rate exhibits an inverse correlation with Gross Motor Function Measure (GMFM) scores [30–32]. Second, dorsal rhizotomy is applicable across various etiologies when chosen carefully. While spastic cerebral palsy at any degree (GMFCS levels 1–5) stands as a preferred candidate, careful consideration may extend its candidacy to other pathologies contributing to spasticity [17, 18, 33, 34]. Third, dorsal rhizotomy does not influence dystonia. In cases where patients exhibit both dystonic features and spasticity, frequently encountered in severe spasticity scenarios, alternative treatment modalities should be considered first. If a patient with severe spasticity demonstrates associated prominent dystonic movements, ITB treatment is recommended as the primary choice [22, 23]. Lastly, dorsal rhizotomy is posited as the most cost-effective procedure for spasticity reduction when indicated and executed appropriately [29]. It enables dorsal rhizotomy as a possible procedure for spasticity control in LMICs.

4.6 Limitations

Dorsal rhizotomy, while effective in reducing spasticity, entails several considerations and limitations that warrant careful assessment. First, it is a surgery to reduce spasticity. It is not a surgery to directly improver motor function. Functional improvement is achieved through postoperative neurorehabilitation, with the extent of improvement constrained by the original degree of CNS damage. Motor function improvement, as measured by a one-level shift in GGMFCS and a GMFM score increase of 10–20 points within a few years post-surgery, may have practical limitations, seldom surpassing a 2-level shift or more than a 20-point gain. Practical goal setting about the motor improvement is important. Secondly, dorsal rhizotomy constitutes a one-time, irreversible surgery. In instances where spasticity reduction is insufficient, additional treatments like BTX or, in selected cases, ITB may be considered. Conversely, excessive dorsal root/rootlet cutting can result in postoperative hypotonia, necessitating careful management. Treatment of postoperative hypotonia remains challenging and should be avoided. Some individuals, particularly adolescents, may utilize spasticity as a supportive factor for motor function (useful spasticity), and reduced spasticity after dorsal rhizotomy in such cases could lead to postoperative deterioration. Thorough preoperative evaluation by a comprehensive multidisciplinary spasticity clinic is imperative. Lastly, dorsal rhizotomy stands as one of the most invasive modalities in spasticity management, requiring meticulous attention to prevent perioperative complications [35–37]. Long-term follow-up is essential to monitor aspects such as spine deformity, spasticity recurrence, and motor function deterioration in adulthood, facilitating ongoing refinement of the procedure in future.

4.7 Summary

Dorsal rhizotomy is a neurosurgical intervention for the management of spasticity, holding a notable position among various treatment modalities dedicated to spasticity reduction. This irreversible procedure is useful in reducing both generalized and focal spasticity in carefully selected cases. Dorsal rhizotomy's distinctive role, when compared to alternative modalities, lies in its efficacy across a spectrum of spasticity severities, applicability to various pathological backgrounds, and its cost-effectiveness due to its one-time nature. Despite certain limitations, meticulous indication by a comprehensive multidisciplinary spasticity clinic can yield satisfactory results in spasticity reduction.

References

1. Sheean G. The pathophysiology of spasticity. Eur J Neurol. 2002;9(Suppl. 1):3–9.
2. Albright AL. Spasticity and movement disorders in cerebral palsy. Childs Nerv Syst. 2023;39:2877–86. https://doi.org/10.1007/s00381-023-06045-5.
3. James HE, Hofrichter PB, Spierre LZ, Aldana PR. Initiating a pediatric spasticity program with multispecialty and multi-institutional support: a preliminary report. Pediatr Neurosurg. 2013;49:11–5. https://doi.org/10.1159/000355125.

4. Abbott R, Forem SL, Johann M. Selective posterior rhizotomy for the treatment of spasticity: a review. Childs Nerv Syst. 1989;5:337–46.
5. Steinbok P. Outcomes after selective dorsal rhizotomy for spastic cerebral palsy. Childs Nerv Syst. 2001;17:1–18.
6. Mclaughlin J, Bjornson K, Temkin N, Steinbok P, Wright V, Roberts T, Drake J, O'Donnell M, Rosenbaum P, Barber J, Ferrel A. Selective dorsal rhizotomy: meta-analysis of three randomized controlled trials. Dev Med Child Neurol. 2002;44:17–25.
7. Steinbok P. Selective dorsal rhizotomy for spastic cerebral palsy: a review. Childs Nerv Syst. 2007;23:981–90.
8. Morota N, Ihara S, Ogiwara H. Neurosurgical management of childhood spasticity: functional posterior rhizotomy and intrathecal baclofen infusion therapy. Neuro Med Chir (Tokyo). 2015;55:624–39.
9. Sargut TA, Haberl H, Wolter S, Tafelski S, van Riesen A, Linhard M, Kaindl AM, Thomale UW, Schulz M. Motor and functional outcome of selective dorsal rhizotomy in children with spastic diplegia at 12 and 24 months of follow-up. Acta Neurochir. 2021;163:2837–44.
10. Gillespie CS, Hall BJ, George AM, Hennigan D, Sneade C, Cawker S, Silva AHD, Vloeberghs M, Aquilina K, Pettorini B. Selective dorsal rhizotomy in non-ambulant children with cerebral palsy: a multi-center prospective study. Childs Nerv Syst. 2024;40:171–80.
11. Mugglestone MA, Eunson P, Murphy MS. The guideline development group: spasticity in children and young people with non-progressive brain disorders: summary of NICE guidance. BMJ. 2012;345:e4845. https://doi.org/10.1136/bmj.e4845.
12. Novak I, Mcityre S, Morgan C, Campbell L, Dark L, Morton N, Stumbles E, Wilson SA, Goldsmith S. A systematic review of interventions for children with cerebral palsy: state of the evidence. Dev Med Child Neurol. 2013;55:885–910.
13. Vadivelu S, Stratton A, Pierce W. Pediatric tone management. Phys Med Rehabil Clin N Am. 2015;26:69–78. https://doi.org/10.1016/j.pmr.2014.09.008.
14. Nahm NJ, Graham HK, Gormley ME Jr, Georgiadis AG. Management of hypertonia in cerebral palsy. Curr Opin Pediatr. 2018;30:57–64. https://doi.org/10.1097/MOP.0000000000000567.
15. Albright AL. Neurosurgical treatment of spasticity and other pediatric movement disorders. J Child Neurol. 2003;18(1 Suppl):S67–78.
16. Roberts A. Surgical management of spasticity. J Child Orthop. 2013;7:389–94. https://doi.org/10.1007/s11832-013-0512-9.
17. Gump WC, Mutchnick IS, Moriarty TM. Selective dorsal rhizotomy for spasticity not associated with cerebral palsy: reconsideration of surgical inclusion criteria. Neurosurg Focus. 2013;35:E6.
18. Lohkamp LN, Coulter I, Ibrahim GM. Selective dorsal rhizotomy for spasticity of genetic etiology. Childs Nerv Syst. 2020;35:1357–65. https://doi.org/10.1007/s00381-020-04601-x.
19. Palisano R, Rosenbaum P, Walter S, et al. Development and reliability of a system to classify gross motor function in children with cerebral palsy. Dev Med Child Neurol. 1997;39:214–23.
20. Narayanan UG. Management of children with ambulatory cerebral palsy: an evidence-based review. J Pediatr Orthop. 2012;32:S172–81.
21. Oki A, Oberg W, Siebert B, Plante D, Walker ML, Gooch JL. Selective dorsal rhizotomy in children with spastic hemiparesis. J Neurosurg Pediatrics. 2010;6:353–8.
22. Albright AL, Barry MJ, Painter MJ, Shultz B. Infusion of intrathecal baclofen for generalized dystonia in cerebral palsy. J Neurosurg. 1998;88:73–8.
23. Motta F, Stignani C, Atonello E. Effect of intrathecal baclofen on dystonia in children with cerebral palsy and the use of functional scales. J Pediatr Orthop. 2008;28:213–7.
24. Hagemann C, Ilka S, Lischetzki G, Kunkel P. Intrathecal baclofen therapy for treatment of spasticity in infants and small children under 6 years of age. Childs Nerv Syst. 2020;36:767–73. https://doi.org/10.1007/s00381-019-04341-7.
25. Flett PJ. Rehabilitation of spasticity and related problems in childhood cerebral palsy. J Paediatr Child Health. 2003;39:6–14.

26. Reynolds MR, Ray WZ, Strom RG, Blackburn SL, Lee A, Park TS. Clinical outcomes after selective dorsal rhizotomy in an adult population. World Neurosurg. 2011;75(1):138–44.
27. Kakodkar P, Fallah A, Tu A. Systematic review on use and efficacy of selective dorsal rhizotomy (SDR) for the management of spasticity in non-pediatric patients. Childs Nerv Syst. 2021;37:1837–47.
28. Sharma J, Bonfield C, Steinbok P. Selective dorsal rhizotomy for hereditary spastic paraparesis in children. Childs Nerv Syst. 2016;32:1489–94.
29. Steinbok P, Daneshvar H, Evans D, Kestle JR. Cost analysis of continuous intrathecal baclofen versus selective functional posterior rhizotomy in the treatment of spastic quadriplegia associated with cerebral palsy. Pediatr Neurosurg. 1995;22:255–64.
30. Russel D, Rosenbaum P, Cadman D, Gowland C, Hardy S, Jarvis S. The gross motor function measure: a means to evaluate the effects of physical therapy. Dev Med Child Neurol. 1989;31:341–52.
31. Morota N. Clinically practical formula for preoperatively estimating the cutting rate of the spinal nerve root in a functional posterior rhizotomy. Childs Nerv Syst. 2019;35:665–72.
32. Xiao B, Constantini S, Browd SR, Zhan Q, Jiang W, Mei R. The role of intra-operative neuroelectrophysiological monitoring in single-level approach selective dorsal rhizotomy. Childs Nerv Syst. 2020;36:1925–33. https://doi.org/10.1007/s00381-019-04408-5.
33. Grunt S, Fieggen AG, Vermeulen RJ, Becher JG, Langerak NG. Selection criteria for selective dorsal rhizotomy in children with spastic cerebral palsy: a systematic review of the literature. Dev Medi Child Neurol. 2014;56:302–12.
34. Ingale H, Ughratdar I, Muquit S, Moussa AA, Vloeberghs MH. Selective dorsal rhizotomy as an alternative to intrathecal baclofen pump replacement in GMFCS grades 4 and 5 children. Childs Nerv Syst. 2016;32:321–5.
35. Tu A, Steinbok P. Long term outcome of selective dorsal rhizotomy for the management of childhood spasticity—functional improvement and complications. Childs Nerv Syst. 2020;36:1985–94.
36. Veerbeek BE, Lamberts RP, Fieggen AG, Mankahla N, de Villiers RVP, Botha E, Langerak NG. A long-term follow-up study of spinal abnormalities and pain in adults with cerebral palsy and spastic diplegia more than 25 years after selective dorsal rhizotomy. J Neurosurg Spine. 2021;34:228–35.
37. Mishra D, Barik S, Raj V, Kandwal P. A systematic review of complications following selective dorsal rhizotomy in cerebral palsy. Neurochirugie. 2023;69:101425. https://doi.org/10.1016/j.neuchi.2023.101425.

Chapter 5
Creating a Selective Dorsal Rhizotomy Team

Benjamin J. Hall, Conor S. Gillespie, Christine Sneade, Alder Hey Children's Hospital Physiotherapy Group, Deborah Quirk, Dawn Hennigan, and Benedetta Pettorini

Abbreviation

6MWT	6-Minute Walk Test
ADL	Activities of daily living
EMG	Electromyography
MAS	Modified Ashworth Scale
MDT	Multidisciplinary team
ODP	Operating department practitioner
OT	Occupational therapist
PT	Physiotherapist
SDR	Selective dorsal rhizotomy
SSEPs	Somatosensory-evoked potentials
TIVA	Total intravenous anaesthesia
TUG	Timed Up and Go

B. J. Hall (✉)
Department of Neurosurgery, Alder Hey Children's Hospital NHS Foundation Trust, Liverpool, UK

Department of Neurosurgery, The Walton Centre NHS Foundation Trust, Liverpool, UK
e-mail: benjaminhall@doctors.org.uk

C. S. Gillespie
Department of Clinical Neurosciences, University of Cambridge, Cambridge, UK
e-mail: conor.gillespie1@nhs.net

C. Sneade · Alder Hey Children's Hospital Physiotherapy Group · D. Quirk · D. Hennigan · B. Pettorini
Department of Neurosurgery, Alder Hey Children's Hospital NHS Foundation Trust, Liverpool, UK
e-mail: Christine.sneade@alderhey.nhs.uk; deborah.quirk@alderhey.nhs.uk; dawn.hennigan@alderhey.nhs.uk; benedetta.pettorini@alderhey.nhs.uk

N. Morota, P. Steinbok (eds.), *Dorsal Rhizotomy: Neurosurgery for Childhood Spasticity*, Advances and Technical Standards in Neurosurgery 51,
https://doi.org/10.1007/978-3-031-86441-4_5

5.1 Introduction

Providing the highest standard of care for children with cerebral palsy and spastic diplegia cannot be achieved in isolation. Creating a multidisciplinary team (MDT) for the provision of selective dorsal rhizotomy (SDR) therefore involves assembling healthcare professionals with diverse skills and expertise (Table 5.1) [1]. The team's composition should reflect the comprehensive and coordinated approach required for successful evaluation, surgery, and rehabilitation [2]. Each team member contributes their unique perspective and plays a crucial role in optimising patient outcomes. This chapter will focus on the breakdown of the individuals that constitute an SDR team, some of the specific skills that they contribute, and the steps involved in coordinating them into a cohesive unit (Fig. 5.1).

Table 5.1 Specialist team members and their critical roles in the management of patients undergoing selective dorsal rhizotomy (SDR)

Specialist	Role
General paediatric medicine	Often the first point of access for either caregivers or primary care practitioners. Paediatricians are either already involved in those patients expected to develop cerebral palsy or are able to recognise those referred with gross motor developmental delays for further assessment. They play a key role in managing medical comorbidities
Neurology	Support and in some circumstances may even take over the responsibilities of the general paediatrician. Neurology have specific expertise in the medical management of spasticity, movement disorders, and epilepsy, ensuring not only that patients are optimised for SDR but that they are suitable for consideration in the first place
Physiotherapy	Provide comprehensive preoperative assessments and determine suitability for SDR, as well as rehabilitation and support in the postoperative phase
Occupational therapy	Assess baseline functional status preoperatively and ensure suitable progress is made following surgery in their ability to adapt to functional changes enacted by SDR
Nursing staff	Support provided during assessment, treatment, and follow-up to ensure patients remain well on the ward as well as during clinic follow-up. Often central figures in the MDT for patients to become more familiar with
Social workers and psychology	Ensure ample support provided to both patient and caregivers during assessment, preparatory, and follow-up periods. Help prepare families for the inevitable impact of SDR on their lives
Anaesthetics	Ensure complex patients are optimised for surgery, deliver safe anaesthesia to facilitate surgery, and monitor postoperative pain and recovery
Neurophysiology	Intraoperative monitoring of root function to aid the neurosurgeon in their surgical technique
Neurosurgery	Ultimately responsible for the patient selection, surgical procedure, and eventual follow-up of all SDR patients. An overarching, leading role amongst the MDT
Orthopaedics	Regular discussion with the SDR multidisciplinary team to assess suitability for additional procedures either following SDR or if not deemed suitable

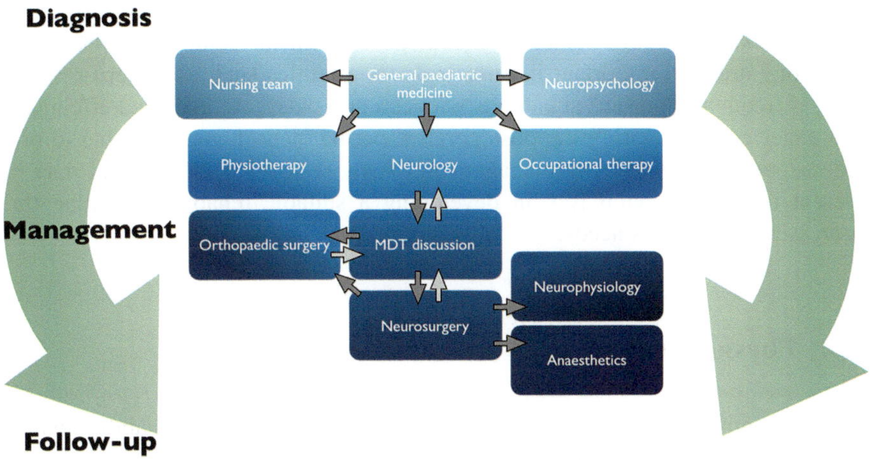

Fig. 5.1 Diagrammatic representation of the patient referral and discussion pathway from diagnosis, through management and into long-term follow-up for patients undergoing SDR. *Note that nursing staff and psychology support are often present throughout the duration of the care pathway*

5.2 General Paediatric Medicine

A paediatrician familiar with the patient's medical history and overall health status plays an important role in the selective dorsal rhizotomy MDT. It is often via a paediatrician that referrals for SDR will be initiated; therefore, they are often best placed to give an idea of the patient's clinical history and contribute their expertise by providing an holistic view of the patient's general health and well-being. Through this holistic lens, they may often highlight clinical information or comorbidities that could impact the undertaking of the surgery or rehabilitation process itself. In some circumstances, it may even by the patient's primary care practitioner that ultimately begins the referral process, remaining engaged in both the preoperative work-up and postoperative recovery phases.

5.3 Neurology

Spasticity is primarily managed by general paediatricians or neurologists. Often, only after climbing multiple tiers of pharmacological interventions and dosing regimens do patients eventually get discussed with the scope of being considered for SDR. As such, it is crucial that a strong and cohesive relationship between neurology and neurosurgery is established early on in the process of developing an SDR team. Through this, neurology are able to support in the initial diagnostic process as many patients may be referred to them as a result of their spasticity in the first instance. This is also a critical opportunity to assess the presence and severity of dystonia that may be affecting the patient, as this may ultimately influence the likelihood of whether they undergo SDR in the future. Preoperatively, neurology are also important in ensuring comorbidities such as epilepsy, which itself is frequently present in patients with cerebral palsy, are managed effectively and under control. During the postoperative period, neurologists are able to provide support in the ongoing management of any residual spasticity that may be present and play a vital role in developing a suitable rehabilitation plan that addresses the patient's needs.

5.4 Physiotherapy

A team of physiotherapists (PTs) specialising in paediatric neurorehabilitation are an essential component of the SDR team. While SDR is the surgical procedure that aims to reduce spasticity, without rigorous physiotherapy support, teams would not be able to deliver the positive outcomes that are recognised. They are responsible for evaluating the patient's motor abilities, gait patterns, muscle tone, and range of motion. This may involve exercises to strengthen weakened muscles, improve balance, and enhance coordination. Gait training is a crucial component to help individuals achieve a more functional and efficient walking pattern. Their expertise is crucial in developing a tailored rehabilitation plan that includes preoperative preparation and postoperative exercises to optimise motor function. The physiotherapy team closely monitors the patient's progress, adjusts therapy techniques as needed, and helps facilitate a successful recovery. While these skills are needed ubiquitously across physiotherapy in healthcare, the pre- and postoperative assessments for SDR patients require particularly close attention. The intensity and duration of postoperative physiotherapy necessitate that the team have a good variety of communication skills and are able to engage patients early on. The must also be familiar with a broad range of metrics, including but not limited to the Modified Ashworth Scale (MAS), Timed Up and Go (TUG), 6-Minute Walk Test (6MWT), and the Gillette Functional Assessment.

Physiotherapists continue to address residual spasticity through targeted stretching exercises and other modalities postoperatively, helping to prevent contractures and improving the overall range of motion. PTs will also be able to design exercise programmes to enhance muscle strength and endurance. This is essential for promoting functional independence in activities of daily living and reducing fatigue. In some circumstances, often with the support of an orthotics department, physiotherapists may be involved in the prescription and management of orthotic devices to support proper alignment, improve stability, and facilitate mobility. Physiotherapists also play a critical role in educating patients and their families on home exercises, adaptive strategies, and techniques to promote ongoing progress. This education empowers individuals to continue their rehabilitation outside of formal therapy sessions.

5.5 Occupational Therapy

Preoperatively occupational therapists (OTs) collaborate with the multidisciplinary team to evaluate the patient's functional abilities, identify specific challenges related to daily activities, and set baseline measurements for future comparison. This assessment helps in tailoring intervention plans to address the unique needs of each patient. Occupational therapists are actively engaged during the perioperative phase, focusing on maintaining or enhancing the individual's functional capabilities. They provide preoperative education to the patient and their family, helping them understand the potential changes in motor function post-surgery and discussing strategies to optimise recovery. Following SDR, occupational therapists play a pivotal role in postoperative rehabilitation. They work closely with other healthcare professionals, such as physical therapists and speech and language specialists, to create a comprehensive rehabilitation plan. The primary goal is to maximise the individual's independence in activities of daily living (ADLs) and improve their overall quality of life. OTs focus on improving fine motor skills, such as hand–eye coordination and manual dexterity. This is particularly important for tasks like dressing, grooming, and feeding. To support patients in honing their fine motor skills, OTs also assess the need for adaptive equipment and assistive technology to enhance the individual's independence; this may include devices to aid in mobility, communication, or activities like writing. OTs may also support in the process of identifying potential home environment modifications that may also facilitate greater independence. This may involve adapting the layout, installing handrails, or making adjustments to facilitate independent living. OTs work closely with family members and caregivers to provide training on how to support the individual in daily activities. This includes teaching adaptive techniques and strategies for optimal care.

5.6 Clinical Nurse Specialists and the Nursing Team

No clinical team in any area of healthcare can succeed without a committed team of nursing staff. Before and after surgery, skilled nurses with a good understanding of the clinical nuances of SDR patients are invaluable. Nurses often spend the greatest proportion of time with patients during inpatient admissions, so the rapport they develop with them can often prove vital to their overall experience. Nurses with a comprehensive understanding of the SDR rehabilitation process can support patients and their caregivers in engaging with therapies, ensuring any pain is managed and that they are able to rehabilitate as effectively as possible. Nurse specialists are also an increasingly integral part of the team and often provide a leading role in the delivery of an SDR service through their intimate understanding of the overarching processes involved. Often, nurse specialists will have met patients early on after referral, following them through to surgery and then forward during postoperative recovery and in some cases for many years after surgery. This continuity of care and central figure provides patients and their families with additional reassurance that can be challenging for other professionals to delivery. Nurse specialists are also often responsible for coordinating logistical aspects of the service delivery: organising clinic appointments and remote follow-up, as well as scoping work to determine how the service can continue to adapt and improve by reflecting on data.

5.7 Social Worker and Psychology Team

The inclusion of a social worker or psychologist on the multidisciplinary team is essential for providing psychosocial support to the patient and their family. They help address emotional, social, and behavioural aspects related to the procedure, as well as lend support when reflecting on the goals that were set preoperatively. They also play a crucial role in the transition to postoperative care and may connect the family with community resources and support networks.

5.8 Anaesthetist and Theatre Staff

Anaesthesia for SDR requires a careful balance between achieving adequate muscle relaxation, analgesia, and monitoring of the patient's neurological status. Intraoperative neuromonitoring is a critical aspect of SDR surgery, wherein anaesthetists must collaborate closely with neurophysiologists to monitor the patient's neural function in real time. In order to do so, a comprehensive understanding and familiarity with total intravenous anaesthesia (TIVA) is required. Achieving appropriate muscle relaxation is essential for the success of SDR; it is similarly crucial to maintain a balance to avoid excessive muscle relaxation that might interfere with neuromonitoring. Anaesthesia providers carefully titrate muscle relaxants to ensure optimal conditions for surgical exposure while preserving the integrity of neuromonitoring signals. Understandably, these add a layer of technical complexity to the anaesthetic role and necessitate the support of operating department practitioners (ODPs) familiar with SDR from a procedural and patient perspective. Anaesthetists may also play a role in the postoperative rehabilitation of the patient through their support in achieving adequate pain relief. Effective pain management is critical in ensuring the patient is quick to engage in the rehabilitation process and occasionally requires the anaesthetist's involvement continues beyond surgery itself.

5.9 Neurophysiology

Neurophysiologists may be involved throughout each phase of SDR delivery. Preoperatively, they are crucial in conducting thorough assessments of the patient's neurological function, including detailed testing of nerve conduction, electromyography (EMG), and other neurophysiological measures to map the neural pathways and identify the specific nerves contributing to spasticity. By understanding the neural anatomy and function, neurophysiologists contribute valuable information to the surgical planning process. During the SDR procedure, neurophysiologists play a critical role in intraoperative neuromonitoring. Monitoring techniques may include somatosensory-evoked potentials (SSEPs) and electromyography (EMG) to assess the integrity of the spinal cord and identify specific nerve roots for selective sectioning. This involves continuously monitoring the electrical activity of the nerves and muscles to ensure the precise identification and selective targeting of the dorsal rootlets responsible for spasticity. This real-time monitoring helps the surgical team navigate the spinal cord safely, minimising the risk of damage to critical neural structures while also ensuring a sufficient degree of cutting is undertaken so as to provide the intended benefit.

5.10 Neurosurgery

A skilled neurosurgeon with experience in performing selective dorsal rhizotomy is a key member of the team and often plays a leading role in coordinating the other team members. The neurosurgeon supports evaluation of the patient's suitability for SDR, performs the surgery, and is ultimately responsible for managing any surgical complications that may arise. Their knowledge of spinal cord anatomy and precise nerve root sectioning is crucial for achieving optimal outcomes. In contemporary SDR surgery, progressively fewer levels are involved and therefore substantially reduce the risk of postoperative pain or complications such as scoliosis. Minimal access surgery however requires greater precision to perform and therefore necessitates a high level of technical ability. Beyond this, the surgeon must have a comprehensive understanding of neurophysiological concepts involved in intraoperative monitoring in order to work cohesively with neurophysiology and ensure sufficient but not excessive nerve root sectioning is performed.

5.11 Orthopaedic Surgery

As discussed elsewhere in this book, orthopaedic surgery can play a critical role in improving the quality of life of patients with spasticity. While it is not typically employed until after more definitive attempts to ameliorate a patient's spasticity, such as SDR, involving orthopaedic colleagues in the multidisciplinary meetings is invariably helpful. This provides additional insight into alternative management options for patients in the immediate setting, as well as potentially help plan for future eventualities.

5.12 Research and Development

After being largely abandoned during the middle of the twentieth century, the last few decades have seen a reemergence of SDR in the treatment of spasticity. With increasing popularity comes the need to ensure that practitioners are delivering the highest possible standard of care to patients, by perpetually seeking to review their outcomes and aspire to improve further. In order to do this, active engagement in both audit and research processes are critical to the success of an effective SDR team. Each individual member of the team should be encouraged to review their own practice and contribution to patient care: in doing so allowing them to recognise where improvements may be made and prompting formal plans to do so. Dedicated 'academic' time to support colleagues in their pursuit of research can be challenging but should ultimately remain the goal in helping a team progress their ideas further. More junior members of the clinical team are often overlooked, but enthusiastic trainee doctors or medical students can be valuable assets. By integrating into the clinical SDR team and learning from seniors, this group are often able to apply their own research skills in reviewing the literature, analysing data, and formulating novel research avenues. Moreover, engaging with trainees at the very start of their careers ensures that they will be able to provide an increasingly high standard of care for their own patients in years to come.

5.13 Steps in Creating an SDR Team

5.13.1 Identify Team Members

Initial identification of healthcare professionals who possess the necessary expertise and experience in their respective fields forms the basis for creating an SDR team. The growing success of SDR as a surgical intervention is only achievable through continued, comprehensive follow-up, and without several key components of the team outlined above to deliver this, the goal of establishing a reliable service is near impossible. The core members of an SDR team then are both intraoperative (neurophysiology, anaesthetics, and the theatre department team) and postoperative (physiotherapy, occupational therapy, and nursing staff), with neurosurgery providing an overarching leadership role. As increased adoption of SDR continues, it should be the aspiration of all units to recruit each member listed in this chapter to their SDR team, but the authors appreciate the logistical and financial challenges this presents. Thus, these core members are recognised as the most fundamental components in the greater machine (Fig. 5.2). Team members may be sought from within the unit, from external units, or from a combination of the two. Enthusiasm and a patient-centred approach should be shared by all members of the team, regardless of their specific role within it.

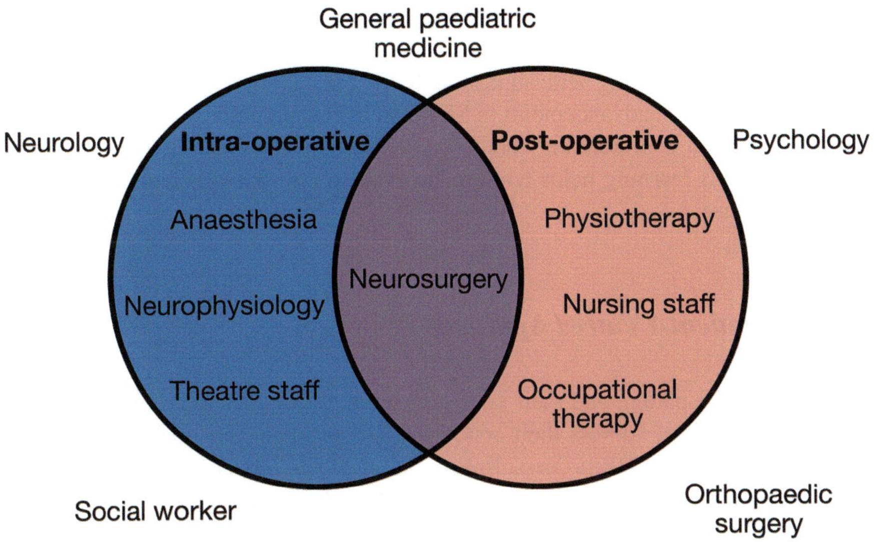

Fig. 5.2 Core members of a selective dorsal rhizotomy (SDR) team required are situated centrally, with additional members surrounding

5.13.2 Collaboration and Communication

Establish open lines of communication and foster collaboration amongst team members. Encourage a culture of respect, mutual learning, and teamwork to optimise patient care. In the modern age of remote teamworking, the tools available to facilitate regular meetings and discussion have never been more accessible and should therefore be utilised. Regular team meetings and case discussions help facilitate information sharing and enhanced decision-making while also ensuring timely discussion of new referrals, complex cases, and postoperative queries submitted by patients and their families during follow-up.

5.13.3 Continuity of Care

Ensure continuity of care by involving team members throughout the patient's journey, from preoperative evaluation to postoperative rehabilitation and follow-up. This approach promotes a comprehensive understanding of the patient's needs, fosters consistent messaging and coordination, and allows for better evaluation of treatment outcomes. By providing a sense of continuity, patients and their families are also more likely to feel comfortable in sharing their questions or concerns.

5.13.4 Training and Education

Provide ongoing training and education for team members to ensure they stay updated on the latest advancements in SDR and its related fields. Encourage participation in relevant conferences, workshops, and continuing education programmes. This continuous learning helps team members refine their skills and expand their knowledge base.

5.13.5 Patient-Centred Approach

Always keep the patient and their family at the centre of decision-making. Involve them in discussions, address their concerns, and consider their goals and expectations throughout the SDR process. Ensure that the team's interventions are aligned with the patient's individual needs and priorities. By assembling a well-rounded multidisciplinary team and fostering effective collaboration, healthcare professionals can provide comprehensive care, individualized treatment plans, and optimize outcomes for individuals undergoing SDR.

5.13.6 Creating Partnerships and Referral Networks

To build a comprehensive SDR team, it's essential to establish partnerships and referral networks with other healthcare institutions and professionals. This allows for collaboration, knowledge sharing, and access to a broader range of expertise. By reaching out to other paediatric neurosurgery centres, rehabilitation facilities, and research institutions, as well as primary care practitioners and general paediatricians who may refer patients, relationships are established that can enhance the broader team's capabilities and resources.

5.13.7 Research and Quality Improvement

Emphasise the importance of research and quality improvement within the multidisciplinary team. Encourage team members to engage in research activities and contribute to the advancement of SDR techniques and rehabilitation approaches. Regularly review outcomes and patient experiences to identify areas for improvement, and implement evidence-based practices. Establish a system for continuous evaluation and team development. Regularly assess the team's performance, patient outcomes, and patient satisfaction. Conduct peer reviews, clinical audits, and quality improvement projects to identify areas for growth and ensure ongoing excellence in delivery of an SDR service.

5.13.8 Patient and Family Education

Develop educational resources and materials to support patients and their families throughout the SDR process. These resources should provide clear information about the procedure, potential outcomes, rehabilitation expectations, and long-term care. Education sessions, informational handouts, and online resources can help families make informed decisions and actively participate in the treatment journey.

5.14 Conclusion

In conclusion, creating a multidisciplinary team for the delivery of SDR involves assembling healthcare professionals with diverse backgrounds, skills, and expertise. Collaboration, communication, and continuity of care are crucial in achieving optimal patient outcomes. Additionally, partnerships, research initiatives, patient education, and continuous service evaluation contribute to the ongoing development of the team and the improvement of patient care.

Acknowledgements Special thanks to Alder Hey Children's Hospital Physiotherapy Group:
Chris Sneade, Beata Migas, Colm MacEoin, Helen Gedrim, Nicola Idowu, Joe Ford, Jamie Loydon, and Ryan Hughes.

References

1. Clinical Commissioning Policy: Selective Dorsal Rhizotomy (SDR) for the treatment of spasticity in Cerebral Palsy (children aged 3–9 years) NHS England Specialised Services Clinical Reference Group for Paediatric Neurosciences, July 2019, call number 170063P.
2. Al-Shaar HA, et al. Selective dorsal rhizotomy: A multidisciplinary approach to treating spastic diplegia. Asian J Neurosurg. 2017;12(3):454–65. https://doi.org/10.4103/1793-5482.175625.

Chapter 6
Selection of Children with Spasticity Other Than Cerebral Palsy: Indications, Long-Term Outcome, and Exclusion Criteria

Pramath Kakodkar, Nooshin Shekari, Madhura Thipse, Debajyoti Datta, and Albert Tu

6.1 Background

Selective dorsal rhizotomy (SDR) is well reported in the management of spasticity in predominantly pediatric patients with cerebral palsy (CP) [1, 2]. There is a significant paucity however in descriptions of SDR for other etiologies of elevated tone such as autoimmune conditions, neurodegenerative disease, and trauma [1, 3–11]. Unmanaged spasticity in these pediatric patients will similarly precipitate significant limitations in ambulation and quality of life. Determining the appropriate utility and treatment response to SDR for non-CP-related spasticity in pediatric patients is not well delineated [12–25]. Therefore, a systematic review was conducted across pediatric patients undergoing SDR for management of spasticity besides cerebral palsy to evaluate functional efficacy and major contributors to appropriate patient selection.

Disclosure: The authors have no personal, financial, or institutional interest in any of the drugs, materials, or devices described in this article.

P. Kakodkar
Diagnostic and Clinical Pathology, University of Saskatchewan, Saskatoon, SK, Canada
e-mail: pramath.kakodkar@saskhealthauthority.ca

N. Shekari
Department of Anatomy, Physiology & Pharmacology, University of Saskatchewan, Saskatoon, SK, Canada
e-mail: cqw946@usask.ca

N. Morota, P. Steinbok (eds.), *Dorsal Rhizotomy: Neurosurgery for Childhood Spasticity*, Advances and Technical Standards in Neurosurgery 51,
https://doi.org/10.1007/978-3-031-86441-4_6

6.2 Methods

A systematic literature review was conducted during August 2023 by authors PK and NS in accordance with PRISMA (2020) guidelines as shown in Fig. 6.1 [26]. The review was restricted to publications between January 1970 and August 2023. Combinations of search terms "selective dorsal rhizotomy" OR "selective posterior rhizotomy" AND "spasticity" were queried on Medline and Embase databases. All studies that were not published in English language and inaccessible via digital or local repository and described adult ($\geq$18 years old) patients or reviews without any original data were excluded. Publications were evaluated for demographic variables, etiology of spasticity, procedural parameters, need for post-procedural intervention, and pre- and post-procedural clinical status (i.e., spasticity, tone, ambulatory status, complications). Additional variables documented were interventions for spasticity (i.e., oral baclofen, intrathecal baclofen, or botulinum A toxin injections) as well as orthopedic procedures (i.e., tendon lengthening, osteotomies, etc.). Follow-up outcomes were documented quantitatively when possible and described qualitatively when not.

M. Thipse
Department of Clinical Research, Children's Hospital of Eastern Ontario, Ottawa, ON, Canada
e-mail: mthipse@cheo.on.ca

D. Datta
Division of Pediatric Neurosurgery, Children's Hospital of Eastern Ontario, Ottawa, ON, Canada
e-mail: DDatta@cheo.on.ca

A. Tu (✉)
Division of Pediatric Neurosurgery, Children's Hospital of Eastern Ontario, Ottawa, ON, Canada

Department of Surgery, University of Ottawa, Ottawa, ON, Canada
e-mail: atu@cheo.on.ca

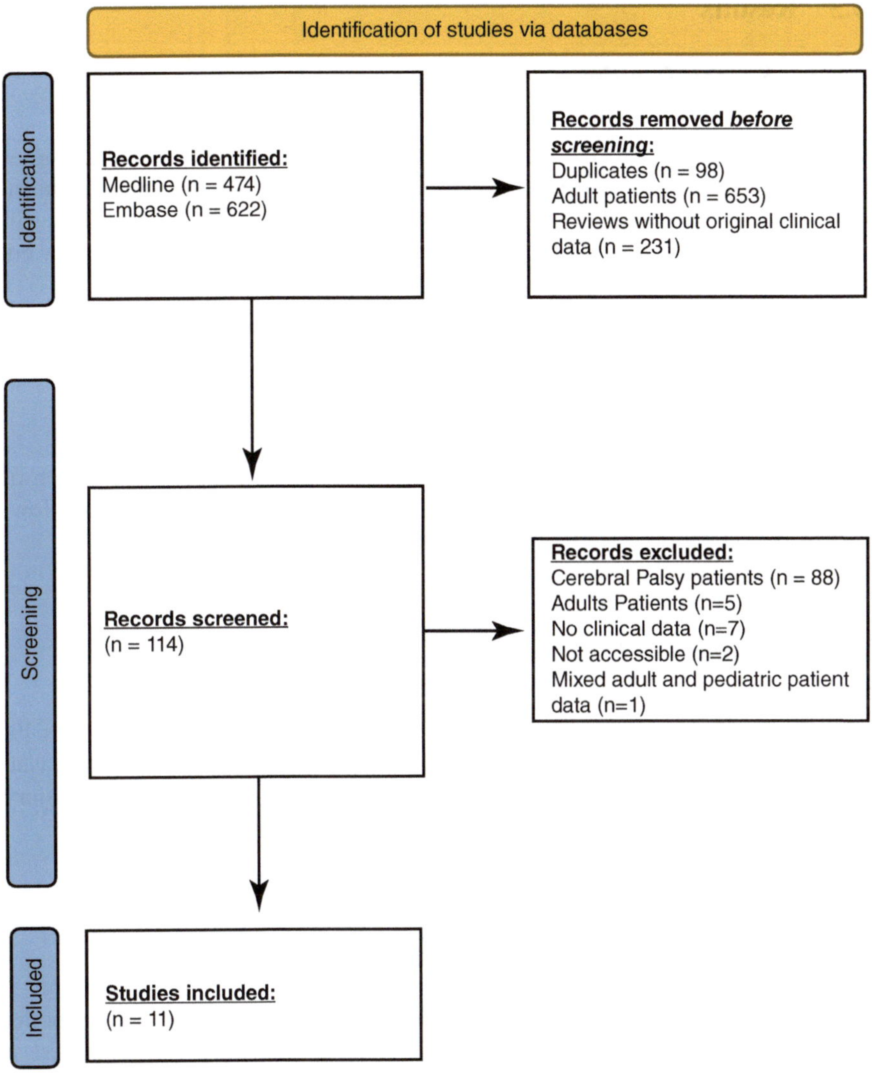

Fig. 6.1 PRISMA-based flowchart for the resultant publications from the search terms, inclusion, and exclusion criteria

6.3 Results

6.3.1 Search Results

Our review criteria yielded a total of 114 potential publications. Excluded studies included those that pertained to CP patients (88 studies), were devoid of clinical data (7 studies), mixed adult and pediatric clinical data (1 study), and were unavailable on digital or local repository (2 studies). The remaining 11 publications were analyzed for use and outcomes of SDR in 127 pediatric patients (Fig. 6.1).

6.3.2 Demographics

The pediatric patient cohort (n = 127 patients) had a mean age at intervention of 8.0 ± 4.3 years with a predilection for male gender (M:F = 1.5:1). The mean follow-up assessment period was 51.2 ± 60.8 months.

6.3.3 Etiology of Spasticity

The clinical data for this patient cohort was obtained from 11 publications [9, 27–36]. The most commonly known etiologies for spasticity were hereditary spastic paraparesis (27.8%, n = 34), congenital syndrome (n = 7), and spinal cord injury (21.9%, n = 6). The remainder of the data is summarized in Table 6.1.

6.3.4 SDR Procedural Parameters

The majority of patients underwent bilateral rhizotomy with documented rootlet resection percentages. The extent of rootlet division ranged from 45% to 62% at each level. Only posterior rootlet division was described. Intraoperative electrophysiological monitoring was utilized in all patients. Multilevel laminectomy (90%, n = 27 out of 30) with rootlet sectioning from L2 to S1 was most commonly selected. A complete breakdown of extent of SDR and surgical approach is shown in Table 6.2.

Table 6.1 Summary of etiology of spasticity in pediatric patients undergoing SDR ($n = 127$)

Etiology	Diagnosis	Mean age (years)	Mean follow-up (months)
Hereditary spastic paraparesis ($n = 34$)	HSP [no mutation testing] ($n = 7$)	11.4 ± 4.7	101.8 ± 68.8
	HSP [ALS2] ($n = 2$)	5.0 ± 2.0	97.0 ± 25.0
	HSP [SPG3A] ($n = 6$)	5.4 ± 3.2	98.0 ± 136.2
	HSP [SPG4] ($n = 11$)	6.7 ± 4.3	29.6 ± 29.7
	HSP [SPG6] ($n = 1$)	15.2	65.0
	HSP [SPG7] ($n = 2$)	6.3 ± 0.85	18
	HSP [SPG10] ($n = 2$)	6.5 ± 1.5	55.5 ± 11.5
	HSP [SPG11] ($n = 1$)	2.7	90.0
	HSP [SPG30] ($n = 1$)	9.6	26.0
	HSP [SPG54] ($n = 1$)	3.6	30.0
Congenital syndrome ($n = 7$)	Pelizaeus–Merzbacher disease ($n = 2$)	12	19
	Epilepsy syndrome ($n = 2$)	7.5 ± 3.5	32.0 ± 20.0
	Laurence–Moon syndrome ($n = 1$)	3	64
	Leigh syndrome ($n = 1$)	13	18
	Sjögren–Larsson syndrome ($n = 1$)	17	19
Spinal cord injury ($n = 6$)	Cervical to lumbar spinal trauma ($n = 4$)	9.7 ± 2.6	22.2 ± 24.1
	T10 lipomatous neoplasm ($n = 1$)	7	15
	C5 transverse myelitis ($n = 1$)	17	18
Congenital malformation ($n = 2$)	Congenital hydrocephalus ($n = 2$)	9.0 ± 1.0	64
Autoimmune ($n = 1$)	Periventricular leukomalacia	5	64
Infection ($n = 1$)	HIV encephalomyelopathy	8	64
Degenerative disease ($n = 1$)	Unknown	11	19
Others ($n = 75$)	Unknown	6.0 ± 0.9	41.7 ± 25.7

Abbreviations: *HSP* hereditary spastic paraparesis, *HIV* human immunodeficiency virus, *T* thoracic, *C* cervical

6.3.5 Measured Outcomes

6.3.5.1 Efficacy of SDR on Tone

The reported preoperative and postoperative change in tone after SDR was expressed qualitatively ($n = 34$) as well as quantitatively ($n = 81$) in this cohort. Figure 6.2 shows that the majority of patients with HSP (97.1%, $n = 33$ out of 34), congenital syndrome (66.7%, $n = 4$ out of 6), and spinal cord injury (100%, $n = 5$ out of 5) attained normalization in their tone at the time of their final follow-up. After SDR,

Table 6.2 Summary of SDR procedural parameters for pediatric patients with non-CP-related spasticity

Etiology	Diagnosis	SDR laminectomy (*n*)	Rootlet levels (*n*)	Range of rootlet cut
Hereditary spastic paraparesis (*n* = 34)	HSP [no mutation testing] (*n* = 7)	Multilevel (4), NA (3)	L2–S1 (4), NA (3)	40–55.5%
	HSP [ALS2] (*n* = 2)	Multilevel (1), limited (1)	L5–S1 (1), L2–S1 (1)	60–67.5%
	HSP [SPG3A] (*n* = 6)	Multilevel (1), NA (5)	L2–S1 (1), NA (5)	NA
	HSP [SPG4] (*n* = 11)	Multilevel (1), NA (10)	L2–S1 (1), NA (10)	NA
	HSP [SPG6] (*n* = 1)	NA	NA	NA
	HSP [SPG7] (*n* = 2)	NA	NA	NA
	HSP [SPG10] (*n* = 2)	NA	NA	NA
	HSP [SPG11] (*n* = 1)	NA	NA	NA
	HSP [SPG30] (*n* = 1)	NA	NA	NA
	HSP [SPG54] (*n* = 1)	NA	NA	NA
Congenital syndrome (*n* = 7)	Pelizaeus–Merzbacher disease (*n* = 2)	Multilevel (2)	L2–S1 (2)	NA
	Epilepsy syndrome (*n* = 2)	Unilateral (2)	L1–S2 (2)	NA
	Laurence–Moon syndrome (*n* = 1)	Multilevel	L2–S1	NA
	Leigh syndrome (*n* = 1)	Multilevel	L2–S1	NA
	Sjögren–Larsson syndrome (*n* = 1)	Multilevel	L2–S1	NA
Spinal cord injury (*n* = 6)	Cervical to lumbar spinal trauma (*n* = 4)	Multilevel (4)	L2–S1 (4)	50–80%
	T10 lipomatous neoplasm (*n* = 1)	Multilevel	L1–S2	40–60%
	C5 transverse myelitis (*n* = 1)	Multilevel	L2–S1	NA
Congenital malformation (*n* = 2)	Congenital hydrocephalus (*n* = 2)	Multilevel (2)	L2–S1 (2)	NA
Autoimmune (*n* = 1)	Periventricular leukomalacia	Multilevel	L2–S1	NA
Infection (*n* = 1)	HIV encephalomyelopathy	Multilevel	L2-S1	NA
Degenerative disease (*n* = 1)	Unknown	Multilevel	L2–S1	NA
Others (*n* = 75)	Unknown	Multilevel (4), NA (71)	L2–S1 (4), NA (71)	50–60%

Abbreviations: *C* cervical, *HSP* hereditary spastic paraparesis, *HIV* human immunodeficiency virus, *L* lumbar, *NA* not available, *S* sacral, *T* thoracic

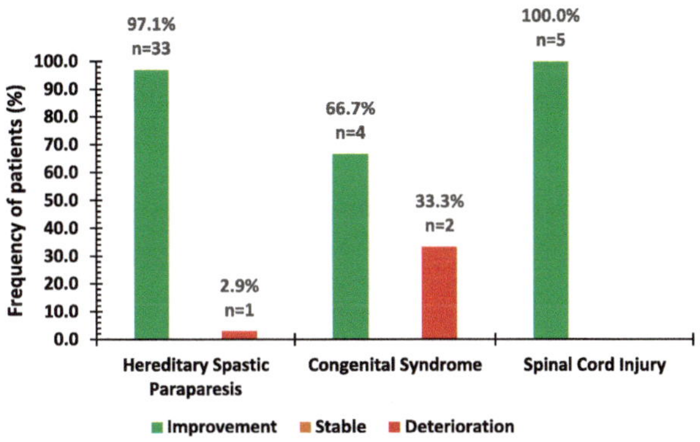

Fig. 6.2 Distribution of various etiologies of spasticity and the change in tone post-SDR relative to the baseline tone (improvement, stable, and deterioration)

deterioration to dystonia at follow-up was seen in patients with the congenital syndrome Pelizaeus–Merzbacher disease (*n* = 2), HSP [SPG4] (*n* = 1), and an unknown neurodegenerative disorder (*n* = 1). [30] Among the patients with reported modified Ashworth score (MAS), the largest mean change in tone after SDR was seen in a Leigh syndrome patient (−4, *n* = 1 out of 1), spinal cord injury cohort (−2.6, *n* = 5 out of 6 patients), and unknown etiology cohort (−2.5, *n* = 71 out of 75 patients) [9, 28, 29, 32, 36]. A comprehensive summary of post-SDR change in tone from baseline is shown in Table 6.3.

6.3.5.2 Efficacy of SDR on Ambulation

After SDR, the change in ambulation status relative to the baseline was recorded using the Gross Motor Function Classification System (GMFCS) (*n* = 118). Overall, SDR in pediatric patients with non-CP-related spasticity predominantly led to improvement (49.2%, *n* = 58) or stability (45.8%, *n* = 54) compared to their baseline (Table 6.4). Deterioration in GMFCS after SDR was only seen in HSP patients (5%, *n* = 6) with the following mutations: ALS2 (2), SPG4 (3), SPG 7 (1), and SPG11 (1) [31, 34]. The rest of the patients with HSP had improvement (32%, *n* = 11) and stability (50%, *n* = 17) in their GMFCS. After SDR, the change in ambulation status was recorded as Gross Motor Function Measure-66 GMFM66 (*n* = 9) at follow-up. The mean baseline GMFM% in patients with congenital hydrocephalus (*n* = 2), PVL (*n* = 1), HIV encephalomyelopathy (*n* = 1), and unknown (*n* = 4) was 62.2 ± 6.6, 52.3, 73.6, and 71.9 ± 7.1, respectively. For these patients with congenital hydrocephalus (*n* = 2), PVL (*n* = 1), HIV encephalomyelopathy (*n* = 1), and unknown (*n* = 4), the corresponding post-SDR change in GMFM improved to a mean of 62.5 ± 6.2, 62.98, 80.5, and 79.3 ± 8.0 at follow-up, respectively. [27]

6.3.5.3 Adjunct Interventions After SDR

The need for adjunct interventions for persistent spasticity after SDR was also available 17 patients (Table 6.5). [30–35] Overall, the majority of patients with congenital syndrome (57.1%, *n* = 4 out of 7) and HSP (38.2%, *n* = 13 out of 34) underwent

Table 6.3 Summary of qualitative change in tone from baseline post-SDR

Etiology	Diagnosis	Change in tone post-SDR relative to baseline		
		Improved (*n*)	Stable (*n*)	Deterioration (*n*)
Hereditary spastic paraparesis (*n* = 34)	HSP [no mutation testing] (*n* = 7)	7	0	0
	HSP [ALS2] (*n* = 2)	2	0	0
	HSP [SPG3A] (*n* = 6)	6	0	0
	HSP [SPG4] (*n* = 11)	10	0	1
	HSP [SPG6] (*n* = 1)	1	0	0
	HSP [SPG7] (*n* = 2)	2	0	0
	HSP [SPG10] (*n* = 2)	2	0	0
	HSP [SPG11] (*n* = 1)	1	0	0
	HSP [SPG30] (*n* = 1)	1	0	0
	HSP [SPG54] (*n* = 1)	1	0	0
Congenital syndrome (*n* = 7)	Pelizaeus–Merzbacher disease (*n* = 2)	0	0	2
	Sturge-Weber syndrome (*n* = 2)	2	0	0
	Laurence–Moon syndrome (*n* = 1)	NA	NA	NA
	Leigh syndrome (*n* = 1)	1	0	0
	Sjögren–Larsson syndrome (*n* = 1)	1	0	0
Spinal cord injury (*n* = 6)	Cervical to lumbar spinal trauma (*n* = 4)	3	0	0
	T10 lipomatous neoplasm (*n* = 1)	1	0	0
	C5 transverse myelitis (*n* = 1)	1	0	0
Congenital malformation (*n* = 2)	Congenital hydrocephalus (*n* = 2)	NA	NA	NA
Autoimmune (*n* = 1)	Periventricular leukomalacia	NA	NA	NA
Infection (*n* = 1)	HIV encephalomyelopathy	NA	NA	NA
Degenerative disease (*n* = 1)	Unknown	0	0	1
Others (*n* = 75)	Unknown	71	0	0

Abbreviations: *C* cervical, *HSP* hereditary spastic paraparesis, *HIV* human immunodeficiency virus, *NA* not available, *T* thoracic

Table 6.4 Change in GMFCS after SDR compared to baseline, stratified by etiology of spasticity

Etiology	Baseline GMFCS	Improvement % (*n*)	Stable % (*n*)	Deterioration % (*n*)
Hereditary spastic paraparesis (*n* = 34)	GMFCS I (*n* = 2)	NA	50% (1)	50% (1)
	GMFCS II (*n* = 16)	37.5% (6)	56.25% (9)	6.25% (1)
	GMFCS III (*n* = 13)	23.1% (3)	53.8% (7)	23.1% (3)
	GMFCS IV (*n* = 2)	50% (1)	–	50% (1)
	GMFCS V (*n* = 1)	100% (1)	–	NA
	Subtotal (*n* = 34)	**32.3% (11)**	**50% (17)**	**17.7% (6)**
Congenital syndrome (*n* = 7)	GMFCS I (*n* = 2)	NA	100% (2)	–
	GMFCS II (*n* = 1)	100% (1)	–	–
	GMFCS IV (*n* = 2)	50% (1)	50% (1)	–
	GMFCS V (*n* = 2)	100% (2)	–	NA
	Subtotal (*n* = 7)	**57.1% (4)**	**42.9% (3)**	**–**
Spinal cord injury (*n* = 6)	GMFCS II (*n* = 1)	100% (1)	–	–
	GMFCS III (*n* = 2)	50% (1)	50% (1)	–
	GMFCS IV (*n* = 1)	–	100% (1)	–
	GMFCS V (*n* = 1)	–	100% (1)	NA
	Subtotal (*n* = 5)	**40.0% (2)**	**60.0% (3)**	**–**
Neurodegeneration (*n* = 1)	GMFCS V (*n* = 1)	–	100% (1)	NA
Unknown (*n* = 75)	GMFCS III (*n* = 21)	100% (21)	–	–
	GMFCS IV (*n* = 26)	76.9% (20)	23.1% (6)	–
	GMFCS V (*n* = 24)	–	100% (24)	NA
	Subtotal (*n* = 71)	**57.7% (41)**	**42.3% (30)**	**–**

Abbreviation: *GMFCS* Gross Motor Function Classification System

Table 6.5 Summary of adjunct interventions post-SDR at follow-up

Etiology	Diagnosis	Adjunct intervention (*n*)
Hereditary spastic paraparesis (*n* = 34)	HSP [no mutation testing] (*n* = 7)	Gabapentin (2)
	HSP [ALS2] (*n* = 2)	Botulinum toxin A injection (1)
	HSP [SPG3A] (*n* = 6)	Adductor lengthening (1)
	HSP [SPG4] (*n* = 11)	ITB (1), Achilles tendon lengthening (2), Hamstring lengthening (1), Adductor lengthening (1), Spinal deformity correction (1)
	HSP [SPG7] (*n* = 2)	Hamstring lengthening (1)
	HSP [SPG11] (*n* = 1)	Achilles tendon lengthening (1)
	HSP [SPG54] (*n* = 1)	Achilles tendon lengthening (1)
Congenital syndrome (*n* = 7)	Pelizaeus–Merzbacher disease (*n* = 2)	ITB (2)
	Epilepsy syndrome (*n* = 2)	Achilles tendon lengthening (2)
Spinal cord injury (*n* = 6)	Cervical to lumbar spinal trauma (*n* = 4)	ITB (1)
Degenerative disease (*n* = 1)	Unknown	ITB (1), spinal deformity correction (1)
Others (*n* = 75)	Unknown	Tendon lengthening (16)

Abbreviation: *ITB* intrathecal baclofen

adjunct interventions with predilection for tendon lengthening surgery (*n* = 10) and intrathecal baclofen pump (ITB) (*n* = 3). Among the HSP cohort, patients with the SPG4 mutation most commonly required adjunct interventions. The need for surgical correction of spinal deformity was only reported in HSP (SPG4) and neurodegenerative disease patients.

6.3.5.4 Complications and Quality of Life After SDR

Complications post-SDR were documented in only nine patients [9, 30, 33, 34]. The patients with Pelizaeus–Merzbacher disease (*n* = 2) and HSP with SPG4 mutation (*n* = 1) developed severe dystonia requiring ITB pump insertion. A small number of patients with HSP treated with SDR developed new-onset sensory dysfunction with hyperesthesia in L3–S1 dermatomes requiring gabapentin (*n* = 2) and hypoesthesia (*n* = 2). Other postoperative events documented were unexplained pyrexia at postoperative day 2 in a patient with Leigh syndrome and delayed wound healing in a patient with Sjögren–Larsson syndrome. Quality of life at baseline and after SDR was documented in seven patients [9, 29, 30, 32, 35, 36]. The quality of life was qualitatively described as substantially improved after SDR in patients with Sjögren–Larsson syndrome ($n = 1$), Leigh syndrome ($n = 1$), Epilepsy syndrome ($n = 2$), transverse myelitis ($n = 1$), debulking of T10 lipomatous neoplasm ($n = 1$), and T2 gunshot leading to spinal cord injury ($n = 1$).

6.4 Discussion

Non-CP-related spasticity can arise from a multitude of pathologic etiologies in pediatric and adult patients [1, 2, 37]. Similar to patients with CP, uncompensated spasticity in non-CP patients can lead to tendon shortening, contractures, and dislocation leading to severely diminished quality of life. Our literature review found that the vast majority of information currently available exclusively describes the use of SDR in CP patients. Guidance related to patient selection for SDR and its utility in managing pediatric patients with non-CP-related spasticity remains highly overlooked.

This systematic review utilized data from 127 pediatric patients with non-CP-related spasticity with a mean age at intervention of 8.0 ± 4.3 years. Results regarding changes in ambulation, tone, adjunct interventions, complications, and quality of life post-SDR are based on a longer follow-up duration (mean: 51.2 ± 60.8 months) which provides long-term efficacy data. Hereditary spastic paraparesis (HSP), spinal cord injury, congenital syndrome, and malformations were identified as frequent causes of non-CP-related spasticity requiring SDR in a pediatric population. Interestingly, our previous study on the common causes for non-CP-related spasticity requiring SDR in the adult population yielded overlapping etiologies such as spinal cord injury, Sjögren–Larsson syndrome, and transverse myelitis [2].

6.4.1 Selecting Candidates for SDR

Appropriate candidate selection for SDR in non-CP-related spasticity management is primarily dependent on the goal for the surgery as well as patient natural history. Given the heterogeneity in genetic mutation and ensuing phenotypic expression, identifying patients for candidacy for SDR by HSP designation alone is inadequate to determine those patients most likely to have a good result. Deterioration in GMFCS and/or development of severe dystonia after SDR was only seen in HSP patients with SPG4 ($n = 4$), ALS2 ($n = 2$), SPG7 ($n = 1$), and SPG11 ($n = 1$) mutations [31, 34]. It is possible that there is a rapid progressive course for HSP with these mutations resulting in a younger mean age of 5.2 ± 1.6 years and a higher baseline GMFCS 3 ± 1 at time of consideration for SDR. In particular, patients with HSP driven by SPG4 mutations required the highest frequency of adjunct interventions as well as surgical correction for spinal deformity. Contrastingly, HSP patients devoid of any known mutations ($n = 7$), SPG3A ($n = 3$), and SPG6 (1) had improved GMFCS and tone normalization post-SDR. [30, 31] This cohort of patients had an older mean age at surgery of 10.2 ± 5.0 years and a lower baseline GMFCS of 2 ± 1 which may be explained by a more insidious clinical course driven by these unique mutations. Taking these findings as a whole, the efficacy of SDR in patients with genetic neurodegenerative disorders may likely be best predicted by their clinical presentation and course prior to treatment. Patients with a nonprogressive course or a mutation known to have periods of long stability may have a much more durable and stable response in comparison to those with an evolving or deteriorating natural history. It is important to note that the sample size for patients with these mutations is small and larger studies are required to make definitive conclusions regarding its contribution to prognosis post-SDR. Furthermore, the documented category of HSP patients devoid of any known common mutations is limited to testing of known HSP genes. This limitation can ideally be resolved by building a larger repository of HSP mutation drivers with whole exome sequencing.

6.4.2 Outcomes After SDR

In our review, pediatric patients with spinal cord injury treated with SDR had overall improvement in ambulation, tone, and quality of life relative to their baseline. Special consideration must be given to patients in this cohort as they often score significantly lower on their baseline quality of life evaluation. Therefore, the goal of SDR should also incorporate individual parameters contributing to the quality-of-life improvement such as personal hygienic care, pain, and fatigue resolution to discern the extent of improvement. Most cases of SCI in our review focused on improvements in function in the form of GMFCS or GFMF and tone as well as qualitatively described improvement in their quality of life after SDR. Overall, this group may achieve significant and persistent tone reduction without as dramatic a change in their functional status, and the benefit of this change should be considered on an individual basis.

Among patients with congenital syndromes, patients with Laurence–Moon syndrome ($n = 1$), Leigh syndrome ($n = 1$), and Sjogren–Larsson syndrome ($n = 1$) had improvement in ambulation, tone, pain, and quality of life relative to their baseline. Contrastingly, neurodegenerative diseases ($n = 1$) and Pelizaeus–Merzbacher disease ($n = 2$) had deterioration in their GMFCS and developed severe dystonia post SDR requiring further intervention, specifically insertion of an ITB pump. It is interesting that Pelizaeus–Merzbacher disease in pediatric patients and multiple sclerosis in adult patients are autoimmune primary demyelination disorders with poor prognosis for spasticity management after SDR [2]. Given the limited treatment options that exist for abating the primary disease in these patients, failure of SDR may potentially be attributable not to a technical failure of the intervention so much as recurrence or progression of their primary disease. This interpretation may be extrapolated to other conditions where primary disease progression has yet been stymied, and SDR in these patients should only be considered with the caveat that outcomes are likely not to be durable and will not change the long-term outcome.

6.4.3 SDR vs. ITB: A Nuanced Choice?

Our review also showed that in the absence of guidance for patient selection, SDR was considered over ITB pump for the management of non-CP-related spasticity. Reported indications for SDR over ITB included continued financial cost associated with ITB pump refills, possible infection nidus, or downstream complications of ITB pump malfunction or blockage. These considerations can result in situations wherein removal of ITB pump and SDR may be performed in a single surgery. As such, latent dystonia initially suppressed by ITB may rebound prominently after SDR when simultaneous ITB removal is opted. This scenario may be avoided by trialing an ITB wean first. This review emphasizes caution when choosing SDR in pediatric patients with congenital syndromes initially managed with ITB.

Based on the results of this review supplemented with our own institutional experience, we believe that the selection of an ideal pediatric non-CP patient for SDR remains multifactorial. Table 6.6 is a summary of our suggestion of possible beneficial and poor prognostication factors for SDR in pediatric non-CP-related spasticity management with a goal focusing on improving ambulatory functionality and spasticity. We would emphasize that SDR utilized in a palliative fashion could still be considered in patients where tone reduction, either temporary or permanent, is desired, regardless of the potential functional or ambulatory benefit.

Table 6.6 Summary of possible beneficial and poor prognostic variable when considering SDR as an option in pediatric non-CP-related spasticity management

Etiologies	Beneficial prognosis post-SDR	Poor prognosis post-SDR
Hereditary spastic paraparesis	HSP without any common gene mutations SPG3A SPG6 Baseline GMFCS ≤ 2 Older age at SDR (10.2 ± 5.0 years) Nonprogressive natural history	SPG4 mutation ALS2 mutation SPG7 mutation SPG11 mutation Baseline GMFCS ≥ 3 Younger age at SDR (5.2 ± 1.6 years) Progressive natural history
Other	Spinal cord injury (trauma/autoimmune) Laurence–Moon syndrome Leigh syndrome Sjogren–Larsson syndrome Autoimmune PVL HIV encephalomyelopathy No ventriculomegaly on preoperative MRI	Pelizaeus–Merzbacher disease Unknown neurodegenerative disorder No ITB wean performed

6.4.4 *Limitations*

The documentation of functional outcome measures after SDR are highly varied with a distribution of noncomparable quantitative and qualitative data. Furthermore, many publications were discarded as only pooled adult and pediatric clinical results were provided. A key limiting factor preventing generalizability is the small sample sizes of understandably rare diseases. Additionally, our review also had 75 patients with unknown non-CP-related spasticity etiology. The identification of the etiology in these patients would increase the accuracy of the classification and analysis. This can be resolved with multicenter prospective trials with standardized outcomes to improve management with SDR.

6.5 Conclusion

The literature on the use and efficacy of SDR in non-CP-related spasticity management in pediatric patients remain sparse. This systematic review found that SDR in this cohort is effective at managing spasticity and improving ambulatory functionality in selected patients including those hereditary spastic paraparesis, spinal cord injury, and congenital syndromes. The authors would emphasize that the best predictor for response would be patients with stable or an only insidiously progressive disease. Patients with mixed tone or progressive conditions are likely not to have durable responses to SDR. With the appropriate patient selection, there is a sustained benefit in functionality and quality of life. Formal prospective study of this technique in non-CP-related spasticity within the pediatric populations should be considered.

References

1. Kakodkar P, Girgis H, Nabhan P, Chee SS, Tu A. Efficacy of selective dorsal rhizotomy and intrathecal baclofen pump in the management of spasticity. Adv Tech Stand Neurosurg. 2022;45:379–403. https://doi.org/10.1007/978-3-030-99166-1_13.
2. Kakodkar P, Fallah A, Tu A. Systematic review on use and efficacy of selective dorsal rhizotomy (SDR) for the management of spasticity in non-pediatric patients. Childs Nerv Syst. 2021;37(6):1837–47. https://doi.org/10.1007/s00381-021-05167-y.
3. Bose P, Hou J, Thompson FJ. Traumatic brain injury (TBI)-induced spasticity: neurobiology, treatment, and rehabilitation. In: Kobeissy FH, editor. Brain neurotrauma: molecular, neuropsychological, and rehabilitation aspects, Frontiers in neuroengineering. Boca Raton: CRC Press; 2015.
4. Pidgeon TS, Ramirez JM, Schiller JR. Orthopaedic management of spasticity. R I Med J (2013). 2015;98(12):26–31.
5. Ravindra VM, Christensen MT, Onwuzulike K, et al. Risk factors for progressive neuromuscular scoliosis requiring posterior spinal fusion after selective dorsal rhizotomy. J Neurosurg Pediatr. 2017;20(5):456–63. https://doi.org/10.3171/2017.5.peds16630.

6. Baagøe SK, Kofoed-Hansen M, Poulsen I, Riberholt CG. Development of muscle contractures and spasticity during subacute rehabilitation after severe acquired brain injury: a prospective cohort study. Brain Inj. 2019;33(11):1460–6. https://doi.org/10.1080/02699052.2019.1646433.
7. Calancie B, Molano MR, Broton JG. Interlimb reflexes and synaptic plasticity become evident months after human spinal cord injury. Brain. 2002;125(Pt 5):1150–61.
8. Foran JR, Steinman S, Barash I, Chambers HG, Lieber RL. Structural and mechanical alterations in spastic skeletal muscle. Dev Med Child Neurol. 2005;47(10):713–7. https://doi.org/10.1017/S0012162205001465.
9. Mazarakis NK, Vloeberghs MH. Spasticity secondary to Leigh syndrome managed with selective dorsal rhizotomy: a case report. Childs Nerv Syst. 2016;32(9):1745–8. https://doi.org/10.1007/s00381-016-3071-9.
10. Shahani BT, Young RR. Human flexor reflexes. J Neurol Neurosurg Psychiatry. 1971;34(5):616–27.
11. Westbom L, Lundkvist Josenby A, Wagner P, Nordmark E. Growth in children with cerebral palsy during five years after selective dorsal rhizotomy: a practice-based study. BMC Neurol. 2010;10:57. https://doi.org/10.1186/1471-2377-10-57.
12. Albright AL, Turner M, Pattisapu JV. Best-practice surgical techniques for intrathecal baclofen therapy. J Neurosurg. 2006;104(4 Suppl):233–9. https://doi.org/10.3171/ped.2006.104.4.233.
13. Aquilina K, Graham D, Wimalasundera N. Selective dorsal rhizotomy: an old treatment re-emerging. Arch Dis Child. 2015;100(8):798–802. https://doi.org/10.1136/archdischild-2014-306874.
14. Awaad Y, Rizk T, Siddiqui I, Roosen N, McIntosh K, Waines GM. Complications of intrathecal baclofen pump: prevention and cure. ISRN Neurol. 2012;2012:575168. https://doi.org/10.5402/2012/575168.
15. Chicoine MR, Park TS, Kaufman BA. Selective dorsal rhizotomy and rates of orthopedic surgery in children with spastic cerebral palsy. J Neurosurg. 1997;86(1):34–9. https://doi.org/10.3171/jns.1997.86.1.0034.
16. Dudley RW, Parolin M, Gagnon B, et al. Long-term functional benefits of selective dorsal rhizotomy for spastic cerebral palsy. J Neurosurg Pediatr. 2013;12(2):142–50. https://doi.org/10.3171/2013.4.peds12539.
17. Farmer J-P, Sabbagh AJ. Selective dorsal rhizotomies in the treatment of spasticity related to cerebral palsy. Childs Nerv Syst. 2007;23(9):991–1002. https://doi.org/10.1007/s00381-007-0398-2.
18. Francisco GE, Hu MM, Boake C, Ivanhoe CB. Efficacy of early use of intrathecal baclofen therapy for treating spastic hypertonia due to acquired brain injury. Brain Inj. 2005;19(5):359–64. https://doi.org/10.1080/02699050400003999.
19. Gigante P, McDowell MM, Bruce SS, et al. Reduction in upper-extremity tone after lumbar selective dorsal rhizotomy in children with spastic cerebral palsy. J Neurosurg Pediatr. 2013;12(6):588–94. https://doi.org/10.3171/2013.9.PEDS12591.
20. Gray N, Morton RE, Brimlow K, Keetley R, Vloeberghs M. Goals and outcomes for non ambulant children receiving continuous infusion of intrathecal baclofen. Eur J Paediatr Neurol. 2012;16(5):443–8. https://doi.org/10.1016/j.ejpn.2012.01.003.
21. Hurvitz EA, Marciniak CM, Daunter AK, et al. Functional outcomes of childhood dorsal rhizotomy in adults and adolescents with cerebral palsy. J Neurosurg Pediatr. 2013;11(4):380–8. https://doi.org/10.3171/2013.1.PEDS12311.
22. Mathur SN, Chu SK, McCormick Z, Chang Chien GC, Marciniak CM. Long-term intrathecal baclofen: outcomes after more than 10 years of treatment. PM R. 2014;6(6):506–513.e1. https://doi.org/10.1016/j.pmrj.2013.12.005.
23. Mittal S, Farmer JP, Al-Atassi B, et al. Impact of selective posterior rhizotomy on fine motor skills. Long-term results using a validated evaluative measure. Pediatr Neurosurg. 2002;36(3):133–41. https://doi.org/10.1159/000048368.

24. Ou C, Kent S, Miller S, Steinbok P. Selective dorsal rhizotomy in children: comparison of outcomes after single-level versus multi-level laminectomy technique. Can J Neurosci Nurs. 2010;32(3):17–24.
25. Park TS, Edwards C, Liu JL, Walter DM, Dobbs MB. Beneficial effects of childhood selective dorsal rhizotomy in adulthood. Cureus. 2017;9(3):e1077. https://doi.org/10.7759/cureus.1077.
26. Matthew JP, Joanne EM, Patrick MB, et al. The PRISMA 2020 statement: an updated guideline for reporting systematic reviews. BMJ. 2021;372:n71. https://doi.org/10.1136/bmj.n71.
27. Grunt S, Becher JG, van Schie P, van Ouwerkerk WJ, Ahmadi M, Vermeulen RJ. Preoperative MRI findings and functional outcome after selective dorsal rhizotomy in children with bilateral spasticity. Childs Nerv Syst. 2010;26(2):191–8. https://doi.org/10.1007/s00381-009-0999-z.
28. Kan P, Gooch J, Amini A, et al. Surgical treatment of spasticity in children: comparison of selective dorsal rhizotomy and intrathecal baclofen pump implantation. Childs Nerv Syst. 2008;24(2):239–43. https://doi.org/10.1007/s00381-007-0457-8.
29. Mazarakis NK, Ughratdar I, Vloeberghs MH. Excellent functional outcome following selective dorsal rhizotomy in a child with spasticity secondary to transverse myelitis. Childs Nerv Syst. 2015;31(11):2189–91. https://doi.org/10.1007/s00381-015-2779-2.
30. Buizer AI, van Schie PEM, Bolster EAM, et al. Effect of selective dorsal rhizotomy on daily care and comfort in non-walking children and adolescents with severe spasticity. Eur J Paediatr Neurol. 2017;21(2):350–7. https://doi.org/10.1016/j.ejpn.2016.09.006.
31. Sharma J, Bonfield C, Steinbok P. Selective dorsal rhizotomy for hereditary spastic paraparesis in children. Childs Nerv Syst. 2016;32(8):1489–94. https://doi.org/10.1007/s00381-016-3122-2.
32. Reynolds RM, Morton RP, Walker ML, Massagli TL, Browd SR. Role of dorsal rhizotomy in spinal cord injury-induced spasticity. J Neurosurg Pediatr. 2014;14(3):266–70. https://doi.org/10.3171/2014.5.peds13459.
33. Grootveld LR, van Schie PE, Buizer AI, et al. Sudden falls as a persistent complication of selective dorsal rhizotomy surgery in children with bilateral spasticity: report of 3 cases. J Neurosurg Pediatr. 2016;18(2):192–5. https://doi.org/10.3171/2016.2.peds15527.
34. Park TS, Joh S, Walter DM, Meyer NL. Selective dorsal rhizotomy for treatment of hereditary spastic paraplegia-associated spasticity in 37 patients. Cureus. 2021;13(9):e17690. https://doi.org/10.7759/cureus.17690.
35. Park TS, Joh S, Smyth MD, Meyer NL, Walter DM. Selective dorsal rhizotomy for treatment of spasticity after hemispherectomy in children: a case report. Cureus. 2023;15(3):e36945. https://doi.org/10.7759/cureus.36945.
36. Ryan M, Flavin M, Oleszek J, Bodkin A, Wilson AM, Wilkinson C. Selective dorsal rhizotomy for spasticity associated with spinal cord injury sustained during surgery for spinal lipomatous malformation: a case report. J Pediatr Rehabil Med. 2022;15(2):377–81. https://doi.org/10.3233/prm-200809.
37. Gump WC, Mutchnick IS, Moriarty TM. Selective dorsal rhizotomy for spasticity not associated with cerebral palsy: reconsideration of surgical inclusion criteria. Neurosurg Focus. 2013;35(5):E6. https://doi.org/10.3171/2013.8.focus13294.

Chapter 7
Preoperative Assessments for Selective Dorsal Rhizotomy

Olivia Shien Hui Lee

7.1 Introduction

Selective dorsal rhizotomy (SDR) is an effective neurosurgical treatment that permanently reduces spasticity in children with cerebral palsy (CP). The primary goals of SDR are to improve gait and function in ambulatory children and to improve care and comfort in nonambulatory children [1]. While international studies have established evidence for long-term spasticity reduction, functional outcomes can vary significantly between different centres [2–16]. This variability highlights the importance of developing a local protocol for preoperative assessments and long-term follow-up. This protocol should evaluate selection criteria, treatment objectives, assessment methodologies, intraoperative techniques, and postoperative rehabilitation programmes specific to the centre [13, 17].

This chapter will discuss (1) the recommended minimal dataset for evaluating patients for SDR and (2) additional preoperative assessments that may be useful in informing treatment outcomes and post-SDR rehabilitation needs and providing a baseline reference for monitoring clinical progress.

7.2 Clinical Evaluation for SDR

The assessment for SDR is not internationally standardised, but key elements are focused on answering several clinical questions for decision-making:

O. S. H. Lee (✉)
The Royal Children's Hospital, Melbourne, Australia
e-mail: Oliviashienhui.lee@rch.org.au

N. Morota, P. Steinbok (eds.), *Dorsal Rhizotomy: Neurosurgery for Childhood Spasticity*, Advances and Technical Standards in Neurosurgery 51,
https://doi.org/10.1007/978-3-031-86441-4_7

1. Is the diagnosis correct?
2. What are the goals of SDR for this child and their family?
3. What is the predominant movement disorder, and how much is it related to spasticity or dystonia?
4. What is the current function of this child, and how will it change once spasticity is removed?
5. How much of the current function is related to weakness or poor selective motor control?
6. What were the previous spasticity management strategies, and how effective were they for this child?
7. When is the best time for SDR for this child?
8. Can the child and family cope with the post-SDR rehabilitation process?
9. How much contracture and bony malalignment must be addressed by the orthopaedic surgeon?
10. Is SDR suitable for this child, and if not, what are the other clinical options?

Where possible, it is best practice to use standardised assessments to analyse these areas, as they provide a framework for service development and allow for a more accurate evaluation of outcomes, particularly given the heterogeneity of cerebral palsy [18]. Education and counselling are essential for families of children even when SDR is unsuitable, ensuring they understand the treatment decisions and do not feel they have "missed out" and that all treatment options have been considered. The assessment process emphasises a personalised approach and shared decision-making to ensure treatment goals align with family expectations through transparent communication [19, 20].

7.3 International Classification of Function (ICF) Framework for SDR Assessments

Early multidimensional assessments are needed for young children with multilevel spasticity who have not responded to the combination of physical therapy, oral tone medications, and botulinum toxin injections. These assessments facilitate the timely consideration of intensive treatments like SDR, orthopaedic surgery, or intrathecal baclofen (ITB).

SDR preop assessments should cover the domains of the *International Classification of Function (ICF-model)* [21, 22]. Multiple appointments are dedicated to preoperative assessments to ensure a manageable process for children and families.

Table 7.1 presents various assessments from published literature, categorised according to ICF domains. These include demographic data and the aetiology of spasticity. "Body structure and function" assessments record Gross Motor Function Classification System (GMFCS), the predominant movement disorder, topography, and musculoskeletal measures. "Activity and participation" assessments evaluate

Table 7.1 Pre-SDR assessments based on ICF domains

Personal and environmental factors (Demographics)
Minimum dataset:
Age
History of Prematurity
Brain Magnetic Resonance Imaging (MRI)—Periventricular Ventricular Leukomalacia (PVL)
Goals Assessment- Canadian Occupational Performance Measure (COPM)
Obtain family and social history
Additional assessments:
CP Quality of Life Questionnaire (CP QOL)
Body structure and function
Minimum dataset:
Gross Motor Function Classification System (GMFCS)
Topography: Hemiplegia, Diplegia, Quadraplegia
Spasticity: Modified Ashworth Scale (MAS), Hypertonia Assessment Tool (HAT)
Muscle Range of Motion
Medical Research Council Manual Muscle Testing (MRC MMT)
Selective Control Assessment of the Lower Extremity (SCALE)
Additional assessments:
Xray: Hip, knees, feet, spine
Pain Scores (intensity, frequency, location, interference)
Activity and participation
Minimum dataset:
Gross Motor Function Measure (GMFM)
Video Gait Analysis
Paediatric Evaluation of Disability Inventory (PEDI)
Functional Independence Measure for Children (WeeFIM)

the child's gait, function, and performance in different settings. "Personal and environmental" factors involve understanding the child's goals, quality of life, and family support.

7.4 Goals of Treatment

Clinical teams need thoughtful ways to involve parents and children in setting realistic and meaningful goals [22]. Parental commitment is essential to supporting the child during the lengthy post-SDR rehabilitation journey. Cultural, socioeconomic, and family functions and support influence a child's capacity to participate in rehabilitation and may impact SDR outcomes [22, 23].

Canadian Occupational Performance Measure (COPM) is a validated tool that relies on the child's (or their parent's) self-perception to identify occupational

Table 7.2 Key points of Canadian Occupational Performance (COPM) [24]

Purpose	To identify and prioritise problems in occupational performance experienced by the patient
Assessment areas	Self-care (personal care, functional mobility) Productivity (school/play) Leisure activity (recreation, sports, socialisation)
Process	Trained administrator is required to administer and interpret results through a semi-structured interview. The manual is purchased Subjective measure based on child/parent self-report
Scoring	*Performance*: rated from 1 (not able to do) to 10 (able to do extremely well) *Satisfaction*: rated from 1 (not satisfied) to 10 (extremely satisfied)

Further information on COPM can be found at https://www.thecopm.ca

performance concerns, facilitating individualised goal setting (Table 7.2) [24, 25]. COPM can detect statistically significant changes over time in response to an intervention [25, 26]. An Australian SDR study identified that SDR-related goals that mattered to families and children were linked to functional mobility [23]. SDR self-care goals included walking, the ability to transfer and balance, and attending to daily tasks. Desired productivity goals included improving fine motor skills, playing, and keeping up with peers. SDR leisure goals were related to sports, playground participation, and organised recreational activities [23]. Children at higher GMFCS levels tended to prioritise self-care goals. Post-SDR, self-care and productivity goals demonstrated greater improvement than leisure goals.

7.5 Navigating Goals for SDR

The literature on SDR outcomes varies by the study centre's selection criteria, which can be "ideal" [7, 17, 27–29], "inclusive" [2, 4, 9], or "broad". The "ideal" approach selects "stronger" patients (GMFCS I–III) focused on improving gait. The "inclusive" approach includes patients with more difficult ambulation (GMFCS III) or wheelchair users (GMFCS IV–V) whose goals are care and comfort. Broader inclusion criteria for other spasticity conditions are also being studied [30–34].

While "ideal" candidates yield better SDR outcomes, clinical discretion is needed for those with less optimal characteristics, particularly when severe spasticity is not responding to conventional treatments. A multidisciplinary panel for joint decision-making, often consisting of a physiotherapist, occupational therapist, rehabilitation physician, neurosurgeon, orthopaedic surgeon, social worker, and psychologist, evaluates multiple factors to balance the surgery's costs, time, and risks against its benefits. For ambulatory children, the decision hinges on whether reducing spasticity will improve gait or reveal the underlying weakness that further impacts ambulation. For nonambulatory children, considerations include improvements in daily care and pain reduction against the risk of developing truncal weakness, which can affect sitting balance.

7.6 Preoperative SDR Assessments for Minimum Dataset

7.6.1 Neuroimaging

Prematurity is associated with white matter injury and periventricular leukomalacia (PVL), where children with CP commonly present with spastic diplegia. In spastic quadriplegia, there is usually more extensive PVL and multicystic cortical encephalomalacia, indicating significant functional and independence limitations [35]. SDR has favourable outcomes in children with PVL MRI features without damage to key areas controlling posture and coordination (Fig. 7.1) [36]. Conversely, SDR is less favourable for children with rigidity, dystonia, or ataxia where MRI reveal cortical, subcortical, deep grey matter involvement, cerebellum injury, or congenital brain malformations [1, 36].

Dystonia is common in children with GMFCS IV/V with bilateral spasticity. Spasticity can mask underlying dystonia that emerges after SDR [37]. Mild positional dystonia with PVL on MRI, without basal ganglia involvement, is usually stable post-SDR (Fig. 7.2) [37]. In contrast, uncontrollable dystonia post-SDR is more likely to occur in congenital disorders or non-PVL-related MRI findings (Fig. 7.3) [37].

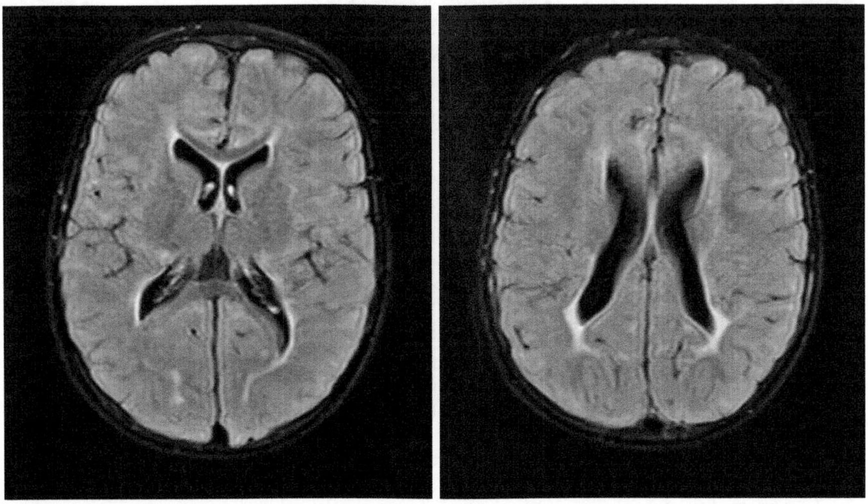

Fig. 7.1 A GMFCS III child with spastic diplegia recommended for SDR to preserve ambulation. MRI shows extensive symmetrical bilateral deep and periventricular white matter signal abnormality on axial T2 FLAIR sequences with volume loss, thinning of the corpus callosum, and crenated appearing lateral ventricles. Basal ganglia are preserved

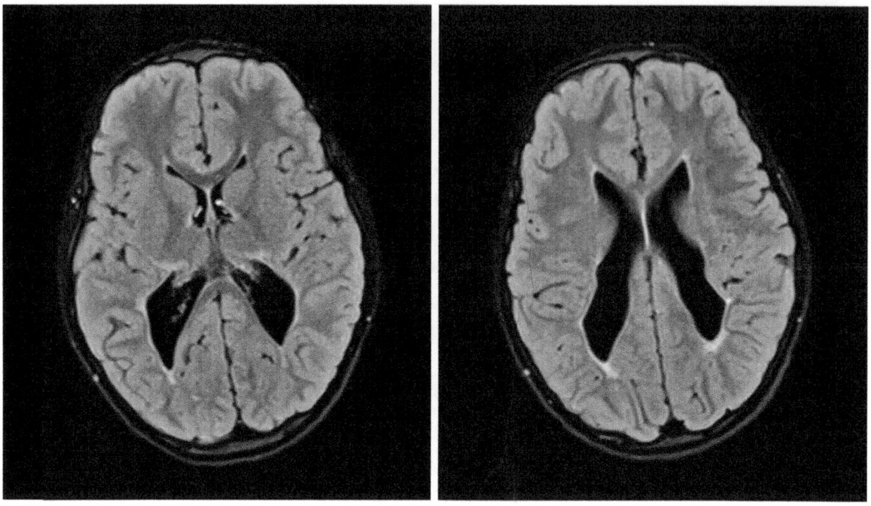

Fig. 7.2 A GMFCS IV child with spastic quadriparesis and mild upper limb dystonia recommended for SDR to ease sitting and daily care. MRI shows extensive white matter injury and ex vacuo dilation of the ventricles due to periventricular volume loss. Basal ganglia are preserved

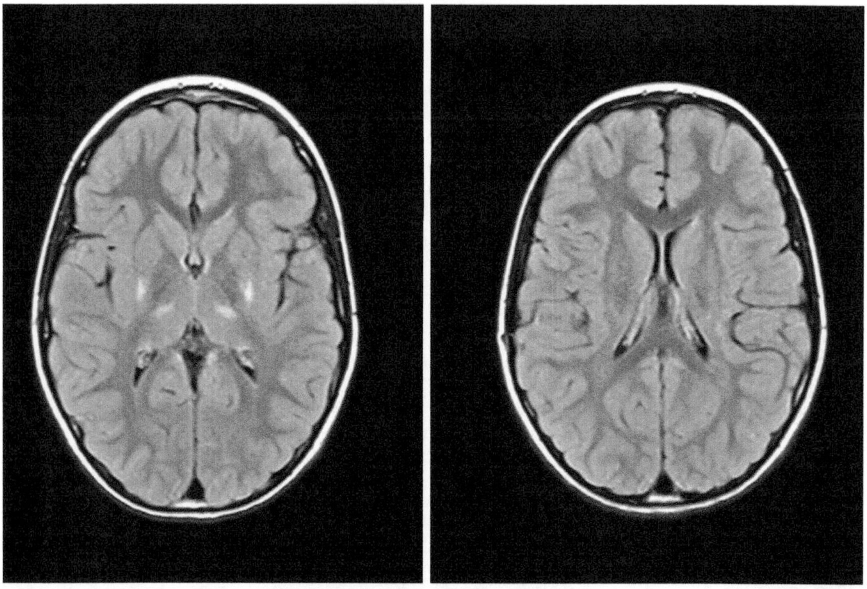

Fig. 7.3 A GMFCS IV child with severe dystonia and spastic quadriplegia from neonatal hypoxic-ischaemic injury. SDR was not recommended, and the child was referred for ITB. MRI shows increased T2 FLAIR signal abnormality in bilateral putamen, anterolateral thalami, and perirolandic areas, corresponding to severe hypoxic-ischemic injury

7.6.2 *Differential Diagnosis of Cerebral Palsy*

Hereditary spastic paraplegia (HSP) can mimic CP and should be considered in children with significant spastic diplegia and a normal brain MRI. While long-term SDR outcomes for HSP children are limited, SDR can be considered if HSP is CP-like, "uncomplicated", and the clinical course is stable and non-regressive. Over 80 genes are linked to HSP, with SPG3, SPG4, SPG5, SPG7, and SPG 11 being the most common genotype and SPG3A and SPG4 most commonly referred for SDR [32, 33]. Children with "complicated" HSP - characterised by seizures, peripheral neuropathy, bladder involvement, or upper limb weakness - should not undergo SDR [33].

7.6.3 *Gross Motor Function Classification Scale (GMFCS)*

The GMFCS categorises children with spastic cerebral palsy (CP) into five levels based on their gross motor skills, ranging from independent walking (GMFCS I) to severe impairment (GMFCS V). Each level describes the gross motor performance [38] and assists in predicting musculoskeletal complications [39].

SDR is most effective in young children functioning at GMFCS levels II and III. Spasticity is most pronounced between ages 3 and 6, and early reduction in spasticity during this period can improve gait and function [17]. In older children, secondary contractures are likely to have developed, limiting the functional gains of SDR but increasing the need for more extensive orthopaedic surgery [2, 14, 40]. For children functioning at GMFCS IV and V, SDR is offered to improve care, increase sitting tolerance, and ease pain [4]. Children functioning at GMFCS I and those with spastic hemiplegia are typically strong functional walkers and are generally not offered SDR [1].

7.6.4 *Physical Assessments*

7.6.4.1 Spasticity

Hypertonicity in CP includes spasticity, rigidity, or dystonia [41]. A systematic neurological examination using validated measures helps identify the type of hypertonicity and determine the appropriate treatments. For SDR, the focus is on measuring spasticity in the hip adductors, rectus femoris, hamstring, and gastrocnemius to determine the levels of muscle involvement [18].

- *Spasticity* is "velocity-dependent resistance" during muscle stretch, often associated with increased reflexes and clonus [41].
- *Rigidity* involves "velocity-independent bidirectional resistance", where agonist and antagonist co-contract simultaneously [41].

Table 7.3 Summary description of MAS [44, 45]

Grade	Description
0	No increase in muscle tone
1	Slight increase in muscle tone with a "catch" and release or minimal resistance at the end of the range of motion (ROM)
1^+	Slight increase in muscle tone with a "catch" followed by minimal resistance throughout the remainder (less than half) of the ROM
2	More marked increase in muscle tone through most of the ROM, but the affected part is easily moved
3	Considerable increase in muscle tone, making passive movement difficult
4	Affected part is rigid in flexion or extension

- *Dystonia* is characterised by "involuntary sustained or intermittent muscle contractions" that lead to twisting, repetitive movements, and abnormal postures [41, 42].

The Modified Ashworth Scale (MAS) is widely used to measure spasticity (Table 7.3) [2, 16, 18]. Suitable SDR candidates typically have a baseline MAS score of 2 or higher in multiple muscle groups [16, 40]. Long-term studies have shown that SDR reduces spasticity in all muscle groups regardless of GMFCS level [2, 40]. *The Hypertonia Assessment Tool (HAT)* is a useful clinical guide to differentiate between dystonia, spasticity, rigidity, or mixed tone [18, 42].

7.6.4.2 Strength and Selective Motor Control

Assessing strength and motor selectivity in severe spasticity is challenging. Staudt and Peacock selected children for SDR by focusing on functional skills like crawling, high kneeling, sitting, and reaching [1]. Importantly, in children with weakness, spasticity may serve a compensatory role for functional tasks such as standing upright [46].

- The *Medical Research Council (MRC)* scale is the most common method for assessing muscle strength against resistance [47]. The MRC provides the following grades: 0, no visible contraction; 1, a flicker or trace of contraction; 2, active movement with gravity eliminated; 3, active movement against gravity; 4, active movement against gravity and resistance; and 5, normal strength. Key muscle power tested for SDR is the flexor and extensor strength of the hips, knees, and ankles.
- The *Selective Control Assessment of the Lower Extremity (SCALE)* evaluates the selective motor control (SMC) of different joints in children with CP [48]. Selective motor control impairment reflects cortical spinal tract dysfunction and is characterised by mass flexion and extension patterns without dissociative movements [48].

In the Oswestry study, "ideal" SDR candidates who have moderate to severe spasticity, moderate strength (MRC $\geq$ 3), and limited SMC impairment, achieved favourable outcomes [17]. Conversely, children unable to high kneel or those with balance impairment showed functional weakness post-SDR. One centre selected children based on hip flexor strength (MRC $\geq$ 3) and the ability to isolate movement at the hips, knees, and ankles without excessive flexion patterns during walking [49]. Another study emphasised the importance of quadriceps strength for maintaining standing and walking, selecting children functioning at GMFCS II and III levels with quadriceps strength of MRC $\geq$ 3 and MRC $\geq$ 2 for higher GMFCS levels [2].

As children with CP grow, their increased body weight can outweigh their strength, posing a challenge for adolescents with significant weakness. In pre- and post-SDR assessments, dietitian involvement is essential for managing the impact of weight gain on ambulation and function, and families need education about this concern [9, 17].

7.6.4.3 Range of Motion

In pre-SDR assessment, the range of motion (ROM) of hip abduction, knee extension, and ankle dorsiflexion is measured [18, 43]. Long-term SDR studies report initial ROM improvement, followed by a decline, indicating the development of contractures with age. Post-SDR contracture is less common in children functioning at GMFCS II, with ROM maintained long term in this group [43].

7.6.5 Functional Measures

7.6.5.1 Gross Motor Function Measure (GMFM)

The Gross Motor Function Measure (GMFM) is the "gold standard" for tracking changes in gross motor function in children with CP [50]. Its use is valuable for selecting children for SDR and predicting their progress relative to their expected trajectory based on the GMFM reference percentiles [16].

- GMFM-88 evaluates a child's ability across five dimensions: lying and rolling, crawling and kneeling, sitting, standing, and walk-run-jump activities. The most challenging items on the scale represent the capacity of a typical 5-year-old [50]. Clinically, GMFM-88 is helpful for descriptive evaluation and for predicting SDR benefits by reviewing performance across these five domains [10].
- GMFM-66, an abbreviated version, evaluates a subset of 66 items ordered by difficulty to track gross motor changes over time [51]. It calculates the interval scores using the Gross Motor Ability Estimator (GMAE). Many SDR follow-up studies use GMFM-66 to track interval progress [7, 52].

The gross motor reference curves for children and youth with CP were created using GMFM-66 scores, plotted by age for each of the five GMFCS levels [53]. Children functioning at GMFCS I and II reach a GMFM-66 stable limit during their adolescent years with no evidence of decline. In contrast, children functioning at GMFCS III–V typically attain peak motor development limits at a younger age, followed by a decline into adulthood. This age-related decline is usually influenced by reduced strength, increased body habitus, and musculoskeletal complications [50, 53]. Post-SDR, GMFM scores typically improve and remain stable at follow-up [3, 9, 10, 13]. However, some long-term studies report a decline in GMFM; yet, without comparisons to reference curves, the impact of SDR remains unclear [4, 5, 50]. SDR studies that used reference curves for comparison have reported positive outcomes [7, 52]. Successful intervention for children functioning at GMFCS III involves preserving ambulation and delaying motor function decline [10, 43].

7.6.5.2 Gait and Function

Instrumental video gait analysis provides a precise and objective stratification of gait pathology severity for children with CP [35]. SDR studies use biplanar video observation or three-dimensional instrumented gait analysis to evaluate the sagittal plane kinematics of the hips, knees, and ankles [40, 54]. *Gait Indices (GI)* such as the *Gillette Gait Index (GGI)*, *Gait Deviation Index (GDI)*, and *Gait Profile Score (GPS)* serve as measures to quantify gait pathology [18, 49, 55–57]. Gait analysis assists clinicians in determining whether SDR can make a difference in sagittal joint kinematics, especially in treating spasticity-related stiff knee gait patterns [17, 49, 58].

Published studies show that SDR improves knee kinematics and overall gait quality. Long-term improvements in step length were observed, and mild crouch gait patterns, when present post-SDR remained stable into adulthood [6, 59, 60]. A long-term matched-control study by Munger et al. (2017) supports SDR's effectiveness in reducing spasticity, with the children receiving SDR showing improved dynamic knee ROM and gait scores. However, their gait improvements were less compared to the non-SDR group, which exhibited better overall gait quality but required more orthopaedic interventions and ongoing need for botulinum toxin injection to manage spasticity [61].

7.6.5.3 Assessments of Self-Care Function

The Functional Independence Measure for Children (WeeFIM) assesses self-care and global performance in children between 6 months and 7 years of age. It is a measure for demonstrating gains in children postintervention, and in SDR studies, the children showed improvement in the self-care domain [62, 63].

The Paediatric Evaluation of Disability Inventory (PEDI) assesses performance across the domains of self-care, mobility, and social function. It shows a strong correlation with WeeFIM in evaluating children within the same age group. Studies on SDR that utilise PEDI concentrate on functional skills, independence in daily living, caregiver assistance measures, and the modifications or adaptive equipment employed. The research indicated that following SDR, there were improvements in self-care and a decrease in caregiver assistance over time, reflecting enhancements in upper extremity function and skills [9, 12, 62].

7.7 Additional Assessments

7.7.1 Orthopaedic Evaluation

Children with spastic diplegic CP commonly develop musculoskeletal deformities in the feet, hips, and spine, which can lead to functional loss [39]. Pre-SDR orthopaedic assessments evaluate soft tissue pathology and bony malalignment through clinical exams and radiological measures. SDR addresses spasticity, while orthopaedic corrections improve lower limb biomechanics. Pre-SDR counselling should inform families about future orthopaedic surgery needs and timing. Studies indicate that 28–94% of children require orthopaedic treatment post-SDR, typically performed at least a year later [2–4, 60, 61, 64].

7.7.2 Scoliosis

Spinal deformities in CP directly correlate with GMFCS level, being most severe in non-ambulant children (GMFCS IV and V) [35]. Baseline spinal assessments identify back deformities, and the frequency of postsurgical monitoring following SDR is based on the future risk of scoliosis and GMFCS level. Clinical examinations are correlated with radiological documentation, commonly using anteroposterior (AP) standing X-rays to evaluate spinal deformities. Some studies employ sitting lateral X-rays to assess lumbar flexibility and lordosis [65]. There are concerns that SDR may accelerate spinal deformity beyond the natural course of the condition [66], particularly in those classified as GMFCS IV and V who exhibit underlying truncal weakness. While ambulatory children generally face a lower risk of developing spinal abnormalities, close monitoring remains essential.

7.7.3 Hips

SDR and alternative treatments are ineffective in preventing hip displacement (HD) [67, 68]. Hip surveillance pre- and post-SDR ensures timely interventions for adductor psoas release, guided growth, or proactive bony reconstruction hip surgery to maintain hip health for long-term functional and care benefits [67, 69]. Hip displacement correlates with GMFCS levels. Ambulant children at GMFCS I–III have a lower risk of HD. Conversely, 60–90% of GMFCS levels IV and V have HD, often causing significant pain and affecting their ability to sit [67, 69, 70].

7.7.4 *Quality of Life Measures*

7.7.4.1 Cerebral Palsy Quality of Life Questionnaire (CP QOL)

The CP QOL is a validated questionnaire used to measure the quality of life (QOL) for children with CP [23, 71]. It covers seven domains of functional and psychosocial QOL and is designed for self-reporting or proxy reporting by parents or caregivers. Studies typically show improvements in functional QOL 2 years after SDR, with no change in psychosocial QOL (social well-being) and a noted decrease in emotional well-being and self-esteem scores [23, 27]. These findings highlight the importance of providing psychosocial support as part of the clinical care for SDR.

7.7.4.2 Pain

Pre- and post-SDR pain assessments aim to determine whether reducing spasticity improves pain in patients with CP. Various tools, such as numerical rating scales, visual analogue scales, and interference scales like the Patient-Reported Outcomes Information System (PROMIS), measure pain intensity and interference [18, 72]. Currently, there is limited consensus on whether SDR reduces pain intensity and interference more than what is experienced by adults with CP [61, 72–74].

7.8 Conclusion

The SDR preoperative assessments involve a thorough evaluation to identify the most suitable spasticity treatment for children whose gait, function, or care and comfort are impacted by spasticity. The ICF framework aids in understanding the factors influencing SDR outcomes and the necessary support thereafter. SDR is a goal-based treatment, with success linked to meaningful, realistic goals, including discussions about uncertainties. Evaluations of physical, functional, and gait aspects are essential for SDR decision-making. The GMFM can serve as both an evaluation and counselling tool for SDR intervention, identifying known factors, anticipated motor trajectories, potential improvements, and areas where limitations might arise.

References

1. Peacock WJ, Staudt LA. Spasticity in cerebral palsy and the selective posterior rhizotomy procedure. J Child Neurol. 1990;5:179–85.
2. Ailon T, Beauchamp R, Miller S, Mortenson P, Kerr JM, Hengel AR, Steinbok P. Long-term outcome after selective dorsal rhizotomy in children with spastic cerebral palsy. Childs Nerv Syst. 2015;31:415–23.

3. Tedroff K, Hägglund G, Miller F. Long-term effects of selective dorsal rhizotomy in children with cerebral palsy: a systematic review. Dev Med Child Neurol. 2020;62:554–62.
4. Tedroff K, Löwing K, Åström E. A prospective cohort study investigating gross motor function, pain, and health-related quality of life 17 years after selective dorsal rhizotomy in cerebral palsy. Dev Med Child Neurol. 2015;57:484–90.
5. Tedroff K, Löwing K, Jacobson DNO, Åström E. Does loss of spasticity matter? A 10-year follow-up after selective dorsal rhizotomy in cerebral palsy. Dev Med Child Neurol. 2011;53:724–9.
6. Langerak NG, Lamberts RP, Fieggen AG, Peter JC, Van Der Merwe L, Peacock WJ, Vaughan CL. A prospective gait analysis study in patients with diplegic cerebral palsy 20 years after selective dorsal rhizotomy. J Neurosurg Pediatr. 2008;1:180–6.
7. Bolster EA, van Schie PE, Becher JG, van Ouwerkerk WJ, Strijers RL, Vermeulen RJ. Long-term effect of selective dorsal rhizotomy on gross motor function in ambulant children with spastic bilateral cerebral palsy, compared with reference centiles. Dev Med Child Neurol. 2013;55:610–6.
8. Mittal S, Farmer J-P, Al-Atassi B, Gibis J, Kennedy E, Galli C, Courchesnes G, Poulin C, Cantin M-A, Benaroch TE. Long-term functional outcome after selective posterior rhizotomy. J Neurosurg. 2002;97:315–25.
9. Nordmark E, Josenby AL, Lagergren J, Andersson G, Strömblad LG, Westbom L. Long-term outcomes five years after selective dorsal rhizotomy. BMC Pediatr. 2008;8 https://doi.org/10.1186/1471-2431-8-54.
10. Dudley RWR, Parolin M, Gagnon B, et al. Long-term functional benefits of selective dorsal rhizotomy for spastic cerebral palsy: clinical article. J Neurosurg Pediatr. 2013;12:142–50.
11. Vermeulen RJ, Becher JG. Long-term outcome in selective dorsal rhizotomy in spastic cerebral palsy: differentiation in mobility levels is needed. Dev Med Child Neurol. 2015;57:408–9.
12. Josenby AL, Wagner P, Jarnlo GB, Westbom L, Nordmark E. Functional performance in self-care and mobility after selective dorsal rhizotomy: a 10-year practice-based follow-up study. Dev Med Child Neurol. 2015;57:286–93.
13. Steinbok P. Outcomes after selective dorsal rhizotomy for spastic cerebral palsy. Childs Nerv Syst. 2001;17:1–18.
14. Steinbok P. Selective dorsal rhizotomy for spastic cerebral palsy: a review. Childs Nerv Syst. 2007;23:981–90.
15. Grunt S, Becher JG, Vermeulen RJ. Long-term outcome and adverse effects of selective dorsal rhizotomy in children with cerebral palsy: a systematic review. Dev Med Child Neurol. 2011;53:490–8.
16. McLaughlin J, Bjornson K, Temkin N, et al. Selective dorsal rhizotomy: meta-analysis of three randomized controlled trials. Dev Med Child Neurol. 2002;44:17–25.
17. Cole GF, Farmer SE, Roberts A, Stewart C, Patrick JH. Selective dorsal rhizotomy for children with cerebral palsy: the Oswestry experience. Arch Dis Child. 2007;92:781–5.
18. Lewis J, Bear N, Baker F, et al. Australian children undergoing selective dorsal rhizotomy: protocol for a national registry of multidimensional outcomes. BMJ Open. 2019;9:e025093. https://doi.org/10.1136/bmjopen-2018-025093.
19. Parent A, Marois P, Letellier G, Raison M, Mercier C, Ballaz L. Experience-based decision-tree process for selective dorsal rhizotomy in children with cerebral palsy. Ann Phys Rehabil Med. 2021;64:101287.
20. Waite G, Chugh D, Cawker S, Oulton K, Wray J, Harniess P. 'Wanting no regrets': parental decision making around selective dorsal rhizotomy. Child Care Health Dev. 2023;49:382–91.
21. Grunt S, Fieggen AG, Vermeulen RJ, Becher JG, Langerak NG. Selection criteria for selective dorsal rhizotomy in children with spastic cerebral palsy: a systematic review of the literature. Dev Med Child Neurol. 2014;56:302–12.
22. Rosenbaum P, Stewart D. The World Health Organization International classification of functioning, disability, and health: a model to guide clinical thinking, practice and research in the field of cerebral palsy. Semin Pediatr Neurol. 2004;11:5–10.

23. Lewis JA, Bear N, Smith N, Baker F, Lee OS, Wynter M, Paget SP. Goal setting, goal attainment and quality of life of children following selective dorsal rhizotomy. Child Care Health Dev. 2023;49:760–8.
24. Law M, Baptiste S, Carswell A, McColl MA, Polatajko H, Pollock N. Canadian occupational performance measure. 5th ed. Altona: COPM Inc.; 2019.
25. Law M, Polatajko H, Pollock N, Mccoll MA, Carswell A, Baptiste S. Pilot testing of the Canadian occupational performance measure: clinical and measurement issues. Can J Occup Ther. 1994;61:191–7.
26. McColl MA, Denis CB, Douglas K-L, Gilmour J, Haveman N, Petersen M, Presswell B, Law M. A clinically significant difference on the COPM: a review. Can J Occup Ther. 2023;90:92–102.
27. Summers J, Coker B, Eddy S, et al. Selective dorsal rhizotomy in ambulant children with cerebral palsy: an observational cohort study. Lancet Child Adolesc Health. 2019;3:455–62.
28. Enslin JMN, Langerak NG, Fieggen AG. The evolution of selective dorsal rhizotomy for the management of spasticity. Neurotherapeutics. 2019;16:3–8.
29. Aquilina K, Graham D, Wimalasundera N. Selective dorsal rhizotomy: an old treatment re-emerging. Arch Dis Child. 2015;100:798–802.
30. Park T, Joh S, Walter DM, Meyer NL, Dobbs MB. Selective dorsal rhizotomy for the treatment of spastic hemiplegic cerebral palsy. Cureus. 2020;12:e9605. https://doi.org/10.7759/cureus.9605.
31. Park T, Joh S, Smyth MD, Meyer NL, Walter DM. Selective dorsal rhizotomy for treatment of spasticity after hemispherectomy in children: a case report. Cureus. 2023;15:e36945. https://doi.org/10.7759/cureus.36945.
32. van de Pol LA, Burgert N, van Schie PEM, Slot KM, Gouw AA, Buizer AI. Surgical treatment options for spasticity in children and adolescents with hereditary spastic paraplegia. Childs Nerv Syst. 2023;40:855. https://doi.org/10.1007/s00381-023-06159-w.
33. Park T, Joh S, Walter DM, Meyer NL. Selective dorsal rhizotomy for treatment of hereditary spastic paraplegia-associated spasticity in 37 Patients. Cureus. 2021;13:e17690. https://doi.org/10.7759/cureus.17690.
34. Reynolds RM, Morton RP, Walker ML, Massagli TL, Browd SR. Role of dorsal rhizotomy in spinal cord injury–induced spasticity. J Neurosurg Pediatr. 2014;14:266–70.
35. Graham HK, Rosenbaum P, Paneth N, et al. Cerebral palsy. Nat Rev Dis Primers. 2016;2:15082. https://doi.org/10.1038/nrdp.2015.82.
36. Graham D, Aquilina K, Mankad K, Wimalasundera N. Selective dorsal rhizotomy: current state of practice and the role of imaging. Quant Imaging Med Surg. 2018;8:209–18.
37. Van De Pol LA, Vermeulen RJ, et al. Risk factors for dystonia after selective dorsal rhizotomy in nonwalking children and adolescents with bilateral spasticity. Neuropediatrics. 2018;49:44–50.
38. Palisano R, Rosenbaum P, Walter S, Russell D, Wood E, Galuppi B. Development and reliability of a system to classify gross motor function in children with cerebral palsy. Dev Med Child Neurol. 1997;39:214–23.
39. Graham HK, Selber P. Musculoskeletal aspects of cerebral palsy. J Bone Joint Surg Ser B. 2003;85:157–66.
40. Wang KK, Munger ME, Chen BP-J, Novacheck TF. Selective dorsal rhizotomy in ambulant children with cerebral palsy. J Child Orthop. 2018;12:413–27.
41. Sanger TD, Delgado MR, Gaebler-Spira D, Hallett M, Mink JW. Classification and definition of disorders causing hypertonia in childhood. Pediatrics. 2003;111:e89–97.
42. Jethwa A, Mink J, Macarthur C, Knights S, Fehlings T, Fehlings D. Development of the hypertonia assessment Tool (HAT): a discriminative tool for hypertonia in children. Dev Med Child Neurol. 2010;52:e83–7.
43. Tu A, Steinbok P. Long term outcome of Selective Dorsal Rhizotomy for the management of childhood spasticity – functional improvement and complications. Childs Nerv Syst. 2020;36:1985–94.

44. Bohannon RW, Smith MB. Interrater reliability of a modified Ashworth scale of muscle spasticity. Phys Ther. 1987;67:206–7.
45. Fosang AL, Galea MP, McCoy AT, Reddihough DS, Story I. Measures of muscle and joint performance in the lower limb of children with cerebral palsy. Dev Med Child Neurol. 2003;45 https://doi.org/10.1017/S0012162203001245.
46. Engsberg JR, Ross SA, Collins DR, Park TS. Effect of selective dorsal rhizotomy in the treatment of children with cerebral palsy. J Neurosurg. 2006;105:8–15.
47. Medical Research Council. Aids to examination of the peripheral nervous system. Memorandum no. 45. London; 1976
48. Fowler EG, Staudt LA, Greenberg MB, Oppenheim WL. Selective control assessment of the lower extremity (SCALE): development, validation, and interrater reliability of a clinical tool for patients with cerebral palsy. Dev Med Child Neurol. 2009;51:607–14.
49. Trost JP, Schwartz MH, Krach LE, Dunn ME, Novacheck TF. Comprehensive short-term outcome assessment of selective dorsal rhizotomy. Dev Med Child Neurol. 2008;50:765–71.
50. Hanna SE, Rosenbaum PL, Bartlett DJ, Palisano RJ, Walter SD, Avery L, Russell DJ. Stability and decline in gross motor function among children and youth with cerebral palsy aged 2 to 21 years. Dev Med Child Neurol. 2009;51:295–302.
51. CanChild. Gross motor function measure (GMFM). In: CanChild; 2019. https://canchild.ca/en/resources/44-gross-motor-function-measure-gmfm. Accessed 22 June 2024.
52. Iorio-Morin C, Yap R, Dudley RWR, Poulin C, Cantin M-A, Benaroch TE, Farmer J-P. Selective dorsal root rhizotomy for spastic cerebral palsy: a longitudinal case-control analysis of functional outcome. Neurosurgery. 2020;87:186–92.
53. Bartlett DJ, Hanna SE, Avery L, Stevenson RD, Galuppi B. Correlates of decline in gross motor capacity in adolescents with cerebral palsy in gross motor function classification system levels III to V: an exploratory study. Dev Med Child Neurol. 2010;52:e155. https://doi.org/10.1111/j.1469-8749.2010.03632.x.
54. Munger ME, Chen BPJ, Macwilliams BA, Mcmulkin ML, Schwartz MH. Comparing the effects of two spasticity management strategies on the long-term outcomes of individuals with bilateral spastic cerebral palsy: a multicentre cohort study protocol. BMJ Open. 2019;9:e027486. https://doi.org/10.1136/bmjopen-2018-027486.
55. McMulkin ML, MacWilliams BA. Application of the Gillette gait index, gait deviation index and gait profile score to multiple clinical pediatric populations. Gait Posture. 2015;41:608–12.
56. Baker R, McGinley JL, Schwartz MH, Beynon S, Rozumalski A, Graham HK, Tirosh O. The gait profile score and movement analysis profile. Gait Posture. 2009;30:265–9.
57. Van Campenhout A, Huenaerts C, Poulussen L, Prinsen SD, Desloovere K. Role of femoral derotation on gait after selective dorsal rhizotomy in children with spastic cerebral palsy. Dev Med Child Neurol. 2019;61:1196–201.
58. Graham HK, Harvey A, Rodda J, Nattrass GR, Pirpiris M. The functional mobility scale (FMS). J Pediatr Orthop. 2004;24:514–20.
59. Langerak NG, Lamberts RP, Fieggen AG, Peter JC, Peacock WJ, Vaughan CL. Selective dorsal rhizotomy: long-term experience from Cape Town. Childs Nerv Syst. 2007;23:1003–6.
60. Langerak NG, Tam N, Vaughan CL, Fieggen AG, Schwartz MH. Gait status 17–26 years after selective dorsal rhizotomy. Gait Posture. 2012;35:244–9.
61. Munger ME, Aldahondo N, Krach LE, Novacheck TF, Schwartz MH. Long-term outcomes after selective dorsal rhizotomy: a retrospective matched cohort study. Dev Med Child Neurol. 2017;59:1196–203.
62. Merckx L, Poncelet F, De Houwer H, Laumen A, Peeters L, Nuttin B, Pauwels P, Van Campenhout A, Ortibus E, De Vloo P. Upper-extremity spasticity and functionality after selective dorsal rhizotomy for cerebral palsy: a systematic review. J Neurosurg Pediatr. 2023;32:1–13.
63. Gigante P, McDowell MM, Bruce SS, et al. Reduction in upper-extremity tone after lumbar selective dorsal rhizotomy in children with spastic cerebral palsy. J Neurosurg Pediatr. 2013;12:588–94.

64. Langerak NG, Veerbeek BE, Fieggen AG, Lamberts RP. Gait status 26–35 years after selective dorsal rhizotomy: a 9 year follow up study. Gait Posture. 2022;91:284–9.
65. Johnson MB, Goldstein L, Thomas SS, Piatt J, Aiona M, Sussman M. Spinal deformity after selective dorsal rhizotomy in ambulatory patients with cerebral palsy. J Pediatr Orthop. 2004;24:529–36.
66. Wheelwright M, Selvey PJ, Steinbok P, Singhal A, Ibrahim G, Fallah A, Weil AG, Halvorson K, Tu A. Systematic review of spinal deformities following multi-level selective dorsal rhizotomy. Child's Nervous Syst. 2020;36:1025–35.
67. Miller SD, Juricic M, Hesketh K, Mclean L, Magnuson S, Gasior S, Schaeffer E, et al. Prevention of hip displacement in children with cerebral palsy: a systematic review. Dev Med Child Neurol. 2017;59:1130–8.
68. Miller SD, Juricic M, Bone JN, Steinbok P, Mulpuri K. The effect of selective dorsal rhizotomy on hip displacement in children with cerebral palsy. J Pediatr Orthop. 2023;43:e701–6.
69. Howard JJ, Willoughby K, Thomason P, Shore BJ, Graham K, Rutz E. Hip surveillance and management of hip displacement in children with cerebral palsy: clinical and ethical dilemmas. J Clin Med. 2023;12 https://doi.org/10.3390/jcm12041651.
70. Soo B. Hip displacement in cerebral palsy. J Bone Joint Surg. 2006;88:121.
71. Waters E, Davis E, Mackinnon A, et al. Psychometric properties of the quality of life questionnaire for children with CP. Dev Med Child Neurol. 2007;49:49–55.
72. Daunter AK, Kratz AL, Hurvitz EA. Long-term impact of childhood selective dorsal rhizotomy on pain, fatigue, and function: a case–control study. Dev Med Child Neurol. 2017;59:1089–95.
73. Hurvitz EA, Marciniak CM, Daunter AK, Haapala HJ, Stibb SM, McCormick SF, Muraszko KM, Gaebler-Spira D. Functional outcomes of childhood dorsal rhizotomy in adults and adolescents with cerebral palsy. J Neurosurg Pediatr. 2013;11:380–8.
74. van der Slot WMA, Benner JL, Brunton L, et al. Pain in adults with cerebral palsy: a systematic review and meta-analysis of individual participant data. Ann Phys Rehabil Med. 2021;64:101359.

Part III
Surgical and Intraoperative Neurophysiological Procedures

Chapter 8
Rhizotomy Surgery at the Conus Medullaris

Kevin Paul Ferraris and Ash Singhal

8.1 Introduction

In this chapter, we will describe the technique of selective dorsal rhizotomy (SDR) at the level of the conus medullaris. We will allude briefly to other main points described in detail in other chapters. Spasticity is a form of velocity-dependent hypertonia that results in resistance to muscle movement, wherein the more rapidly the muscle is stretched, the more likely the muscle is to "catch" during the neurologic examination [1]. Spasticity in children typically accompanies the clinical diagnosis of cerebral palsy, due to damage to either the developing brain or to the spinal cord. In simplified terms, spasticity results from an imbalance of the excitatory and inhibitory neural signals with a relative deficiency of the inhibitory neurotransmitter gamma aminobutyric acid (GABA). This pathophysiology informs the basis for SDR in becoming a durable procedure in addressing spasticity: by selectively cutting the dorsal sensory roots in the lumbosacral region, the input to the poorly inhibited spinal reflex neurons are reduced, thereby reducing spasticity. After the first description of the modern SDR procedure by Peacock in 1987 [2], the procedure has been modified by Park and colleagues [3, 4]. Since then, many groups went on to have other variations of the procedure in terms of anatomical level, extent of bony exposure, and manner of nerve root identification [5–7]. Park and colleagues advocate a minimal exposure at the level of the conus medullaris—a similar technique to that which we are describing herein.

K. P. Ferraris · A. Singhal (✉)
Faculty of Medicine, Division of Pediatric Neurosurgery, British Columbia Children's Hospital, and Division of Neurosurgery, The University of British Columbia, Vancouver, BC, Canada

N. Morota, P. Steinbok (eds.), *Dorsal Rhizotomy: Neurosurgery for Childhood Spasticity*, Advances and Technical Standards in Neurosurgery 51,
https://doi.org/10.1007/978-3-031-86441-4_8

8.2 Patient Selection

It can be argued that the most important step for surgery would be patient selection. Children with spasticity can have impairment of their daily functioning and in their quality of life as well as that of their caregivers. The ideal candidate would be a child in the younger age bracket of about 4–8 years with spastic diplegia inhibiting ambulation, with good motor strength in the lower limbs and with mild contractures only, for which overlapping dystonia, athetosis, and truncal weakness are ruled out. This usually corresponds to a Gross Motor Function Classification System (GMFCS) score of II–III. A subset of patients may benefit from SDR despite being non-ambulant. For children with spasticity who have pain and poor weight gain, durable treatment of their spasticity by surgical means may be an option. Not all children with spasticity, however, qualify for surgical treatment. Variable degrees of spasticity help with tone and upright posture and may even augment the contraction of weak muscles, therefore posing no interference to usual daily function. Treatment goals need to be clarified before taking the surgical option especially since there are potential complications [8, 9]. The natural history of spasticity over time in children with cerebral palsy must also be taken into account. Untreated spasticity often results in an eventual lack of desire for weightbearing and walking even with assistance, a decrease in daily functioning, and the development of contractures. Often, the goals of surgery are improving function, facilitating better ease of care, preventing or minimizing contractures, and reducing painful muscle spasms [1].

In terms of the conduct of the surgical procedure, frequent practical questions on the mind of the neurosurgeon would be: How much of each root to cut? Can you select out the rootlets most involved in the spastic process and cut them selectively? Shall I cut at the level of the root exit foramina or at the level of the conus? We answer these questions alongside the following description of the technique for SDR at the level of the conus.

8.3 Surgical Technique

8.3.1 *Localization and Exposure*

After the induction of anesthesia and insertion of an indwelling Foley catheter, the patient is placed on prone position with adequate padding of pressure points. The needle electrodes for the intraoperative physiologic neuromonitoring are inserted. In children, the conus medullaris of the spinal cord terminates anywhere between the T12 and L3 levels. Minimal bony exposure as in a single-level laminectomy or laminotomy is facilitated by proper identification of the corresponding level of the conus deep to the planned incision. A localizing intraoperative radiograph is taken to mark the center of the laminectomy, which should correspond to the posterior arch overlying the anatomic level of the conus medullaris based on the preoperative magnetic resonance images (MRI). Careful study of the sagittal views of the preoperative MRI entails estimating the degree of angulation of the spinous process in relation to the intradural contents, with the conus as the most discernible landmark. In much younger children, ultrasonography through the skin and paraspinal muscles can also aid in localization. This is facilitated by the ultrasound probe positioned off lateral to the spinous process to obtain axial views of intradural structures; however, the surgeon should not be discouraged if the conus is not readily identified via ultrasound as that can frequently be the case. With time and experience, ultrasound localization of the conus can improve somewhat, but the bony anatomy can still impose limitations. Inclining the operating table with the feet and the operative site relatively elevated above the head (Trendelenburg position) may decrease cerebrospinal fluid (CSF) loss from the intracranial compartment.

Following antiseptic skin preparation, draping, and application of local anesthetic that contains epinephrine in a concentration of 1:400,000, a midline incision is made and carried down to identify the level of the spinous process of interest and proceeding to dissect the interlaminar space, all while doing muscular dissection of the bilateral paraspinal muscles. The ultrasound probe is then brought to identify the conus in relation to the extradural tissues, which should determine whether there is a need to expose additionally rostrally and caudally. With the spinous process and interspinous ligament removed, a foot-plated craniotome (a Midas Rex B5 footplate or reasonable equivalent) may be used to facilitate a single-level laminectomy following dissection of the cephalad and caudal portions of the laminae on either side, immediately medial to the facet joints. If the single-level laminectomy is felt to be too tight for the intradural work later on, the rostral or caudal laminae can be undermined with a Kerrison punch and a partial laminectomy performed upward or downward half a laminar level. Extradural hemostasis is then ensured by way of judicious bipolar cautery and/or tucking small matchstick-sized (length and width) pieces of Gelfoam laterally. It must be emphasized that thorough epidural hemostasis is essential to visualization of the subsequent aspects of this operation and therefore to the patient's wellbeing and the surgeon's sanity. Intraoperative ultrasonography on the sagittal plane can then confirm the level of the conus and the adequacy of the surgical field exposure (Fig. 8.1). A hypoechoic region within the center of the rostral portion of the conus can sometimes be found, which corresponds to a ventriculus terminalis.

8.3.2 Separation of Dorsal from Ventral Roots

The dura is then opened in the midline and the edges are tacked up laterally. We find that tacking up the dural edge using a 5–0 NUROLON stitch, secured laterally to the paraspinal muscles or lumbodorsal fascia, provides the best visualization of the intradural contents by properly everting the dural edge. Under the operating microscope, the surgical anatomy becomes better appreciated. If the laminectomy done earlier is wide enough, the neural foramina where the roots exit can be visualized.

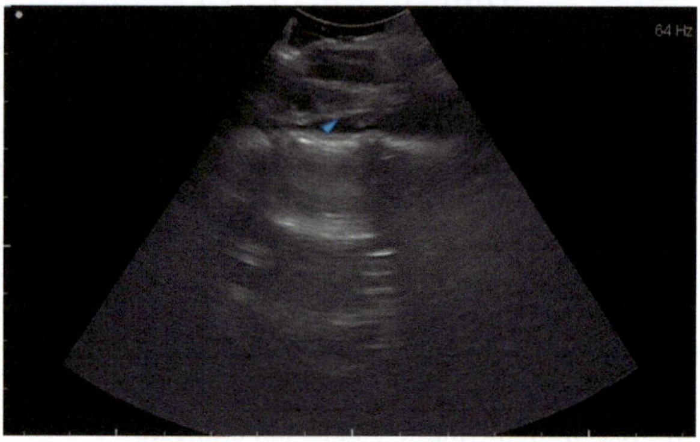

Fig. 8.1 After bony removal but before dural opening, intraoperative ultrasonography can demonstrate the level of the conus medullaris floating in the hypoechoic subarachnoid spaces dorsally and ventrally. This represents a sagittal ultrasound, and the tapering of the spinal cord toward the tip of the conus is shown with a blue arrowhead

Fig. 8.2 Illustrative diagram showing adequate exposure just medial to the facets laterally and generous exposure of the interlaminar spaces craniocaudally. The dural leaflets are tacked dorsolaterally to the fascia to maximize intradural visualization

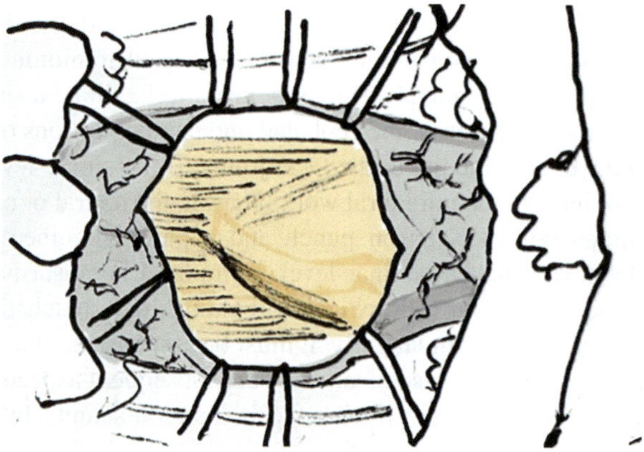

The tip of the conus, the cephalad portion of the filum terminale, and the root exit zones ought to be seen at this point (Fig. 8.2). Arachnoid dissection is then done. Often, cutting away the arachnoid bands and resecting them rather than opening them up results in better visualization of the roots coming out of the conus (Fig. 8.3). Two anatomic landmarks should then be found in order to proceed with separating the dorsal from ventral roots: a relatively large neural foramen and the dorsal root entry zone (DREZ). Initially, it can be a little daunting to look for the DREZ hidden beneath the numerous bundle of nerve roots. The most commonly identified superficial neural foramen in the vicinity of the conus is where the L2 dorsal root exits [4] (Fig. 8.4). This root also looks more robust than other exiting roots. The patient's bed can be rotated by some degree to one side in order to facilitate adequate and

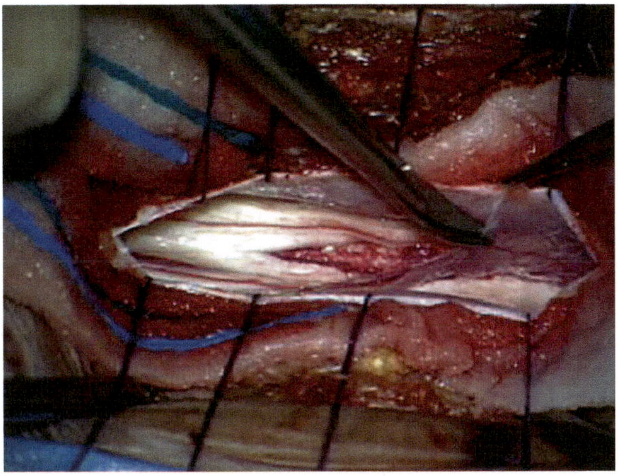

Fig. 8.3 During arachnoid dissection, it is often helpful to resect as much arachnoid as possible, in order to afford better visualization and exposure of the nerve roots

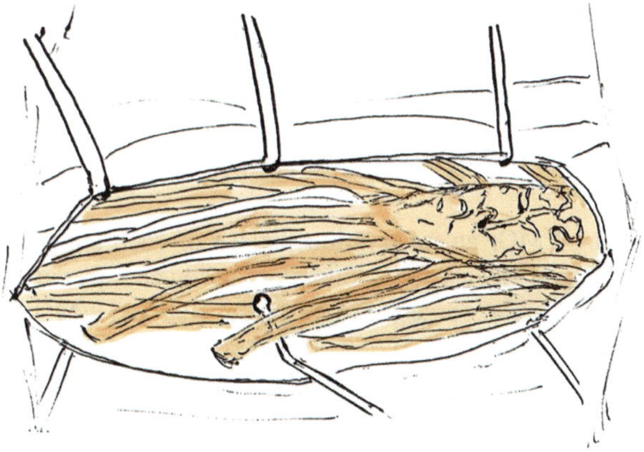

Fig. 8.4 After slightly rotating the patient to the decubitus position toward the surgeon for adequate visualization of the neural foramina, the robust L2 root is identified from its distal portion and followed more proximally to reach the cleft of the DREZ at the side of the conus

ergonomic visualization of the L2 root foramen. The L2 root exiting into the foramen is then followed more proximally to locate the DREZ. The superficial bundle of nerve roots from L2 to S2 are often so close together that unequivocal identification of individual root levels is difficult. This is acceptable as long as the dorsal roots are clearly identified and separated from their ventral counterparts. Close scrutiny of the operative anatomy can be facilitated by the use of a Rhoton spatula and hook, wherein one side of the conus is identified early to discern the outline of the DREZ. Free-run EMG is continuously performed throughout as stretching and traction of ventral roots but not of the dorsal roots produce non-reassuring electrophysiological signals. Further, the exact neurologic level is assessed using intraoperative neurophysiologic feedback with the use of a stimulator probe. Care is taken not to coagulate any vessel unnecessarily.

8.3.3 Guidance from Anatomical Landmarks and Features

With careful dissection, the length of the DREZ allows development of the cleft separating the ventral and dorsal roots anywhere from S2 to L2. An intervening material such as a cottonoid patty can be initially used to protect the ventral roots (Fig. 8.5). Certain anatomic features can give some clues as to the level of the dorsal root: L1 and L2 roots go toward their vertebral foramina below the L1 and L2 vertebral bodies, respectively, whereas S2 forms as a single fascicle laterally to the more caudal thin roots of S3–S5. Among the most caudal set of roots presumed to be the sacral roots, the S1 root is the largest, whereas the S2 root is then markedly decreased in size caudal to it. In contrast, S3–S5 appear as thin threads and whose dorsal and ventral roots are difficult to distinguish from one another [4]; therefore, these are often left intact. Furthermore, roots below the level of L2 are organized more medial to L2 by location. A Silastic sheet, which has the advantage of having less friction and providing visual contrast, can then replace the initial cottonoid patty so as to encompass the whole cleft after identification of the dorsal L2–S2 roots.

8.3.4 Subdividing the Dorsal Roots

Using EMG, an innervation pattern of each stimulated root is identified at each level, and electrical responses of the lower-extremity muscle groups to a threshold voltage are recorded. Single pulse-triggered EMG differentiates motor (ventral) from sensory (dorsal) roots based on the fact that the sensory threshold is higher by several orders of magnitude than the motor. With the use of a blunt tip such as a ball-tipped probe or hook, each dorsal root is then subdivided into three to five, or

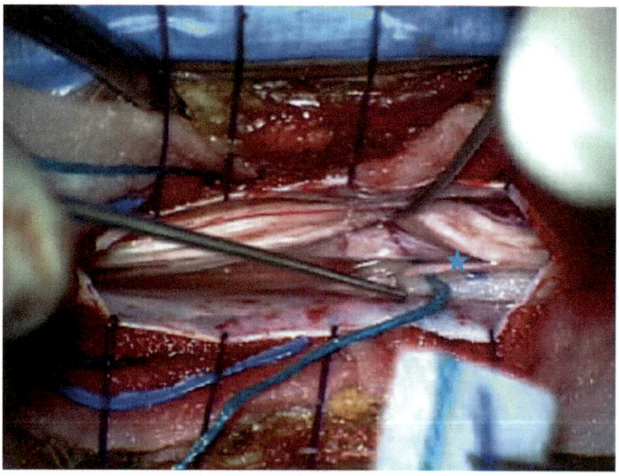

Fig. 8.5 The cleft of the DREZ (blue star) is a useful landmark that can facilitate the anatomical differentiation of the dorsal roots from the ventral roots

up to even ten parts (i.e., rootlets) of equal size. The subdivided rootlets are then tested individually with the monitoring probe. Precise separation of rootlets is often not possible; fortunately, innervation of a particular muscle group comes from several root segments.

8.3.5 Guidance from Electrophysiological Monitoring

Aside from EMG, other physiological neuromonitoring techniques employed during SDR are threshold stimulation and tetanic stimulation [10]. At this point, the surgeon will have isolated the root for electrophysiological interrogation by way of suspending it with the electrode probe with no contact to fluid or nearby roots as much as possible. For threshold stimulation, the initially used settings are the following: a constant-current square wave pulse of 0.1 ms duration, a low intensity of 0.1 mA, and a stimulus frequency of 0.5–1.0 Hz. By starting with 0.1 mA, the intensity is gradually increased to 0.2 mA, at which the ventral root trigger level is almost always reached [11]. The electroclinical responses from the needle electrodes inserted in the patient's muscles are visualized in a software platform, and the surgeon is alerted by the neurophysiology team. The recorded potential shows which root and side it belongs to. The identified dorsal root threshold will be used for the subsequent tetanic stimulation at 50 Hz [10, 11]. Tetanic stimulation elicits rootlet responses that are representative of the hyperactive reflexes of spasticity. These responses are graded ordinally by scales such as the SDR Reflex Grading Criteria and the Park Classification (Table 8.1) [4, 10–12]. For example, a grade 3+ or 4+ response to tetanic stimulation suggests pathologic reflexes and would warrant cutting of the rootlet, whereas a grade 0 would definitely warrant sparing. Clinical judgment of the surgeon in conjunction with the observations of the monitoring team still remains paramount, however.

Table 8.1 The EMG classification of responses during electrophysiological monitoring [4, 12]

Grade	Response
0	Non-sustained or single discharge to a train of stimuli
1+	Sustained discharges from muscles innervated through the segment stimulated in the ipsilateral lower extremity
2+	Sustained discharges from muscles innervated through the stimulated and immediately adjacent segments
3+	Sustained discharges from segmentally innervated muscles and muscles innervated through segments distant from the one stimulated
4+	Sustained discharges from contralateral muscles with or without sustained discharges from the ipsilateral muscles

8.3.6 Sectioning the Rootlets

The rootlets with abnormal responses (grades 3 and 4) are sectioned, attempting to preserve at least 1/3 of each posterior root (Fig. 8.6). This process is conducted from L2 to S2 and then repeated on the other side. In terms of the extent of dorsal root sectioning, the most rootlets are cut at L2, L3, L5, and S1, with a target of 65%. It is notable that there is disagreement on this point, with some surgeons targeting a 50% dorsal root sectioning. While we cut 50–65% of L4 roots, others would aim to cut 25–50% with a rationale to preserve more of knee extension. While we do not cut S2 routinely, others might reasonably advise cutting 25–50%, but those surgeons will acknowledge that might slightly increase the risk of causing bladder dysfunction in the continent child. A detailed clinical examination not only rules out the associated movement disorders (i.e., dystonia and athetosis) that SDR will unmask but also allows clear identification of the most problematic muscle groups in terms of spasticity: quadriceps, tibialis anterior, hamstring, gastrocnemius, tibialis posterior, or combinations thereof. Specific weakness, degree of spasticity, reflexes, and other upper motor neuron signs of particular muscle groups that have been appreciated during the clinical examination can inform surgical decision-making. In order to address certain more problematic patterns of spasticity, for example, certain root levels may be the target of more sectioning, and the percentages of sectioned rootlets can be modified (Table 8.2) [13]. The percentage of rootlets that have been cut and the major intraoperative electrophysiological monitoring results are recorded in a sample table (Table 8.3).

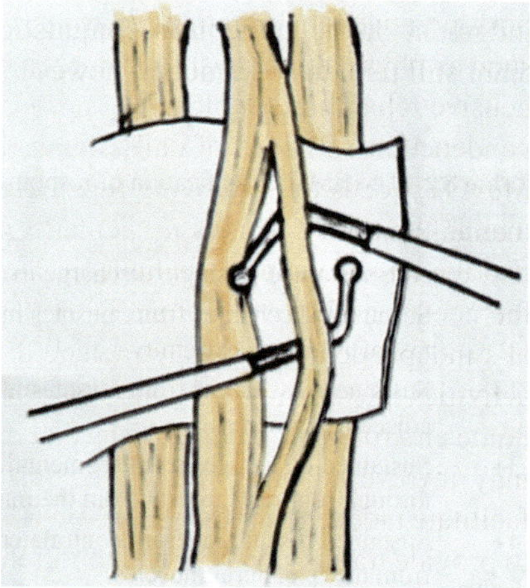

Fig. 8.6 The dorsal root of interest is placed on top of the silastic sheet and is further subdivided into rootlets of which a certain percentage is sectioned after electrophysiological stimulation

Table 8.2 Planning form for percentage of rootlets to be sectioned alongside the muscles involved and nerve roots to be targeted according to clinical pattern for spasticity in the lower limbs [13]

Clinical pattern	Muscle(s) involved	Nerve	Roots of origin	Sectioning quantification
Flexed hip	Iliopsoas	Branch from lumbar plexus	L2–L3	
	Rectus femoris	Femoral	L3–L4	
Adducted thigh	Adductors (longus brevis, magnus), gracilis, obturator externus, pectineus)	Obturator	L2–L3	
Extended knee	Quadriceps (rectus femoris, vastus intermedius, vastus medialis, vastus lateralis)	Femoral	L3–L4	
Flexed knee	Hamstring (biceps femoris, semitendinosus, semimembranosus)	Sciatic	L5–S2	
Equinus of foot	Gastrocnemius, soleus, popliteal	Tibial	S1	
Varus of foot	Tibialis posterior			
Claw toes	Flexor digitorum longus and brevis	Tibial	S1–S2	
Hitchhiker's great toe	Extensor hallucis longus	Peroneal	L4–L5	

8.3.7 Closure and Complications

Following the satisfactory transection of the expected percentage of rootlets per level on either side, the intradural space is irrigated with saline solution. Hemostasis is ensured, and the dura is closed in a watertight manner with running stitches using nylon 4–0 suture. The lumbodorsal fascia and muscles as well as the skin are then closed in the usual fashion.

The limited removal of the spinal posterior elements in this version of the SDR focused on the conus is thought to be better than multilevel bony exposures in terms of specific complications, namely, postoperative spinal deformity including scoliosis [8, 9]. It must be noted, however, that even without surgery, spastic cerebral palsy results in spinal deformity in the majority of cases due to its natural history. Also, limited data exist with regards to head-to-head comparison of the various exposure techniques in terms of complications, although a retrospective study comparing conus-level versus cauda equina-level exposures showed that similar short-term outcomes except in ankle kinematics at follow-up. The cauda group exhibited a large improvement toward dorsiflexion, while there was residual equinus in the conus group despite Ashworth Scale scores normalizing equally in both groups [14]. Other major but rare complications of SDR include paraplegia, sensory loss, bladder and bowel incontinence, CSF leakage, and infection [4].

Table 8.3 Sample form for the record of electrophysiological monitoring results and the percentage of rootlets

Left						Right					
Root	Threshold	Rating	Response	C/S	% Cut	Root	Threshold	Rating	Response	C/S	% Cut
S1						S1					
Rootlet 1						Rootlet 1					
Rootlet 2						Rootlet 2					
Rootlet 3						Rootlet 3					
Rootlet 4						Rootlet 4					
Rootlet 5						Rootlet 5					
Rootlet 6						Rootlet 6					
L5						L5					
Rootlet 1						Rootlet 1					
Rootlet 2						Rootlet 2					
Rootlet 3						Rootlet 3					
Rootlet 4						Rootlet 4					
Rootlet 5						Rootlet 5					
Rootlet 6						Rootlet 6					
L4						L4					
Rootlet 1						Rootlet 1					
Rootlet 2						Rootlet 2					
Rootlet 3						Rootlet 3					
Rootlet 4						Rootlet 4					
Rootlet 5						Rootlet 5					
Rootlet 6						Rootlet 6					
L3						L3					
Rootlet 1						Rootlet 1					
Rootlet 2						Rootlet 2					
Rootlet 3						Rootlet 3					

Rootlet 4						Rootlet 4					
Rootlet 5						Rootlet 5					
Rootlet 6						Rootlet 6					
L2						L2					
Rootlet 1						Rootlet 1					
Rootlet 2						Rootlet 2					
Rootlet 3						Rootlet 3					
Rootlet 4						Rootlet 4					
Rootlet 5						Rootlet 5					
Rootlet 6						Rootlet 6					

Response: incremental/decremental/clonic/flat. Rating scale: 1, one muscle; 2, adjacent muscles; 3, entire leg; 4, bilateral spread

8.3.8 Beyond Electrophysiological Monitoring

Variation in electrophysiological monitoring exists among different neurosurgical centers [15]. From the experience at the British Columbia Children's Hospital, Steinbok and colleagues described three "phases" to reflect the spectrum of differentially weighted electrophysiological guidance being considered during the decision to transect the rootlets [16]. In Phase 1, the initial electrophysiological criteria used to define a transectable dorsal nerve rootlet included the following: (1) a low threshold to a single stimulus, (2) a sustained response to a 50-Hz tetanic stimulus, and (3) diffusion of the response to muscle groups not involved in the rootlet's segmental distribution. These criteria later on evolved into Phase 2, where there was a conscious effort to save more of the L3 and L4 nerve roots in the hope of preserving quadriceps strength that is often lost in the first few weeks postoperatively. In Phase 3, the culminating criterion was the extent of response spread to the contralateral lower limb muscles and to the muscles of the upper limb, neck, and face. The presence of a sustained response to 50-Hz stimulation and the threshold at which the response occurred were purposely ignored. There remains a deliberate effort to spare more of the L3 and L4 nerve roots. While shifting through the three phases, the percentage of dorsal rootlets being transected decreased to an average of 52% from a previous average of 66%. Despite cutting less, however, spasticity was reduced significantly, and in terms of outcomes such as the increase in range of lower limb movement and functional improvement, there were no statistically significant differences among the three phases.

Building on from this experience, Steinbok and colleagues later published a series of patients who underwent dorsal rhizotomy with no electrophysiological guidance in comparison with historical controls who had SDR with intraoperative monitoring [17]. They found that at 1 year after rhizotomy, there were no differences between the two groups in the incidence of complications or outcome measures. In a quite similar manner of execution in a resource-scarce environment, Warf and colleagues showed that a partial dorsal rhizotomy technique without neurophysiological monitoring may equally result in beneficial outcomes [18]. On the other end of the spectrum, nonselective dorsal–ventral rhizotomy for the management of hypertonia is a palliative option for nonambulatory children with mixed hypertonia–dystonia or severe cerebral palsy [19].

8.4 Conclusion

Rhizotomy by means of either predetermined partial dorsal transection or selective with the aid of electrophysiological guidance remains a durable cornerstone in the surgical management of childhood spasticity. Often, a single-level laminectomy will suffice for adequate operative field exposure, and ultrasonography can aid in finding the conus medullaris. The separation of the dorsal roots from their ventral counterparts is the most important step. This is ensured by identification of the L2 root neural foramina and the cleft corresponding to the DREZ. The more intertwined S3–S5 roots are always left intact. Following subdividing the dorsal roots into rootlets, a certain percentage of the rootlets of interest are sectioned depending on correlative findings from the preoperative clinical examination and intraoperative electrophysiological monitoring. Intraoperative physiological neuromonitoring provides real-time feedback and aids surgical decision-making, but it cannot entirely supplant a robust preoperative plan of rootlet transection that is based on good clinical judgment and solid clinical examination. Therefore, the lack of neuromonitoring capabilities should not preclude the adoption of SDR even in resource-challenged settings.

References

1. Brandenburg JE, Rabatin AE, Driscoll SW. Spasticity interventions. Pediatr Clin N Am. 2023;70(3):483–500. https://doi.org/10.1016/j.pcl.2023.01.005.
2. Enslin JMN, Langerak NG, Fieggen AG. The evolution of selective dorsal rhizotomy for the management of spasticity. Neurotherapeutics. 2019;16(1):3–8. https://doi.org/10.1007/s13311-018-00690-4.
3. Park TS, Gaffney PE, Kaufman BA, Molleston MC. Selective lumbosacral dorsal rhizotomy immediately caudal to the conus medullaris for cerebral palsy spasticity. Neurosurgery. 1993;33(5):929.
4. Park TS, Johnston JM. Surgical techniques of selective dorsal rhizotomy for spastic cerebral palsy. Neurosurg Focus. 2006;21 https://doi.org/10.3171/foc.2006.21.2.8.
5. Warsi NM, Tailor J, Coulter IC, et al. Selective dorsal rhizotomy: an illustrated review of operative techniques. J Neurosurg Pediatr. 2020;25(5):540–7. https://doi.org/10.3171/2019.12.PEDS19629.
6. Barolat G. Dorsal selective rhizotomy through a limited exposure of the cauda equina at L-1. J Neurosurg Pediatr. 1991;75(5):804–7. https://doi.org/10.3171/jns.1991.75.5.0804.
7. Bales J, Apkon S, Osorio M, et al. Infra-conus single-level laminectomy for selective dorsal rhizotomy: technical advance. Pediatr Neurosurg. 2016;51(6):284–91. https://doi.org/10.1159/000448046.
8. Steinbok P, Schrag C. Complications after selective posterior rhizotomy for spasticity in children with cerebral palsy. Pediatr Neurosurg. 1998;28(6):300–13. https://doi.org/10.1159/000028668.
9. Steinbok P, Hicdonmez T, Sawatzky B, Beauchamp R, Wickenheiser D. Spinal deformities after selective dorsal rhizotomy for spastic cerebral palsy. J Neurosurg Pediatr. 2005;102(4):363–73. https://doi.org/10.3171/ped.2005.102.4.0363.
10. Turner RP. Neurophysiologic intraoperative monitoring during selective dorsal rhizotomy. J Clin Neurophysiol. 2009;26(2):82. https://doi.org/10.1097/WNP.0b013e31819f9077.
11. Marrone CD, Bedin A, Hoppe AM, D'Aviz CS, Bizzi JWJ. Selective dorsal rhizotomy and intraoperative neurophysiological monitoring: theory to practice. In: Verst SM, Barros MR, Maldaun MVC, editors. Intraoperative monitoring: neurophysiology and surgical approaches. Springer International Publishing; 2022. p. 565–85. https://doi.org/10.1007/978-3-030-95730-8_26.
12. Phillips LH II, Park TS. Electrophysiologic studies of selective posterior rhizotomy patients. In: Park TS, editor. Management of spasticity in cerebral palsy and spinal cord injury. Philadelphia: Hanley & Belfus; 1989. p. 459–70.

13. Sindou M, Georgoulis G, Mertens P, editors. Neurosurgery for spasticity: a practical guide for treating children and adults. Springer International Publishing; 2014. p. 243.
14. Duffy EA, Hornung AL, Chen BPJ, Munger ME, Aldahondo N, Krach LE, Novacheck TF, Schwartz MH. Comparing short-term outcomes between conus medullaris and cauda equina surgical techniques of selective dorsal rhizotomy. Dev Med Child Neurol. 2020;63(3):336–42. https://doi.org/10.1111/dmcn.14716.
15. Steinbok P, Kestle JR. Variation between centers in electrophysiologic techniques used in lumbosacral selective dorsal rhizotomy for spastic cerebral palsy. Pediatr Neurosurg. 2008;25(5):233–9. https://doi.org/10.1159/000121131.
16. Steinbok P, Gustavsson B, Kestle JRW, Reiner A, Cochrane DD. Relationship of intraoperative electrophysiological criteria to outcome after selective functional posterior rhizotomy. J Neurosurg. 1995;83(1):18–26. https://doi.org/10.3171/jns.1995.83.1.0018.
17. Steinbok P, Tidemann AJ, Miller S, Mortenson P, Bowen-Roberts T. Electrophysiologically guided versus non-electrophysiologically guided selective dorsal rhizotomy for spastic cerebral palsy: a comparison of outcomes. Childs Nerv Syst. 2009;25(9):1091–6. https://doi.org/10.1007/s00381-009-0908-5.
18. Sacco DJ, Tylkowski CM, Warf BC. nonselective partial dorsal rhizotomy: a clinical experience with 1-year follow-up. Pediatr Neurosurg. 2000;32(3):114–8. https://doi.org/10.1159/000028914.
19. Abdelmageed S, Dalmage M, Mossner JM, Trierweiler R, Krater T, Raskin JS. Nonselective lumbosacral ventral-dorsal rhizotomy for the management of lower-limb hypertonia in nonambulatory children with cerebral palsy. Neurosurg Focus. 2024;1:E9. https://doi.org/10.3171/2024.3.FOCUS2472.

Chapter 9
Cauda Equina-Level Selective Dorsal Rhizotomy

J. M. N. Enslin

9.1 Introduction

Surgery for spasticity has a long, illustrious history from the late 1800s when people like Abbe and Bennet started sectioning sensory nerve rootlets to treat pain and spasticity [1]. Foerster started performing dorsal rhizotomies for spasticity in 1913. This was followed by Gros in 1960 when he began partially sectioning dorsal roots. In 1976, Fasano and colleagues described the use of electrical stimulation of these dorsal roots to define sectioning landmarks [1].

Today, two leading schools of thought regarding surgical approach and level of surgery are colloquially known as the "Peacock method" and the "Park method" [1]. These two surgeons were not the first to develop their respective approaches, but they are the modern faces and doyens of modern selective dorsal rhizotomy (SDR). For clarity and to better describe the difference between these two approaches, it is better to describe it as a *cauda equina approach* ("Peacock approach") and a *conus medullaris approach* ("Park approach") [1]. In the cauda equina-level approach, the surgeon performs a laminotomy (initially, they performed laminectomy) to allow exposure of the nerve roots from L2 to S2, where they exit the neural foramina. It is, therefore, an approach that relies on identifying the exiting nerve and, thereby, its corresponding innervation level (e.g., L5 nerve root exits between L5 and S1). In the conus approach, the surgeon performs a laminotomy, or laminectomy, over the thoracolumbar junction (usually T10–T12 and commonly uses some form of imaging,

J. M. N. Enslin (✉)
Division of Neurosurgery, Groote Schuur Hospital, University of Cape Town, Observatory, Cape Town, South Africa

Red Cross War Memorial Children's Hospital, Rondebosch, Cape Town, South Africa

Neuroscience Institute, University of Cape Town, Observatory, Cape Town, South Africa
e-mail: johannes.enslin@uct.ac.za

N. Morota, P. Steinbok (eds.), *Dorsal Rhizotomy: Neurosurgery for Childhood Spasticity*, Advances and Technical Standards in Neurosurgery 51,
https://doi.org/10.1007/978-3-031-86441-4_9

e.g., ultrasound, to determine this level) to allow exposure and identification of the nerve roots at the point where they originate from the spinal cord. Usually, this also allows for easy separation between dorsal and ventral roots before they join into one nerve bundle.

In the early 1900s, Foerster started performing the first documented rhizotomies [1], in which he performed complete sectioning of the dorsal root from the T12 level to the S2 level, with the sparing of the L4 root [2, 3]. At this early stage, he had already used basic electrophysiological techniques to differentiate the afferent from the efferent root [4]. However, many complications have been reported with this technique. The most common were problematic sensory denervation in the legs, urinary problems, loss of proprioception, and skin trophic changes [3, 5, 6]. As a result, the technique was used infrequently. The group in Montpellier, under the lead of Gros, revived it with the refining of the technique by sectioning a part of the dorsal root only (four-fifths reportedly) [6, 7]. Gros and colleagues also used a conus approach from T11 to L1 via a laminectomy [3]. Some patients undergoing this technique, however, still had postoperative spasticity remaining, and there were concerns about unpredictable weakness after surgery [6]. During the procedure, this team also started using electromyography (EMG) to identify the rootlets that contribute mainly to normal postural control and gait so that they could be spared [3]. The rest was sectioned [3]. This was the first attempt at being more selective in the rhizotomy procedure by selectively sparing some fascicles identified on EMG to be of functional gait and postural importance [1, 3]. The group of Gros paid significant attention to their clinical evaluation preoperatively. Also, they used a physiotherapist intraoperatively to help identify the muscle and rootlet/fascicle combinations to be sectioned or spared [3]. Each rhizotomy was individualized in this manner. Fasano and his colleagues published a more detailed study on the use of intraoperative electrophysiology during their rhizotomy procedures, and this further developed the selectivity of their selective dorsal rhizotomy method [8, 9]. These principles were then adopted by Gross and later Sindou, as well as most other surgeons that followed.

Until this point (late 1970s), all the above surgeons performed a conus-level approach [1, 10]. Warwick Peacock was concerned about the bladder and bowel complications reported by the predecessors [11]. Attempts at reducing this risk led him to emphasize the correct nerve root level by observing the exiting nerve root at the cauda equina level. In doing this, he maintained that he could better ensure safety for the lower sacral nerve roots and avoid bladder and bowel complications [11]. This necessitated a long-segment laminectomy (L2–L5 level) [11]. So, the cauda equina level SDR was described [1].

9.2 The Technique

The patient is positioned prone on bolsters underneath the shoulders and hips, keeping the abdomen free and preventing pressure on the bony prominences and face. The subdermal needle electrodes are placed into the muscles that will be monitored during the operation (Table 9.1).

At the same time, we also monitor the following sensory evoked potentials: N medianus and N posterior tibialis. Figure 9.1 shows the intraoperative theatre setup, position, and incision marking on the lower back.

The author makes a skin incision in the midline from the L1 to S2 level, and subperiosteal dissection is performed to preserve the muscle fascia as much as possible. I aim to keep the supraspinous ligament intact and then perform a laminotomy with the high-speed drill from S1 to L2 levels on both sides while paying meticulous attention to remain medial to the facet joints and capsule as well as not injuring the thecal sac (see Fig. 9.2). The laminotomy is kept attached at the rostral end, and the ligaments between L1 and L2 are not sectioned (see Fig. 9.2b). I then reflect the laminotomy rostrally like a "lobster tail" (see Fig. 9.3). Careful hemostasis is obtained with bone wax on the bony edges and Surgicel™ strips into the lateral gutters. A midline durotomy is then performed—usually in two stages—with the arachnoid preserved initially to prevent nerve root herniation during opening and restrict intradural blood. Careful hitching is done to the dural edges, and hemostasis is ensured.

A stepwise nerve mapping protocol is then followed (Table 9.2).

There are multiple methods used to confirm dorsal vs. ventral root at the exit foramen:

- The ventral root is often more irritable and may cause muscle contraction when manipulated.
- The ventral root is often more reddish when compared to the dorsal root.
- There is most often one large motor root (ventral) and two smaller dorsal roots.
- The ventral root is situated most ventral in the foramen and is separated from the dorsal roots by an evident sulcus that is easily seen under magnification (Fig. 9.4).

Table 9.1 Muscles that are monitored with electromyography during the procedure (both sides are constantly monitored)

M abductor pollicis brevis
M vastus medialis
M vastus lateralis
M adductor magnus
M hamstrings (M semimembranosis)
M gastrocnemius
M soleus
M tibialis anterior
M adductor hallucis
Anal sphincter

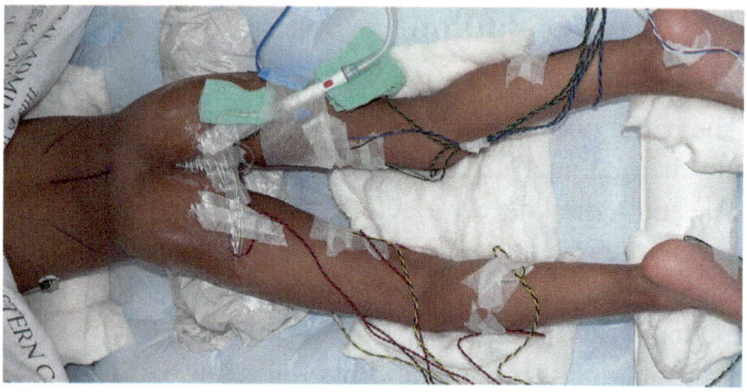

Fig. 9.1 The patient is prone, and subdermal needle electrodes are placed in the muscle groups to be monitored during surgery. The skin incision markings are also shown

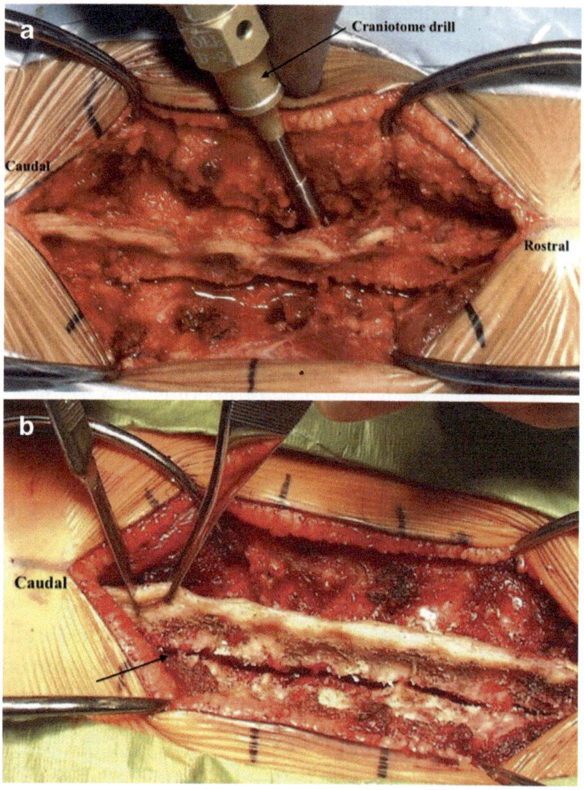

Fig. 9.2 (**a**) Intraoperative photograph where the craniotome drill is used to perform a laminotomy from L2 to S1 level in the patient. (Credit Steinbok, P, personal intraoperative image, used with permission). (**b**) Intraoperative photograph after craniotome drill was used to perform laminotomy from L2 to S1 on both sides. The caudal supraspinous ligament are sectioned, prior to rostral reflection of the laminotomy "flap." The black arrow shows the right side laminotomy sectioning line. (Credit Steinbok, P, personal intraoperative image. Used with permission)

- Electrical stimulation shows a clear difference between ventral roots and dorsal roots:
  - Ventral/motor = Shorter latency and higher amplitude at 0.1 mA direct stimulation
  - Dorsal/sensory = Longer latency and lower amplitude at 0.1 mA direct stimulation

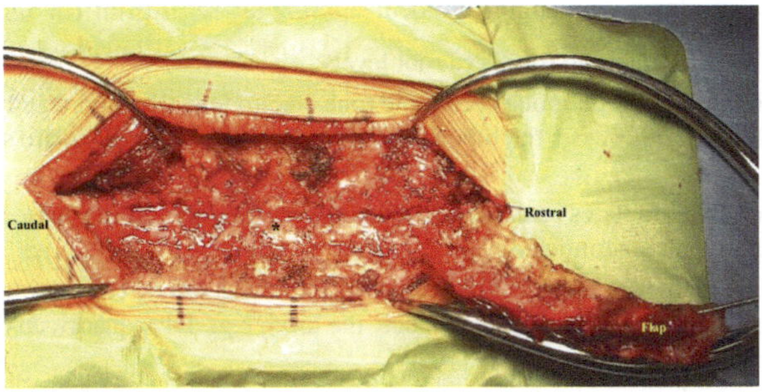

Fig. 9.3 Intraoperative picture where the laminotomy is kept attached at the rostral end and reflected as a "lobster tail." Rostral and caudal ends labelled, and * identifies thecal sac and epidural fat exposed. (Credit Steinbok, P, personal intraoperative image. Used with permission)

In our unit, we have never included S2 in the dorsal rhizotomy out of fear of injury to the pudendal plexus [1, 11]. However, there is a chance that the patient does not have adequate spasticity release in S2 contribution to the triceps surae muscles and may, therefore, remain toe walking. Abbott and colleagues have described their technique of preserving the pudendal plexus using specific bulbocavernosis mapping techniques to circumvent this problem [12]. I prefer to limit my SDR to L2–S1. I will add a selective peripheral neurotomy a few months later, if needed, in which I can then specifically target the offending muscle that remains spastic post-SDR. I can individualize the procedure much more in this manner.

The details around selecting fascicles for sectioning will be discussed in a separate chapter of this book, but here are the main principles that we use.

In general, all our neurophysiological monitoring is based on four goals:

- Confirming the nerve root level and muscles, therefore, innervated by the specific root
- Confirming dorsal and ventral roots
- Identifying the nerve root dorsal fascicles that seem to contribute mainly to the abnormal physiological responses in a specific muscle
- Confirming sufficient inhibition of the abnormal reflex activity by the sectioned number or percentage of the dorsal root.

The "abnormal dorsal fascicles" are identified using most of Fasano's principles [13, 14]. The dorsal root is separated into four to five fascicles, as described above, and each is stimulated separately (I use 0.5 mA current to do this stimulation initially). Regular dorsal nerve fascicle stimulation has a specific latency and amplitude of the CMAP that is recorded. There is a predictable pattern of muscle activation and limited spread to other muscles, which is to be expected. Abnormal spread on electrical stimulation is an indication to cut a specific fascicle. An example is M abductor hallucis activity with L2 nerve root stimulation, or if there is clonus elicited or spread to the contralateral limb or upper limbs, or there is an abnormal brisk or violent clinical contraction of the muscle or joint palpated or seen under the surgical drapes. All of these will be abnormal responces to stimulation of an L2

Table 9.2 Stepwise nerve root mapping protocol

1. Electrophysiological mapping for nerve root levels:
(a) If available, the dual monopolar technique (one electrode is the anode, and the other is the cathode) is used; otherwise, the bipolar technique is used. Train of square stimuli at 50 Hz is used
(b) 0.1 mA current stimulates each nerve root at its exit foramen. At the start, X-ray screening confirms the exact anatomical level
(c) Each visible nerve root is then stimulated (whole bundle—dorsal and ventral root) to confirm the muscles innervated and, hence, the level, e.g., L4 = quadriceps and M tibialis anterior
(d) The level of each root is confirmed by a combination of the direct visualization of the exiting nerve, the initial X-ray screening level, and the corresponding muscle involved (myotome)
2. Confirm left side vs. right side (especially the lower nerve roots in the midline, which may easily be confused at this level)
(a) The above mapping technique and EMG are monitored to confirm the sides.
Once the above is confirmed, I label the nerve roots with silastic vessel loops and proceed with the surgery
3. It is my habit to start with the S1 nerve root on the right-hand side
(a) Microsurgical separation of the dorsal root from the ventral root at the exit foramen level (Fig. 9.4, b)
(b) Electrical stimulation at 0.1 mA to confirm motor vs. sensory roots
(c) Clearly label the ventral root with a vessel loop, and protect it throughout the surgery (Fig. 9.5)
(d) Stimulate the dorsal roots at 0.1 mA also to confirm their sensory nature
(e) The operation then focuses on these dorsal rootlets only
(f)I then typically split the dorsal root into three to four bundles
(g) Each of these dorsal bundles is then stimulated at 0.5 mA, and the compound muscle action potential (CMAP) is recorded and compared to the clinical response to stimulation
4. A decision is then made on what percentage of these bundles/fascicles should be sectioned
(a) This decision is based on:
(i) The preoperative clinical assessment and plan
(ii) Electrophysiological response
(iii) Clinical muscle response
(iv) Preoperative – and intraoperative – decisions on which muscles to preserve
(b) Typically, I would section 50–75% of the dorsal root at a specific level, but it may also be only 30%, and sometimes, I decide to avoid sectioning entirely at a particular level, based on the above assessment
(c) I section the dorsal fascicle and resect a 5 mm piece, and then, bipolar cauterize the sectioned ends of all sectioned fascicles
5. I typically do a proximal-to-section stimulation, as well as a distal-to-sectioning stimulation to confirm adequate suppression of the abnormal hyperactivity – both clinical and electrophysiological
6. This process is repeated for L5–L2 on the right, and then, I do the same on the left side from S1 to L2

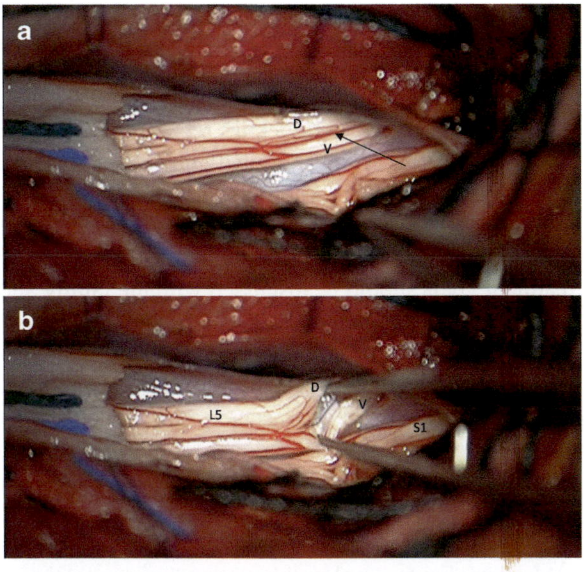

Fig. 9.4 (**a**) Microsurgical dissection is performed, and the dorsal root is separated from the ventral root. This is the L5 nerve root at the exit foramen. D is the dorsal root, and V is the ventral root. The black arrow indicated the sulcus between the ventral and dorsal roots close to the exit foramen. (**b**) Microsurgical dissection is performed, and the dorsal root is separated from the ventral root. This is the L5 nerve root at the exit foramen. D is the dorsal root, and V is the ventral root

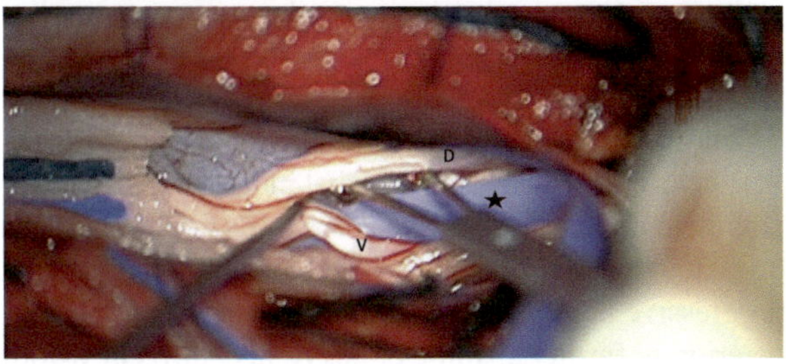

Fig. 9.5 The ventral root is clearly separated from the dorsal root (D), and a silastic vessel loop (black star) is used to label the ventral root (V) and protect it throughout

fascicle, and this fascicle should be sectioned. I also make clinical decisions preoperatively, where I will decide, for example, to preserve quadriceps power but reduce adductor spasticity more selectively, if possible. During the procedure on the L3 nerve root, I will then split the dorsal root and its fascicles and stimulate each, as above. I will then section the fascicle that causes hip adductor muscle contraction (CMAP) but spare the fascicles where the quadriceps are involved.

After surgery, we rinse the thecal sac and confirm that all blood clots and inflammatory cytokines are rinsed out. Thorough rinsing lessens the rate of post-SDR fever in most children. We then perform a watertight dural closure and place a collagen sponge onlay graft. I then reposition the laminotomy and use nonabsorbable sutures to secure the laminoplasty back in place. Leaving the rostral end attached throughout the surgery prevents a typical subsidence that creates a step deformity if one does not do this. We have never used any form of bracing postoperatively, and our long-term results support this practice of not bracing after SDR [15].

We then perform a multilayered and subcuticular skin closure and apply a pressure dressing. Our patients are kept flat in bed and prone/side-lying only, for 5 days, before mobilizing out of bed.

9.3 Selection Process

Previous publications have examined the selection criteria used in children before SDR [16–18]. The basic principles remain the same throughout: In children, where walking is the goal, good antigravity power and the ability to kneel (stand on knees) and bridge (lift buttocks when supine) is essential. In children who are not walking, SDR may also be beneficial in improving seated positioning, nursing care, and better sleeping position and preventing hip problems in the future. In these patients, treatment goals should be discussed with the family and rehab team before surgery.

In my practice, I prefer to see children more than once over a few years and rely on physical therapists, neurologists, parents, and their videos to select surgery cases. I use selective injection with targeted Botox into selected muscle groups to help decision-making. I will, for instance, inject the hip adductors selectively with Botox and evaluate the effect on functional gait in a walking child (GMFCS 2). This allows me to assess what the contribution of adductor spasticity is to the standing posture of an individual spastic diplegic child. In this manner, we can form a biomechanical image of each child before we selectively target spasticity with SDR. The use of IOM allows us to employ this targeted and selective approach during the surgery and, in so doing, individualizing the surgery to each patient. Individualized treatment and surgery are of the utmost importance for patients with function-impairing spasticity.

Through the last 43 years of following up with patients operated by Warwick Peacock, we have also learned that motivated children and driven parents, with good cognitive abilities and easy access to postoperative rehabilitation, are the ones who do best in the long run after SDR. Care should also be taken to evaluate patients for progressive neurological conditions. These patients may benefit in the short run but deteriorate further at some point. Hence, diligent workup and more extended evaluation periods are needed. This also underscores the need to be slow to decide when to operate. We think the ideal age is around 5–8 years old. Younger than this may not allow the children who may still improve and get stronger to improve, and progressive conditions may be missed. In children older than 10 years, the gait pattern is often so ingrained that they benefit less from SDR, although there are many units with good experience in doing SDR in older patients. We will have to see how they perform in the long run. In our series, these older patients often did not do as well in the long term.

9.4 Outcomes with the Cauda Equina Technique of SDR

The group in Cape Town, mainly under Langerak's research lead, has been prospectively following up on patients who underwent SDR with this cauda equina technique (all done by Warwick Peacock) since 1980. Various publications have reported on this, the most extended follow-up series in the world [19–24]. This group is currently reviewing the 40-year follow-up outcomes.

In summary, over 35 years, patients have shown gait stability and improvement in gait after SDR [21–23]. They also remain in the same GMFCS category as the one to which they improved after SDR [19, 20]. Most patients had no loss of function and no spinal deformity [15, 24] or long-term complications reported in this cohort [19, 20].

Selective dorsal rhizotomy, using the cauda equina exposure technique, is safe and effective in improving functional outcomes in children with cerebral palsy and function-impairing spasticity over the long term.

9.5 Conclusion

Selective dorsal rhizotomy, using the cauda equina approach (as described by Peacock in 1980), is a safe and effective technique in managing children with cerebral palsy in whom spasticity impairs their function. Careful selection and emphasis on postoperative rehabilitation are essential, impacting success and expectations. The benefit of this approach is that the surgeon can verify the nerve root operated on, the fascicles can easily be separated, and selective electrophysiological mapping and sectioning is possible. In this way, the risk of pudendal plexus injury and errors in sectioning can be avoided.

It is essential, however, to remind the family and patients that surgery for spasticity is not curative. There is no magic bullet, and we can only aid in a selective, permanent reduction in spasticity. If we choose the targeted muscles carefully, we can help with functional improvement and long-term stability of this improvement in our patients.

References

1. Enslin JMN, Langerak NG, Fieggen AG. The evolution of selective dorsal rhizotomy for the management of spasticity. Neurotherapeutics. 2019;16:3–8. https://doi.org/10.1007/s13311-018-00690-4.
2. Foerster O. Resection of the posterior spinal nerve-roots in the treatment of gastric crises and spastic paralysis. SAGE Publications; 1911.
3. Privat J, Benezech J, Frerebeau P, Gros C. Sectorial posterior rhizotomy, a new technique of surgical treatment for spasticity. Acta Neurochir. 1976;35:181–95.
4. Foerster O. On the indications and results of the excision of posterior spinal nerve roots in men. Surg Gynecol Obstet. 1913;16:463–75.
5. Gros C, Ouaknine G, Vlahovitch B, Frerebeau P. La radicotomie sélective postérieure dans le traitement neuro-chirurgical de lhypertonie pyramidale. Neurochirurgie. 1967;13:505–+.
6. Smyth MD, Peacock WJ. The surgical treatment of spasticity. Muscle Nerve. 2000;23:153–63.
7. Gros C. Spasticity – clinical classification and surgical treatment, advances and technical standards in neurosurgery. Springer; 1979. p. 55–97.

8. Fasano V, Broggi G, Barolat-Romana G, Sguazzi A. Surgical treatment of spasticity in cerebral palsy. Pediatr Neurosurg. 1978;4:289–305.
9. Fasano VA, Barolat-Romana G, Zeme S, Sguazzi A. Electrophysiological assessment of spinal circuits in spasticity by direct dorsal root stimulation. Neurosurgery. 1979;4:146–51.
10. Barolat G. Dorsal selective rhizotomy through a limited exposure of the cauda equina at L-1. J Neurosurg. 1991;75:804–7.
11. Peacock WJ, Staudt LA. Selective posterior rhizotomy: evolution of theory and practice. Pediatr Neurosurg. 1991;17:128–34.
12. Huang JC, Deletis V, Vodusek DB, Abbott R. Preservation of pudendal afferents in sacral rhizotomies. Neurosurgery. 1997;41(2):411–5. https://doi.org/10.1097/00006123-199708000-00015.
13. Fasano VA, Barolat-Romana G, Ivaldi A, Sguazzi A. La radicotomie postérieure fonctionnelle dans le traitement de la spasticité cérébrale Premieres observations sur la stimulation électrique peropératoire des racines postérieures, et leur utilisation dans le choix des racines ã sectionner [Functional posterior radiculotomy, in the treatment of cerebral spasticity. peroperative electric stimulation of posterior roots and its use in the choice of the roots to be sectioned]. Neurochirurgie. 1976;22(1):23–34.
14. Fasano VA, Broggi G, Zeme S. Intraoperative electrical stimulation for functional posterior rhizotomy. Scand J Rehabil Med Suppl. 1988;17:149–54.
15. Veerbeek BE, Lamberts RP, Fieggen AG, Mankahla N, de Villiers RVP, Botha E, Langerak NG. A long-term follow-up study of spinal abnormalities and pain in adults with cerebral palsy and spastic diplegia more than 25 years after selective dorsal rhizotomy. J Neurosurg Spine. 2020;34(2):228–35. https://doi.org/10.3171/2020.6.SPINE20751.
16. Grunt S, Fieggen AG, Vermeulen RJ, Becher JG, Langerak NG. Selection criteria for selective dorsal rhizotomy in children with spastic cerebral palsy: a systematic review of the literature. Dev Med Child Neurol. 2014;56(4):302–12.
17. Aquilina K, Graham D, Wimalasundera N. Selective dorsal rhizotomy: an old treatment re-emerging. Arch Dis Child. 2015;100(8):798–802.
18. Nicolini-Panisson RD, Tedesco AP, Folle MR, Donadio MV. Selective dorsal rhizotomy in cerebral palsy: selection criteria and post-operative physical therapy protocols. Rev Paul Pediatr. 2018;15(36):100–8.
19. Langerak NG, Lamberts RP, Fieggen AG, Peter JC, Peacock WJ, Vaughan CL. Selective dorsal rhizotomy: long-term experience from Cape Town. Childs Nerv Syst. 2007;23:1003–6.
20. Langerak NG, Vaughan CL, Peter JC, Fieggen AG, Peacock WJ. Long-term outcomes of dorsal rhizotomy. J Neurosurg Pediatr. 2013;12(6):664–5.
21. Langerak NG, Veerbeek BE, Fieggen AG, Lamberts RP. Gait status 26–35 years after selective dorsal rhizotomy: a 9 year follow up study. Gait Posture. 2022;1(91):284–9.
22. Langerak NG, Tam N, Vaughan CL, Fieggen AG, Schwartz MH. Gait status 17–26 years after selective dorsal rhizotomy. Gait Posture. 2012;35(2):244–9.
23. Langerak NG, Lamberts RP, Fieggen AG, Peter JC, van der Merwe L, Peacock WJ, Vaughan CL. A prospective gait analysis study in patients with diplegic cerebral palsy 20 years after selective dorsal rhizotomy. J Neurosurg Pediatr. 2008;1(3):180–6.
24. Langerak NG, Vaughan CL, Hoffman EB, Figaji AA, Fieggen AG, Peter JC. Incidence of spinal abnormalities in patients with spastic diplegia 17 to 26 years after selective dorsal rhizotomy. Childs Nerv Syst. 2009;25:1593–603.

Chapter 10
Rootlet Selection by Crescendo Single-Pulse Evoked Compound Muscle Action Potential Interpretation During Selective Dorsal Rhizotomy

Bo Xiao

The current understanding of the pathophysiological underpinnings of spasticity remains incomplete. It is hypothesized that α motor neurons, located in the anterior horn of the spinal cord, are primarily regulated through an integration of descending motor pathway inputs, local spinal circuitry, and sensory afferent feedback from muscle spindles, relayed through the spinal dorsal roots. The efferent signals from these α motor neurons are conveyed via spinal motor nerves to specific muscle groups, maintaining muscle tone vital for posture, stability, and prompt responses [1–3]. In children with spastic cerebral palsy (CP), impairments in descending inhibitory motor signals contrast with unaltered sensory feedback from the dorsal roots, leading to the overactivity of α motor neurons. This hyperactivity results in excessive efferent output to the respective muscles, culminating in heightened muscle tone and spasticity [3–6].

Selective dorsal rhizotomy (SDR) aims to alleviate this condition by selectively severing sensory nerve roots in the lumbar and sacral regions of the spinal cord, which are implicated in lower limb spasticity. This intervention reduces the excitation of α motor neurons, thereby diminishing muscle tone in affected muscle groups and ameliorating the spastic condition [7–14]. However, the irreversible nature of SDR poses a clinical challenge: accurately identifying the sensory dorsal roots that contribute to muscle spasm is critical (Fig. 10.1).

To address the pathogenesis of spasticity, our center has developed an innovative approach to select dorsal nerve roots for sectioning. By analyzing patterns of electromyographic activity (EMG) elicited in the lower limbs through electrical stimulation, we can identify roots that are more responsive to spastic triggers [15–17]. This method complements the traditional EMG response grading system by incorporating a crescendo single-pulse stimulation protocol to evoke compound muscle

B. Xiao (✉)
Shanghai Children's Medical Center, National Children' Medical Center, Shanghai, China

N. Morota, P. Steinbok (eds.), *Dorsal Rhizotomy: Neurosurgery for Childhood Spasticity*, Advances and Technical Standards in Neurosurgery 51,
https://doi.org/10.1007/978-3-031-86441-4_10

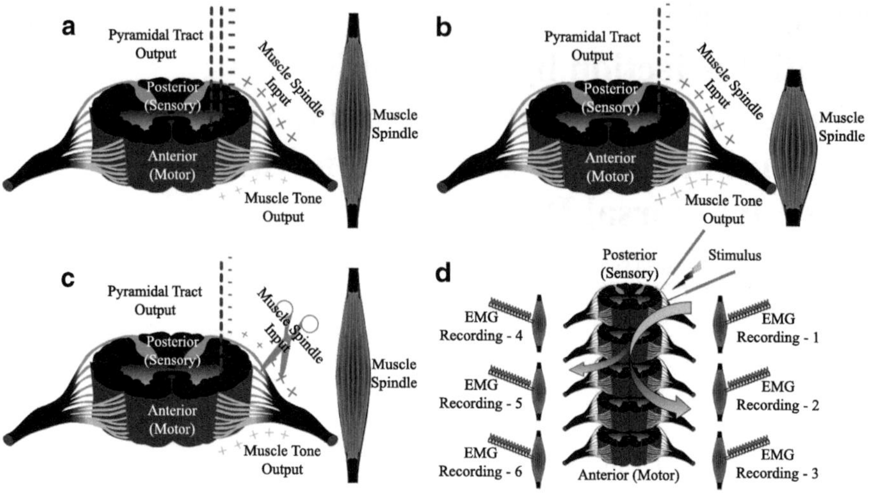

Fig. 10.1 Scheme of muscle tone modulation in the spinal cord and neurophysiological basis for selective dorsal rhizotomy for cases with spastic cerebral palsy. (**a**) Normal muscle tone maintenance. (**b**) Muscle tone increases in cases with spastic cerebral palsy when input via descending motor pathway to the spinal cord decreases. (**c**) Increased muscle tone decreases in cases with spastic cerebral palsy when partially cutting sensory nerve roots on which input from muscle spindles could trigger activation to those α motor neurons at the anterior horn in the spinal cord, causing them overactivated, which exert excessive innovations to the corresponding muscles, resulting into their spasticity. (**d**) Demonstrating EMG evoked and recorded in muscles being innovated by multiple segments of the spinal cord when electrically stimulation is given on one of those dorsal roots during selective dorsal rhizotomy

action potentials (CMAPs) in the monitored muscles. Dorsal roots are selected for cutting when stimulation induces a CMAP amplitude that reaches a predefined threshold (200 μV) first in muscles with a tone ≥ grade 2 on the Modified Ashworth Scale, as assessed preoperatively by our rehabilitation team (Fig. 10.2).

Clinical practice has demonstrated that SDR surgery, following this protocol, could be performed through a single-level approach and has the capability to effectively reduce muscle tone in targeted groups where spasticity is pronounced. Patients exhibited significant improvements in motor function following intensive postoperative rehabilitation. Furthermore, the protocol's built-in redundancy safeguards against potential complications, such as impairment of sphincter function, making surgical complications exceedingly rare [15–19].

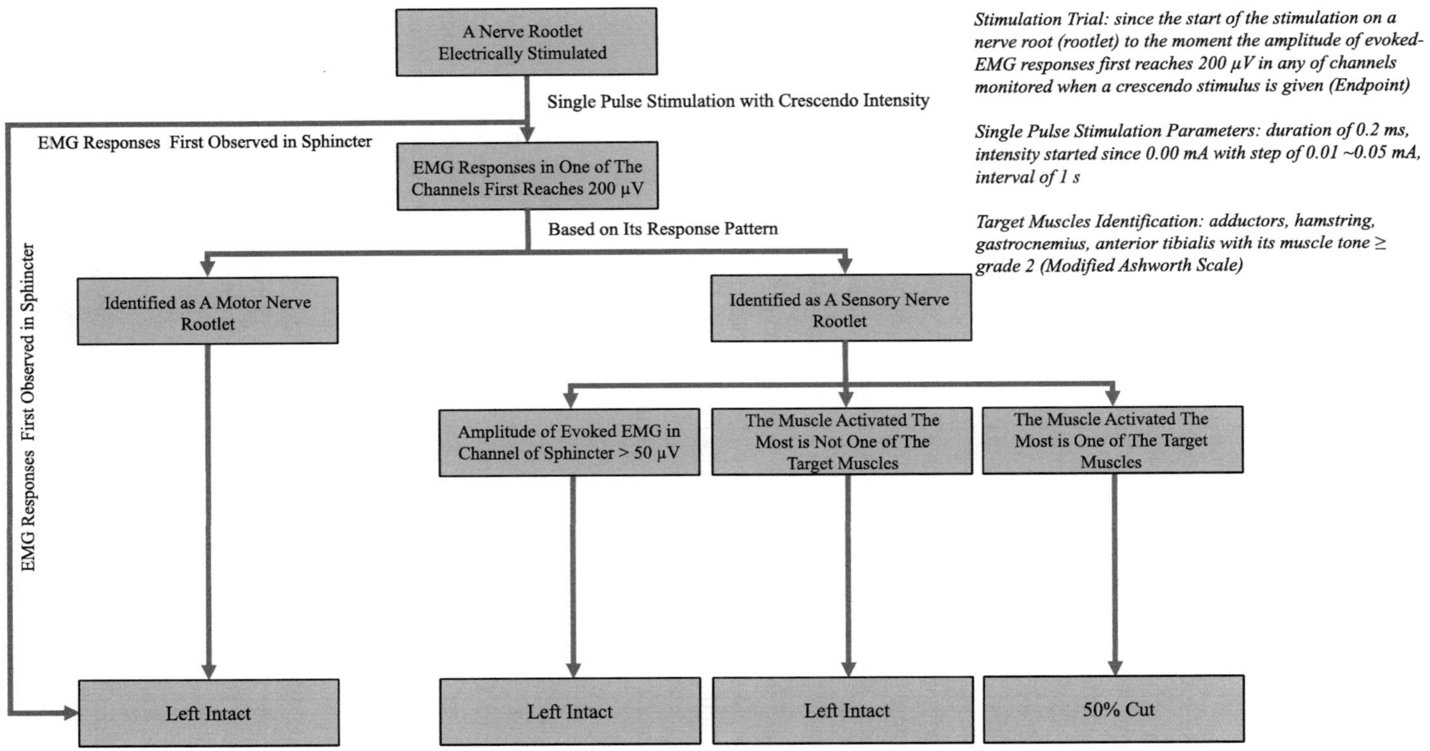

Fig. 10.2 Scheme of root selection in selective dorsal rhizotomy when being guided via EMG pattern interpretation evoked by crescendo single-pulse stimulation

10.1 Setup of Crescendo Single-Pulse Stimulation-Guided SDR

1. Preoperative Spastic Target Muscle Group Identification.

Recently, the accurate identification of dorsal nerve roots contributing to spasticity cannot rely solely on the interpretation of CMAP patterns during crescendo single-pulse stimulation, as per our protocol. Consequently, it is imperative to preoperatively delineate those lower limb muscle groups exhibiting pronounced spasticity as target muscles for the SDR procedure. This task is meticulously carried out by our rehabilitation team.

We employ the Modified Ashworth Scale (MAS) to evaluate muscle tone in patients. Major muscles in the lower extremities such as the adductors, hamstrings, gastrocnemius, soleus, and tibialis anterior are designated as target muscles when their tone is assessed to be grade 2 or higher. Muscles with tone below grade 2 are classified as nontarget muscle groups. Given the crucial weight-bearing role of the rectus femoris in standing and walking, it is typically not targeted for SDR in our practice, even if its tone meets or exceeds grade 2.

2. Intraoperative Neurophysiological Monitoring Channels.

The selection of muscles for intraoperative monitoring is aligned with the preoperative muscle tone assessment while also considering the practicality of monitoring. Our standard protocol includes monitoring 15 channels, which cover bilateral adductors, rectus femoris, hamstrings, tibialis anterior, medial and lateral gastrocnemius, peroneus longus, and the anal sphincter.

3. Intraoperative Neurophysiological Monitoring Setup.

For intraoperative monitoring, our facility utilizes the Cadwell Cascade Intraoperative Monitoring System (Cadwell Laboratories, Kennewick, WA) equipped with Cascade Software Version 3.1. The stimulation parameters are set as follows: a single-pulse stimulus with a pulse width of 0.2 ms; stimulation intensity begins at 0.00 mA and increases incrementally by 0.01–0.05 mA, with a maximum intensity of 5.00 mA. Stimuli are delivered at 1-s intervals.

The acquisition settings for the 15 monitoring channels are configured with a sweep of 10 ms, gain at 200 μV/Div, hi-cut filter at 3000 Hz, and lo-cut filter at 30 Hz. In the EMG thresholds setup, the threshold is set at 1 μV, with features like wave/beep upon threshold crossing, autocapture on threshold, and store on autocapture enabled. This setup is designed to capture comprehensive EMG data throughout the SDR procedure for subsequent analysis.

4. Surgical Approach.

The surgical procedure is conducted under general anesthesia. The patient is positioned prone with the head slightly inclined downward. Following sterile draping, an incision of about 4.0 cm is made at the L2 level. A single-level laminectomy is then performed to expose the cauda equina by opening the dura and arachnoid membranes. A Silastic sheet, approximately 0.5 cm in width, is placed around the nerve roots in the cauda equina, sparing those at the L2 level. This strategy allows neurophysiologists to differentiate neurophysiological characteristics between motor and sensory nerve roots through visual identification at the L2 intervertebral foramen. Understanding this distinction at the initial stage of the SDR procedure is essential, as the operation depends entirely on the interpretation of evoked EMG responses. Stimulation of the nerve roots at the L2 level—typically beginning on the right side for surgical convenience—helps establish the threshold range for motor and sensory nerve roots (Fig. 10.3).

5. Stimulation Protocol and Spinal Nerve Definitions.

The crescendo single-pulse stimulation protocol implemented at our center consists of continuous stimulation at 1-s intervals. Stimulation intensity starts at 0.00 mA and increases incrementally by 0.01 up to 0.20 mA, then by 0.01–0.05 mA thereafter, with a maximum intensity of 5.00 mA.

A complete stimulation trial is defined as the process following this protocol from 0.00 mA to the point where a stable evoked EMG amplitude greater than 200 μV is observed in any monitoring channel (endpoint).

Motor Nerve: A nerve is classified as a motor nerve if stimulating it evokes an EMG response greater than 200 μV in the corresponding muscle group at a stimulus current intensity below 0.2 mA, the EMG amplitude noticeably increases with an

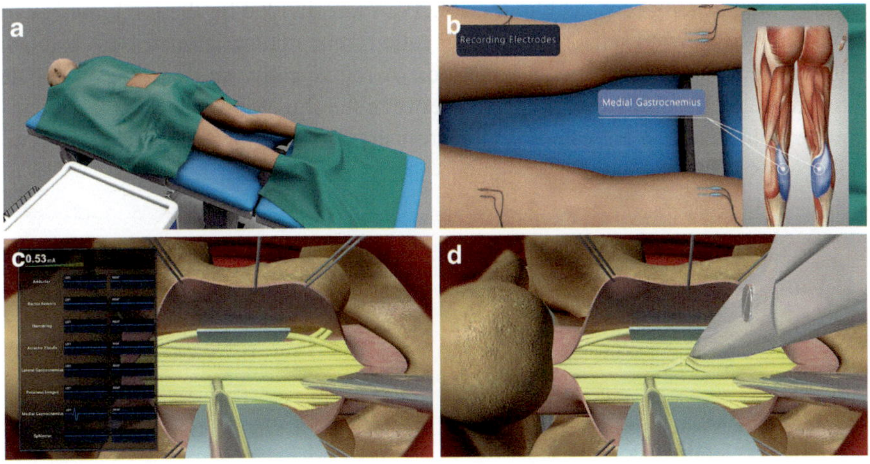

Fig. 10.3 Screenshots from 3D animation showing the main steps how selective dorsal rhizotomy via single-level laminectomy is conducted when evoked CMAP interpretation is applied to guide rootlet selection. (**a**) Patient positioning. (**b**) Fifteen channels are monitored, including the anal sphincter. (**c**) Root matches rhizotomy criteria when evoked EMG amplitude first stably reaches 200 μV in the channel monitoring muscle group with its muscle tone ≥ grade 2 (Modified Ashworth Scale), which has been marked as the target muscle before surgery. (**d**) The root (the same shown in (**c**) is cut for about 50%. CMAP, compound muscle action potential

additional 0.01 mA, and there is significant spread of the EMG activities across the monitored muscles on the same side.

Sphincter-Associated Sensory Nerve: A nerve is identified as sphincter-associated if, upon increasing stimulus current, identifiable stable evoked EMGs with a consistent delay initially appear in the sphincter channel or if the evoked EMG does not initially manifest in the sphincter channel but achieves an amplitude ≥50 μV at the endpoint.

Sensory Nerve for the Lower Limbs: Any spinal nerve among the cauda equina not fitting the criteria for the previous two nerve types is classified as a lower limb-associated sensory nerve (Fig. 10.4).

6. Nerve Root Selection and Rhizotomy Ratio.

Our rhizotomy protocol dictates that when a stimulation trial on a lower limb-associated sensory nerve reaches its endpoint and the maximal evoked EMG amplitude corresponds to a target muscle's channel, the nerve root is considered predominantly responsible for the spastic tone in that muscle group; identified as a "spasticity responsible dorsal nerve root," it is then sectioned by 50% (Fig. 10.5). Otherwise, it will be spared (Fig. 10.6).

From our database of 821 cases of SDR across all 5 levels of the Gross Motor Function Classification System (GMFCS) in children with spastic CP, including 78 cases of hemiplegia, we've observed that the number of lower limb-associated nerve roots varies from 15 to 33 (average 25.3 ± 5.8), with 1–21 nerve roots (average 9.2 ± 3.8) being identified as spasticity responsible. To quantify the extent of rhizotomy performed on each patient, we calculate a "rhizotomy ratio," which is the number of spasticity responsible dorsal nerve roots divided by the total number of lower limb-associated sensory ones. This ratio offers a potential metric to correlate with the severity of our patients' condition. A retrospective study of the 821 SDR cases revealed a significant correlation between the rhizotomy ratio and the preoperative motor function assessment scores from the Gross Motor Function Measure-66 (GMFM-66) (Fig. 10.7).

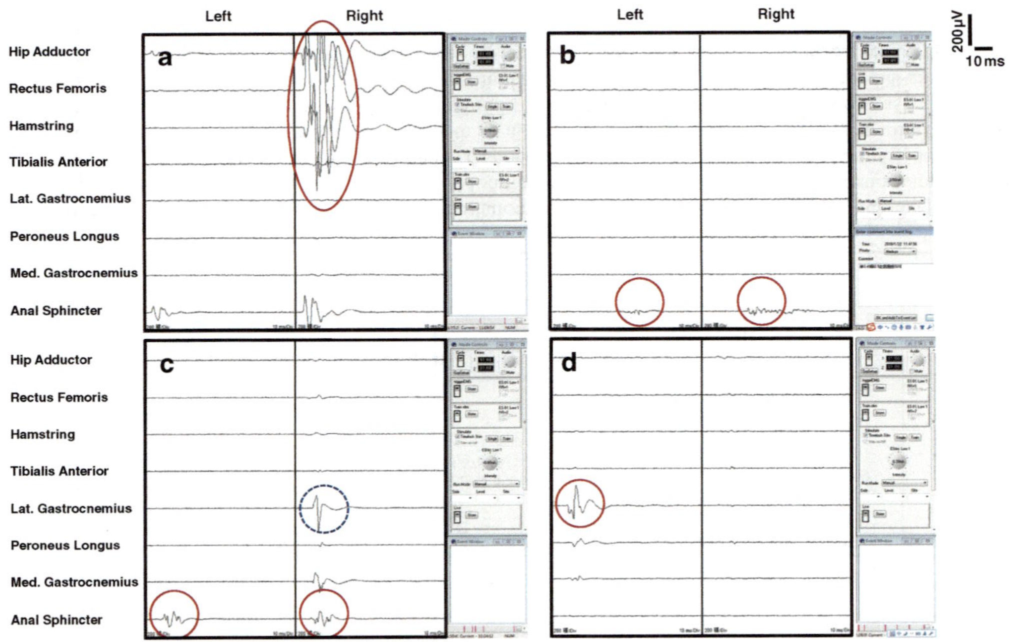

Fig. 10.4 Examples of different evoked CMAP patterns in motor-, anal sphincter-, and lower limb-associated sensory nerve root. (**a**) Motor nerve root: amplitude of evoked CMAP observed in channels of Rt. adductor and rectus femoris was huge (red ellipse)when intensity of stimulus was 0.09 mA. (**b**) Anal sphincter-associated sensory nerve: evoked CMAP first appeared on the channel of the anal sphincter (red circle, amplitude is 56 μV, intensity of stimulus was 0.50 mA). (**c**) Anal sphincter-associated sensory nerve: though at the endpoint of stimulation trial on one nerve root (intensity of stimulus is 0.80 mA), evoked CMAP in the channel of Rt. lateral gastrocnemius first reached 200 μV (blue dash circle), due to the reason that amplitude of evoked CMAP in the channel of the anal sphincter was 76 μV (≥ 50 μV) (red circle). The root was still categorized into group of anal sphincter-associated sensory nerve. (**d**) Lower limb-associated sensory nerve: intensity of stimulus is 0.30 mA. Evoked CMAP in the channel of Lt. lateral gastrocnemius reached 200 μV with almost zero innovation in the channel of the anal sphincter. CMAP, compound muscle action potential

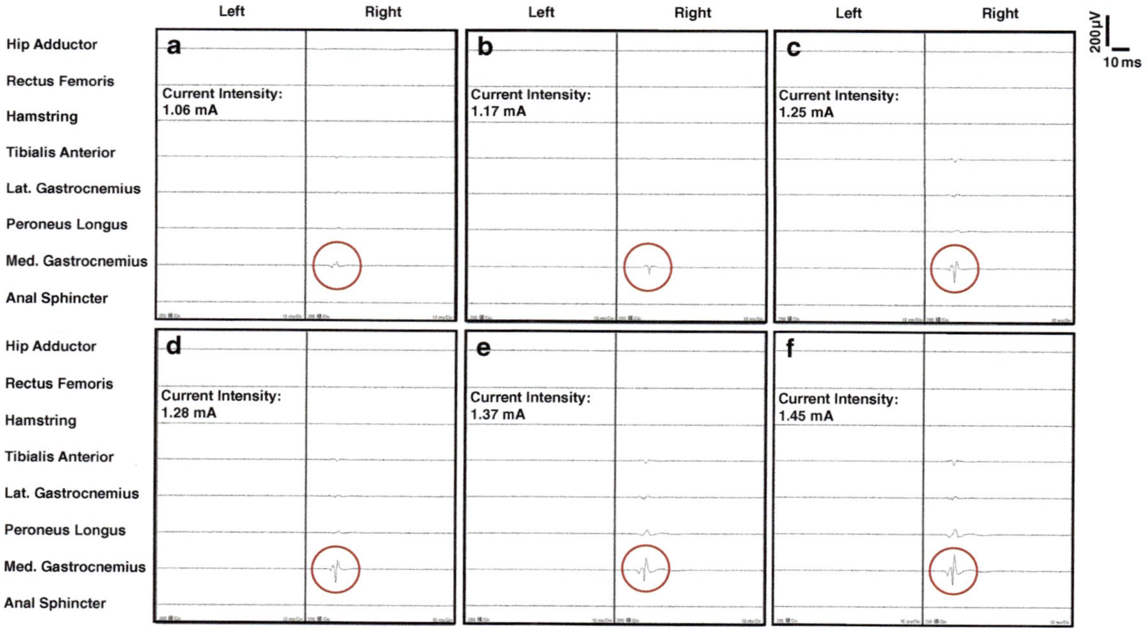

Fig. 10.5 Six representative screenshots during a sensory nerve stimulation trial until it reached its endpoint, which fits rhizotomy criteria. Rt. gastrocnemius was marked as the target muscle since its muscle tone was grade 4 (Modified Ashworth Scale) (channel with greatest amplitude of evoked EMG was marked in red circle). The root was cut by 50%. (**a**) Rt. medial gastrocnemius responded the most with its evoked EMG amplitude of 37 μV when stimulation intensity was 1.06 mA. (**b**) Rt. medial gastrocnemius responded the most with its evoked EMG amplitude of 45 μV when stimulation intensity was 1.17 mA. (**c**) Rt. medial gastrocnemius responded the most with its evoked EMG amplitude of 133 μV when stimulation intensity was 1.25 mA. (**d**) Rt. medial gastrocnemius responded the most with its evoked EMG amplitude of 139 μV when stimulation intensity was 1.28 mA. (**e**) Rt. medial gastrocnemius responded the most with its evoked EMG amplitude of 167 μV when stimulation intensity was 1.37 mA. (**f**) Rt. medial gastrocnemius responded the most with its evoked EMG amplitude of 212 μV when stimulation intensity was 1.45 mA

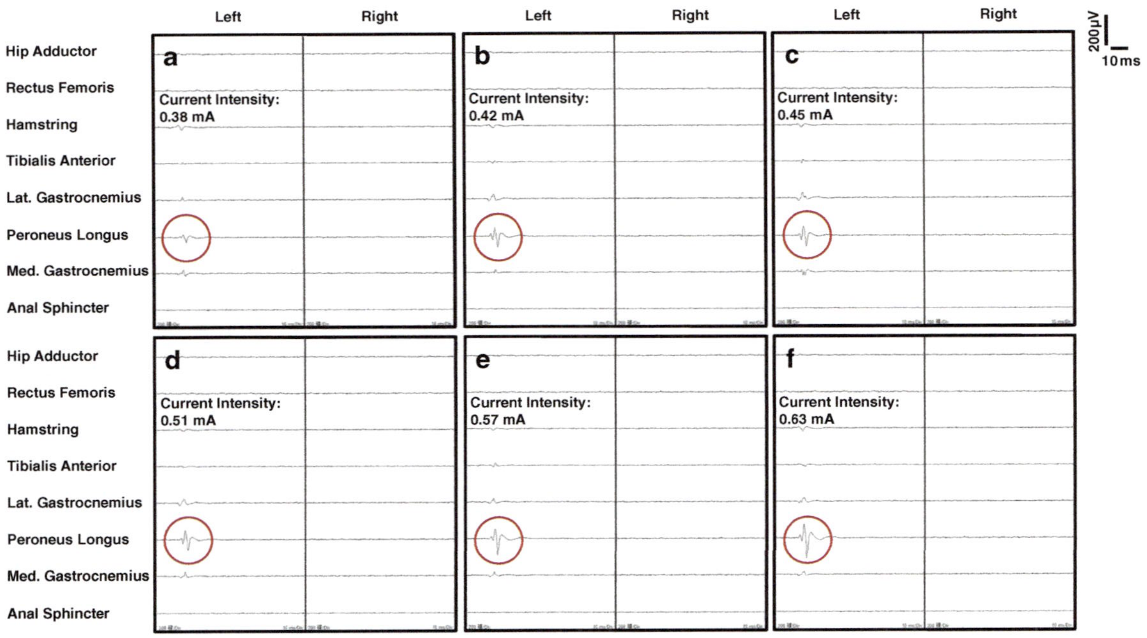

Fig. 10.6 Six representative screenshots during a sensory nerve stimulation trial until it reached its endpoint, which did not fit rhizotomy criteria. Lt. peroneus longus was not the target muscle since its muscle tone was 0 (Modified Ashworth Scale), which was normal (channel with greatest amplitude of evoked EMG was marked in red circle). The root was spared. (**a**) Lt. peroneus longus responded the most with its evoked EMG amplitude of 35 μV when stimulation intensity was 0.38 mA. (**b**) Lt. peroneus longus responded the most with its evoked EMG amplitude of 107 μV when stimulation intensity was 0.42 mA. (**c**) Lt. peroneus longus responded the most with its evoked EMG amplitude of 125 μV when stimulation intensity was 0.45 mA. (**d**) Lt. peroneus longus responded the most with its evoked EMG amplitude of 131 μV when stimulation intensity was 0.51 mA. (**e**) Lt. peroneus longus responded the most with its evoked EMG amplitude of 181 μV when stimulation intensity was 0.57 mA. (**f**) Rt. peroneus longus responded the most with its evoked EMG amplitude of 223 μV when stimulation intensity was 0.63 mA

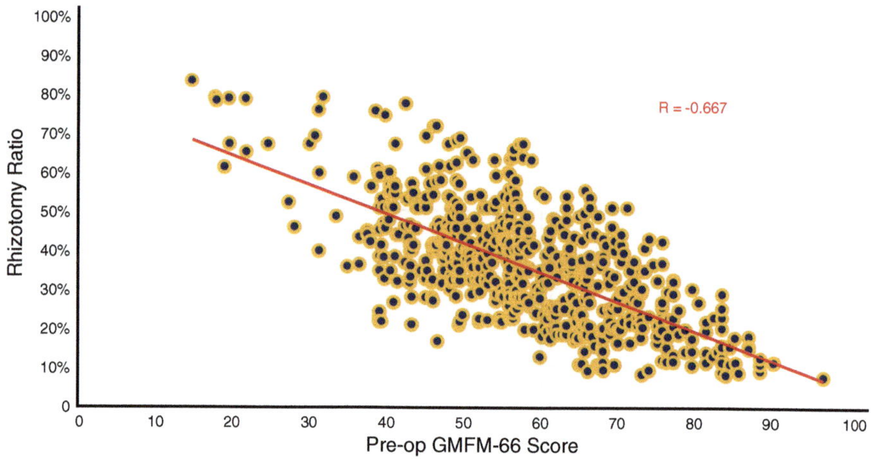

Fig. 10.7 Correlation between rhizotomy ratio and preop GMFM-66 score. Rhizotomy ratio: number of roots being cut/number of lower limb-associated sensory nerve in one case. *GMFM* gross motor function measure

10.2 Midterm Outcomes Following Crescendo Single-Pulse Stimulation-Guided SDR

1. Postoperative Changes in Muscle Tone and Surgery-Related Complications.

After SDR surgery, there's typically a moderate reduction in muscle tone of the treated spastic muscle groups. This reduction is observed immediately postoperative and tends to further decrease during subsequent rehabilitation therapy. Among the 481 children who have a minimum of 2 years of postop follow-up (with the longest being 5 years), muscle tone in the spastic muscle groups decreased by approximately 1.0 grade at around 2 weeks postoperatively and continued to decrease by an additional 0.8 grade by the last follow-up.

Among the 821 cases treated with this surgical approach, no midterm surgery-related complications have been documented to date. However, 11 cases experienced mild weakness in the proximal right lower limb following the surgery, which generally resolved within 6–8 weeks.

2. Postoperative Rehabilitation Strategies and Current Midterm Outcomes.

The tailored postoperative rehabilitation strategies developed by our team cater to the gradual reduction in muscle tone experienced by children with spastic CP following SDR surgery (Fig. 10.8). These strategies are crucial for optimizing motor function improvements postoperatively. In a retrospective analysis of 481 children who underwent at least 2 years of postoperative rehabilitation therapy, significant enhancements in motor functions were recorded.

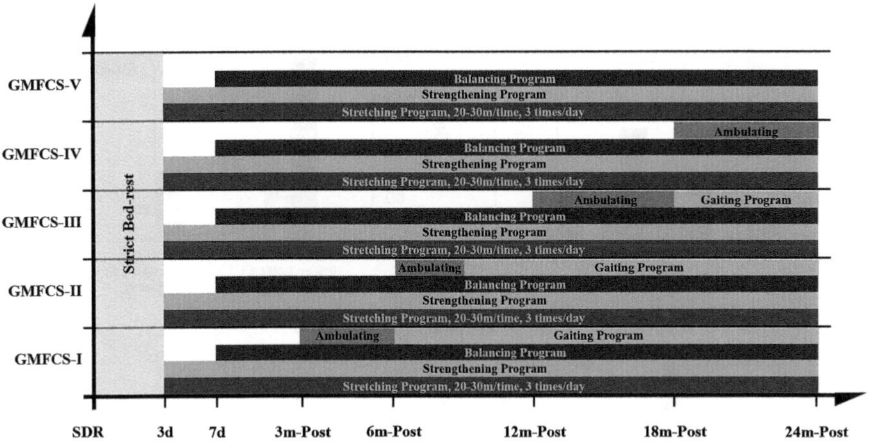

Fig. 10.8 Preop GMFCS level-based postop rehabilitation protocol

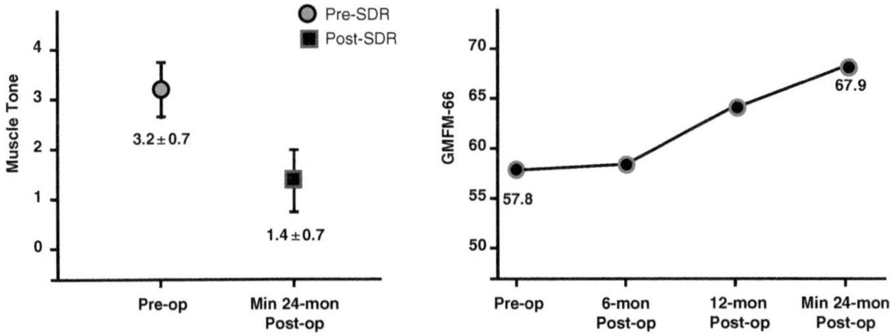

Fig. 10.9 Improvement of muscle tone and the GMFM-66 score in 481 cases with minimally 2 years postoperative rehabilitation therapy (3.0 ± 0.8 years)

At an average follow-up of 3.0 (± 0.8) years postop, the GMFM-66 score saw an average increase of 10.1 (± 5.0). Notably, in the cohort of 432 children initially classed as GMFCS levels II–V, approximately 31.0% advanced by one level and about 8.1% by two levels in the GMFCS classification. GMFCS level improvement is not applicable for those preoperatively at level I; thus, 49 cases were excluded from this data set. The greatest improvements were observed in children who underwent surgery before the age of six and those with less severe motor impairments preoperatively (Figs. 10.9 and 10.10). Gait analysis in 32 mild cases indicated an increase in the gait deviation index post-SDR (right side, 65.8 ± 8.8 vs. 60.1 ± 10.7; left side, 63.5 ± 10.1 vs. 57.0 ± 9.9), suggesting improved walking patterns after SDR procedure [18].

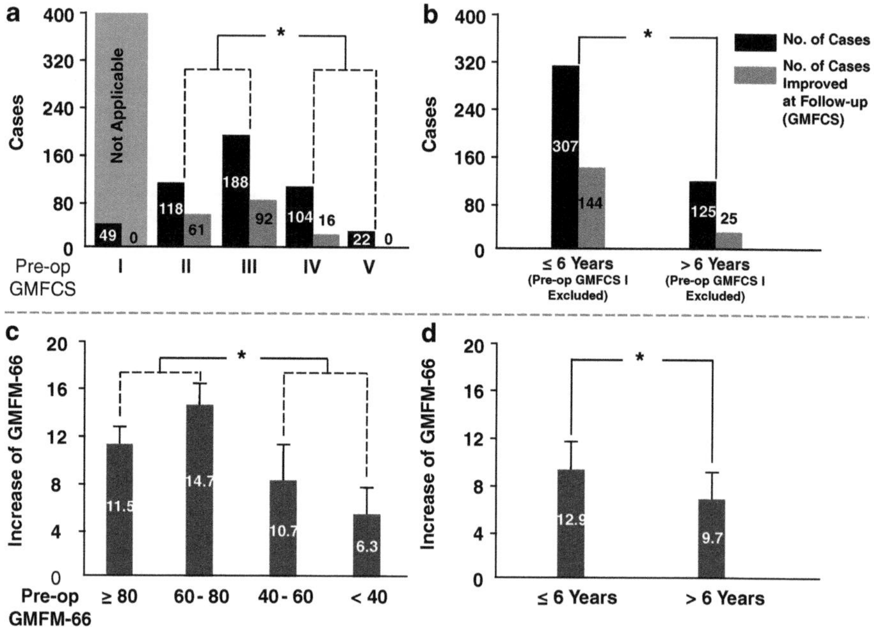

Fig. 10.10 Association between outcomes and preoperative status in 481 cases included. (**a**) Better results were observed in cases with preop GMFCS levels II and III. (**b**) Cases younger than 6 years of age had more chance to upgrade (432 cases with their preop GMFCS levels II–V). (**c**) Score increased more in cases with preop GMFM-66 ≥ 60 than those with score below. (**d**) Cases younger than 6 years of age improved more with regard to score increase of GMFM-66 after SDR. Asterisk indicates statistically significant difference obtained with $p < 0.01$

A retrospective study of 148 cases with spastic CP and preoperative tibial torsion showed that out of 261 affected limbs, 240 (92.0%) demonstrated major improvements post-SDR, with 20.0% returning to normal ranges (Fig. 10.11) [20].

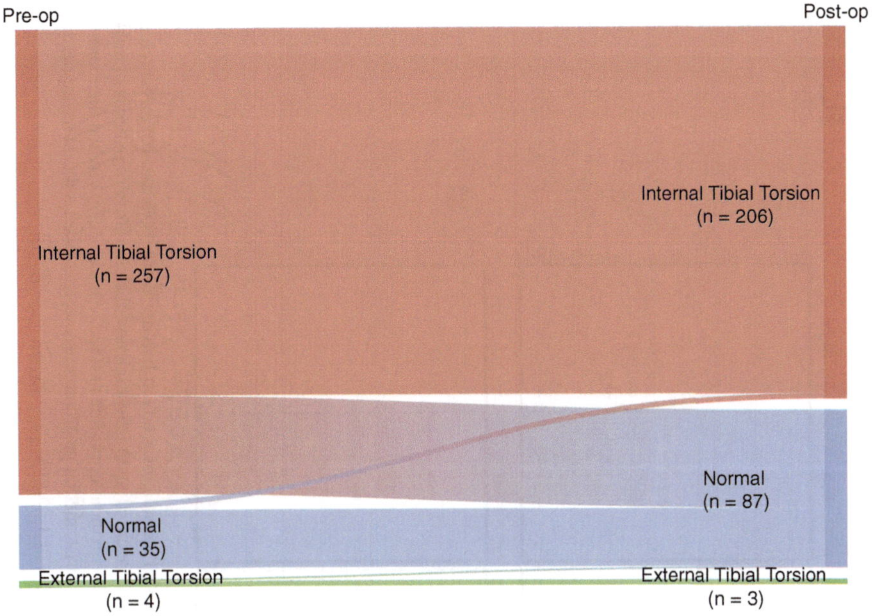

Fig. 10.11 Change of transmalleolar angle (TMA) in 296 limbs involved (148 cases) after SDR

10.3 Potential Evoked EMG Data Analysis

Our clinical practice demonstrates that evoked EMG responses to single-pulse stimulation are remarkably consistent and specific, as illustrated in Fig. 10.12. This reproducibility may form the foundation for future studies using intraoperative paired electrophysiological input–output data, particularly when combined with preoperative status of patients. Such a methodological framework may serve as a tool to explore the variations in neuronal circuit characteristics across different severities and ages in cerebral palsy, potentially enriching our understanding of neuronal network functionality in this patient population.

One of the pivotal challenges in neurophysiological monitoring is the presence of background electrical noise. By adhering to a stringent anesthesia protocol, we aim to mitigate such interference. Nevertheless, to develop a standardized, precise filtering technique and a comprehensive system for analyzing evoked EMG data—including amplitude and waveform characteristics—remains a crucial objective. Achieving this would significantly advance our ability to comprehensively investigate the neurophysiological underpinnings of spasticity and the effects of SDR.

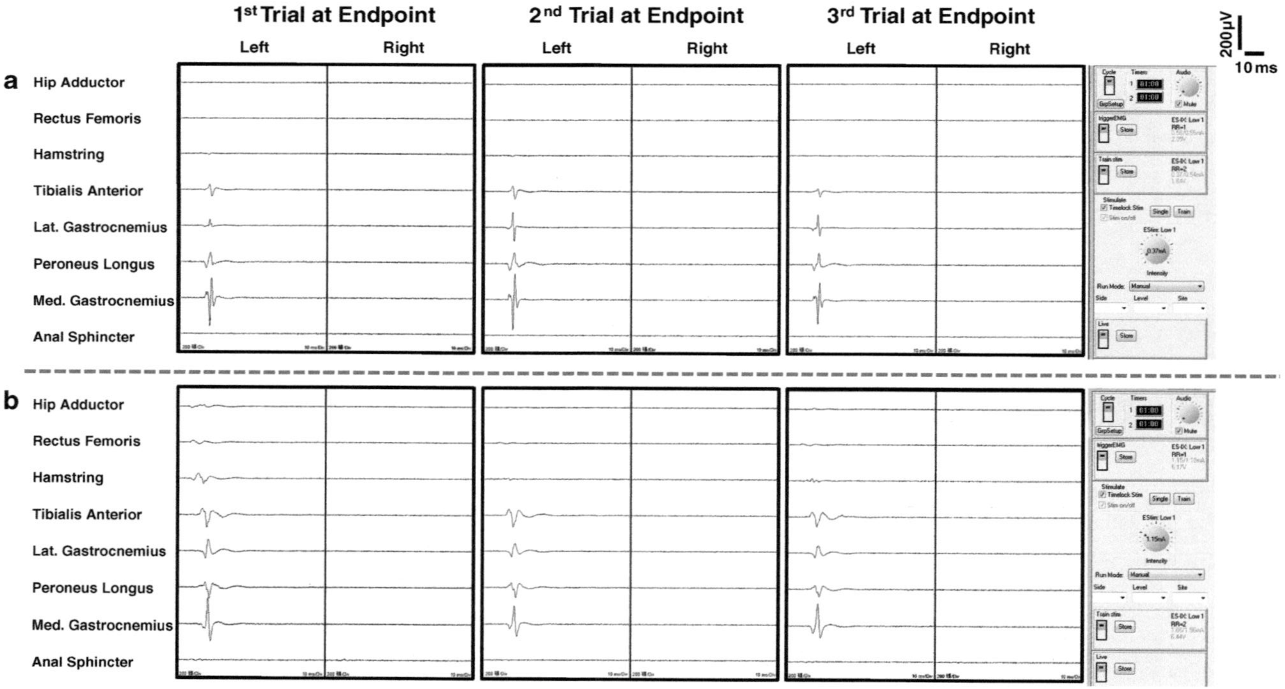

Fig. 10.12 Example of reproducibility in single-pulse stimulus evoked CMAP at endpoints of stimulation trials in two dorsal roots (**a** and **b**), on which crescendo stimulation was carried out three times, 2 mins apart, not only the same channel always responding the most but also the similarity of patterns of evoked CAMPs in those channels. (**a**) EMGs in the channel of Lt. medial gastrocnemius were evoked with their amplitude of 252, 279, and 227 µV when their stimulation trials have reached endpoints with input intensity of 0.37 mA. (**b**) EMGs in the channel of Lt. medial gastrocnemius were evoked with their amplitude of 245, 202, and 214 µV when their stimulation trials have reached endpoints with input intensity of 1.15 mA

10.4 Conclusion

The crescendo single-pulse evoked compound muscle action potential (CMAP) interpretation method provides a novel approach to achieving rootlet selection in SDR procedure for children with spastic cerebral palsy, which offers several key advantages:

1. Quantitative and standardized selection: By utilizing a crescendo stimulation protocol and defined CMAP thresholds, this method provides a more objective and reproducible means of identifying dorsal nerve roots contributing to spasticity.
2. Improved targeting: The preoperative identification of spastic muscle groups, combined with intraoperative neurophysiological monitoring, allows for more precise targeting of problematic nerve roots while sparing those not significantly contributing to spasticity.
3. Enhanced safety: The protocol's built-in redundancies, such as monitoring sphincter function, help minimize potential complications associated with SDR.
4. Correlation with clinical severity: The introduced "rhizotomy ratio" offers a potential metric for quantifying the extent of the procedure and correlating it with preoperative motor function.
5. Promising outcomes: Midterm follow-up data demonstrate significant improvements in motor function and GMFCS levels for many patients, particularly when combined with tailored postoperative rehabilitation strategies.

While long-term studies are still needed to fully assess the efficacy and safety of this approach, the crescendo single-pulse evoked CMAP interpretation method for SDR shows great promise in improving outcomes for children with spastic cerebral palsy. As we continue to refine our understanding of spasticity pathophysiology and surgical techniques, this method provides a valuable tool for neurosurgeons seeking to optimize functional outcomes and quality of life for their patients.

References

1. Brown P. Pathophysiology of spasticity. J Neurol Neurosurg Psychiatry. 1994;57(7):773–7. https://doi.org/10.1136/jnnp.57.7.773.
2. Sheean G. The pathophysiology of spasticity. Eur J Neurol. 2002;9(Suppl 1):3–9. https://doi.org/10.1046/j.1468-1331.2002.0090s1003.x.
3. Trompetto C, Marinelli L, Mori L, et al. Pathophysiology of spasticity: implications for neurorehabilitation. Biomed Res Int. 2014;2014:354906. https://doi.org/10.1155/2014/354906. Epub 2014 Oct 30
4. Bar-On L, Molenaers G, Aertbeliën E, et al. Spasticity and its contribution to hypertonia in cerebral palsy. Biomed Res Int. 2015;2015:317047. https://doi.org/10.1155/2015/317047. Epub 2015 Jan 11
5. Evans SH, Cameron MW, Burton JM, et al. Hypertonia. Curr Probl Pediatr Adolesc Health Care. 2017;47(7):161–6. https://doi.org/10.1016/j.cppeds.2017.06.005. Epub 2017 Jul 15

6. Marsden J, Stevenson V, Jarrett L. Treatment of spasticity. Handb Clin Neurol. 2023;196:497–521. https://doi.org/10.1016/B978-0-323-98817-9.00010-7.
7. Morota N, Abbott R, Kofler M, Epstein FJ. Residual spasticity after selective posterior rhizotomy. Childs Nerv Syst. 1995;11(3):161–5. https://doi.org/10.1007/BF00570257.
8. Steinbok P. Outcomes after selective dorsal rhizotomy for spastic cerebral palsy. Childs Nerv Syst. 2001;17(1–2):1–18. https://doi.org/10.1007/pl00013722.
9. Morota N. Functional posterior rhizotomy: the Tokyo experience. Childs Nerv Syst. 2007;23(9):1007–14. https://doi.org/10.1007/s00381-007-0381-y. Epub 2007 Jul 26
10. Steinbok P. Selective dorsal rhizotomy for spastic cerebral palsy: a review. Childs Nerv Syst. 2007;23(9):981–90. https://doi.org/10.1007/s00381-007-0379-5. Epub 2007 Jun 6
11. Park TS, Dobbs MB, Cho J. Evidence supporting selective dorsal rhizotomy for treatment of spastic cerebral palsy. Cureus. 2018;10(10):e3466. https://doi.org/10.7759/cureus.3466.
12. Wheelwright M, Selvey PJ, Steinbok P, et al. Systematic review of spinal deformities following multi-level selective dorsal rhizotomy. Childs Nerv Syst. 2020;36(5):1025–35. https://doi.org/10.1007/s00381-019-04375-x. Epub 2019 Oct 8
13. Tu A, Steinbok P. Long term outcome of selective dorsal rhizotomy for the management of childhood spasticity-functional improvement and complications. Childs Nerv Syst. 2020;36(9):1985–94. https://doi.org/10.1007/s00381-020-04747-8. Epub 2020 Jun 23
14. Sindou M, Joud A, Georgoulis G. How I do it: selective dorsal rhizotomy, using interlaminar approaches, for spastic diplegia/quadriplegia in children with cerebral palsy. Acta Neurochir. 2021;163(10):2845–51. https://doi.org/10.1007/s00701-021-04770-x. Epub 2021 Feb
15. Zhan Q, Tang L, Wang Y, et al. Feasibility and effectiveness of a newly modified protocol-guided selective dorsal rhizotomy via single-level approach to treat spastic hemiplegia in pediatric cases with cerebral palsy. Childs Nerv Syst. 2019;35(11):2171–8. https://doi.org/10.1007/s00381-019-04194-0. Epub 2019 May 29
16. Zhan Q, Yu X, Jiang W, et al. Whether the newly modified rhizotomy protocol is applicable to guide single-level approach SDR to treat spastic quadriplegia and diplegia in pediatric patients with cerebral palsy? Childs Nerv Syst. 2020;36(9):1935–43. https://doi.org/10.1007/s00381-019-04368-w. Epub 2019 Sep 9
17. Xiao B, Constatntini S, Browd SR, et al. The role of intra-operative neuroelectrophysiological monitoring in single-level approach selective dorsal rhizotomy. Childs Nerv Syst. 2020;36(9):1925–33. https://doi.org/10.1007/s00381-019-04408-5. Epub 2019 Nov 4
18. Jiang W, Jiang S, Yu Y, Zhan Q, et al. Improvement of the gait pattern after selective dorsal rhizotomy derives from changes of kinematic parameters in the sagittal plane. Front Pediatr. 2022;10:1047227. https://doi.org/10.3389/fped.2022.1047227.
19. Hou X, Yan Y, Zhan Q, et al. Unsupervised machine learning effectively clusters pediatric spastic cerebral palsy patients for determination of optimal responders to selective dorsal rhizotomy. Sci Rep. 2023;13(1):8095. https://doi.org/10.1038/s41598-023-35021-x.
20. Wang R, Jiang W, Wei M, et al. Short-term change of tibial torsion in children with spastic cerebral palsy after selective dorsal rhizotomy. Transl Pediatr. 2023;12(12):2131–41. https://doi.org/10.21037/tp-23-339.

Chapter 11
Dorsal Rhizotomy at the Intradural Juxtaforaminal Zone

George Georgoulis, Anthony Joud, and Marc Sindou

11.1 Introduction

The theoretical background of dorsal rhizotomy traces back to 1898 when Sherrington demonstrated that division of the dorsal roots reduced tone in decerebrated cats [1]. Building upon this groundwork, Foerster applied the technique to address human spasticity and published a review in 1913 detailing dorsal root resections in 159 children with cerebral palsy [2]. Foerster's method involved sectioning the entire dorsal roots from L2 to S2, excluding the L4 root, known as the "antigravity root," while utilizing intraoperative electrical stimulation to discern segmental levels and differentiate between ventral and dorsal roots.

In the 1960s, Gros in Montpellier, France, further developed the technique by dissecting dorsal roots into rootlets and performing rhizotomy with nonselective sectioning of 80% of the rootlets of each root to mitigate postoperative sensory deficits [3]. Subsequently, the Montpellier school introduced the "sectorial" dorsal rhizotomy, aiming to limit sectioning to roots corresponding to segmental metameres carrying persistent "disabling" spasticity, as opposed to "useful" spasticity that aids

G. Georgoulis (✉)
Department of Neurosurgery, General Hospital of Athens "G. Gennimatas", Athens, Greece

A. Joud
Department of Pediatric Neurosurgery Centre Hospitalo-Universitaire de Nancy, Nancy, France
e-mail: a.joud@chru-nancy.fr

M. Sindou
University of Lyon, Lyon, France

Groupe ELSAN, Clinique Bretéché, Nantes, France
e-mail: marc.sindou@orange.fr

N. Morota, P. Steinbok (eds.), *Dorsal Rhizotomy: Neurosurgery for Childhood Spasticity*, Advances and Technical Standards in Neurosurgery 51,
https://doi.org/10.1007/978-3-031-86441-4_11

weak lower limbs in extension against gravity [4]. The Montpellier method identified roots based on their topographic muscle responses.

In 1976, Fasano in Torino introduced the concept of "functional" posterior rhizotomy, which identified "abnormal" muscle responses to electrical stimulation of roots and rootlets [5]. Abnormal responses were characterized by repetitive stimulation producing continuous, tetanic responses in corresponding segmental muscles, often spreading ipsilaterally or contralaterally. Fasano's technique involved a limited laminectomy.

In the early 1980s, Peacock and Arens expanded exposure to entire lumbar and sacral roots with extended laminectomy from the first lumbar to the first sacral vertebra [6]. To achieve greater precision and selectivity, various technical approaches have since emerged [7–9].

In the same period, dorsal rhizotomy fell down into decline due to its invasiveness and emergence of alternative methods: botulinum toxin injections, orthopedic measures including surgical ones, and intrathecal baclofen (ITB) therapy.

However, since the early 2000s, it appeared a progressive awareness among the pediatric rehabilitation community that, besides their immense usefulness, the abovementioned methods reveal limits to control underlying spasticity. A growing consensus came to estimate that dorsal rhizotomy could be an effective way to reduce the excess of hypertonia, provided its main component is of the spastic mechanism over the frequently associated dystonic component [7]. Nevertheless, there remains important elements of controversy concerning pros and cons of the various possible modalities of dorsal hizotomy [8, 9]. Still persisting dilemmas are the following:

- Which spine approach is better? Extended L1–S1 laminectomies/laminotomies to directly expose all lumbosacral roots or limited ones to a few or even a single vertebral level(s) to limit invasiveness of the approach.
- Which deployment of intraoperative neurophysiology (ION) should be used? None—relying on anatomical/radiological landmarks [10, 11]—or full neurophysiological exploration for mapping and testing, individually, all lumbosacral ventral and dorsal roots [12].
- What amount of the dorsal roots/rootlets to cut (from 30% to 80%)? Actually, there is an empirical consensus to divide on average 60% of the total number of the L2–S1 (S2) roots.
- At what time to indicate dorsal rhizotomy within the course of childhood and for which indication? There is a discussion about the (limited) interest to indicate surgery in patients with irreducible deformities. Furthermore, age for ideal timing is the object of important controversies.

Based on our initial past experience and thorough evaluation of the various modalities available, considering their respective advantages and disadvantages, the following strategy with its different (recommended) steps was chosen [13]:

1. Expose and identify all lumbar to sacral roots from L2 to S2 (included) intradurally at proximity of their corresponding foramen; then, confirm their respective anatomical levels on electrical stimulation of the VR with observation of the corresponding muscular responses.

2. List the muscular groups corresponding to every stimulated VR to establish its territory of innervation (i.e., its myotome). This anatomical mapping seemed to us the more so important as there exists an individual variability from one patient to another for identical radicular levels [14].
3. Explore the degree of excitability of each of the exposed dorsal roots using electrical stimulation to determine the extent of the territories of diffusion of the elicited muscle responses. Quantification of the rootlets' cutting is adjusted according to this physiological testing [15, 16].

This method was named Keyhole Interlaminar Dorsal rhizotomy (KIDr), because the approach consists in enlarged interlaminar openings with respect of the spinous processes and their interspinous ligaments, so preserving the spine posterior architecture.

11.1.1 The Keyhole Interlaminar Dorsal Rhizotomy Technique (KIDr)

11.1.1.1 Surgical Procedure [17]

This "multistaged" interlaminar approach was designed to further reduce invasiveness while maintaining precision, depending on the roots to be accessed [17, 18] (Figs. 11.1 and 11.2). Description is the following:

The lumbar midline skin incision and corresponding detachment of the paraspinal muscles are extended according to the selected interlaminar levels to be opened, generally from L1 to S1 when all roots must be targeted.

Access to L2 and L3 roots can be achieved through a L1–L2 interlaminar opening, L4 and L5 roots through a L3–L4 interlaminar opening, and S1–S2 roots through a L5–S1 interlaminar opening, as illustrated in Fig. 11.2. Spinous processes are preserved along with the interspinous ligaments. After removal of the ligamentum flavum at the selected interlaminar spaces, the space is enlarged as much as possible by resection of the lower two-thirds of the upper lamina and three-quarters of the lower lamina. The dura and arachnoid are then opened in the midline for at least 2 cm at each of the selected interspaces. The surgeon, with the optical axis of the microscope at 45°, focuses on the accessed opposite pair of roots under the bridge of the preserved midline spinous ligament (Fig. 11.3). That is, if the surgeon is on the right of the patient, the left roots are targeted, and if on the left, the right roots. In the pair of roots, the upper root is relatively easily located intradurally before entering its dural sheath, while, for the lower one, a large resection of three-quarters of the lower lamina is required to visualize it.

To avoid the (rare) complication of paraplegia from eventual extradural hemostatic coagulation or intradural rupture of the Adamkiewicz artery, it is important that this major radiculomedullary is recognized and protected.

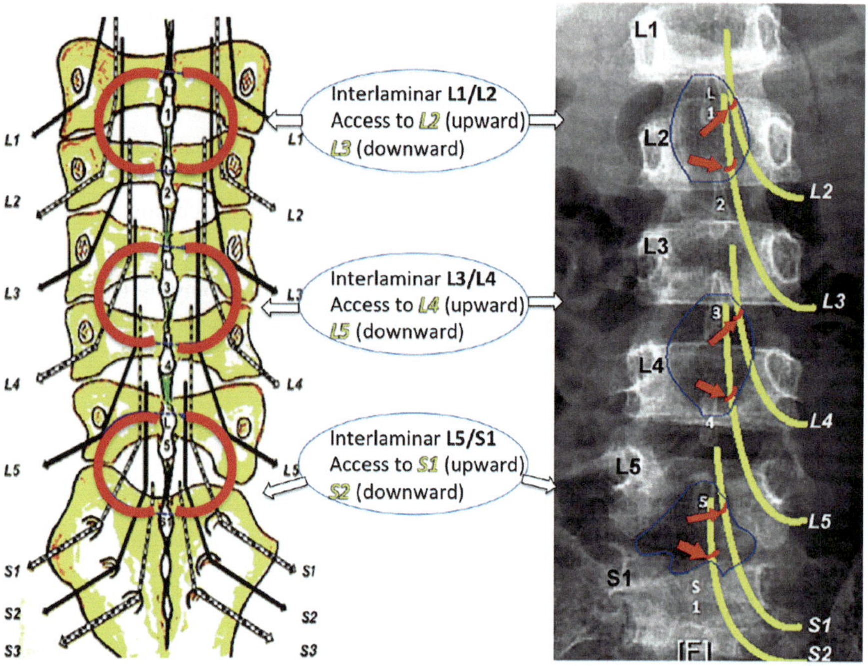

Fig. 11.1 Principles of the Keyhole Interlaminar Dorsal rhizotomy (KIDr) procedure. Schematic representation of the intervertebral spaces where the roots are targeted according to preoperative planning. The image shows the postoperative anterolateral X-ray. The enlarged interlaminar spaces are outlined in brown: L1–L2, L3–L4, and L5–S1, with preservation of the spinous processes and interspinous ligaments at all levels. As seen on the X-ray: The pair of *L2* and *L3* roots are targeted at the L1–L2 interlaminar space (for the treatment of spastic hip and thigh in flexion–adduction). The pair of *L4* and *L5* roots are targeted at the L3–L4 interlaminar space (for the treatment of spastic quadriceps with patella elevation). The pair of S1 and S2 roots are targeted at the L5–S1 interlaminar space (for the treatment of spastic equinism and spastic hamstrings)

The dorsal root (with an average of five rootlets per root) is identified under the microscope posteriorly to the ventral root. It appears thicker, compared to the ventral root. Sometimes, the dorsal root is separated from the ventral root by an arachnoid fold, which eases their differentiation. Most often, their separation requires meticulous microsurgical dissection as winding between them makes them a single root unit, especially at the S1 and S2 levels.

Then, with a bipolar stimulator to avoid current spreading, muscle responses are elicited, first from the ventral roots (for myotomal mapping) and second from the dorsal root/rootlets (for segmental excitability testing). Noteworthy, the threshold for eliciting muscle responses with dorsal root stimulation is generally three to four times higher than that for responses to corresponding ventral root stimulation. After their identification, the dorsal roots to be targeted are prepared to be sectioned according to the percentage of rootlets' cutting indicated in the preoperative chart and subsequently adjusted from the intraoperative neurophysiology information,

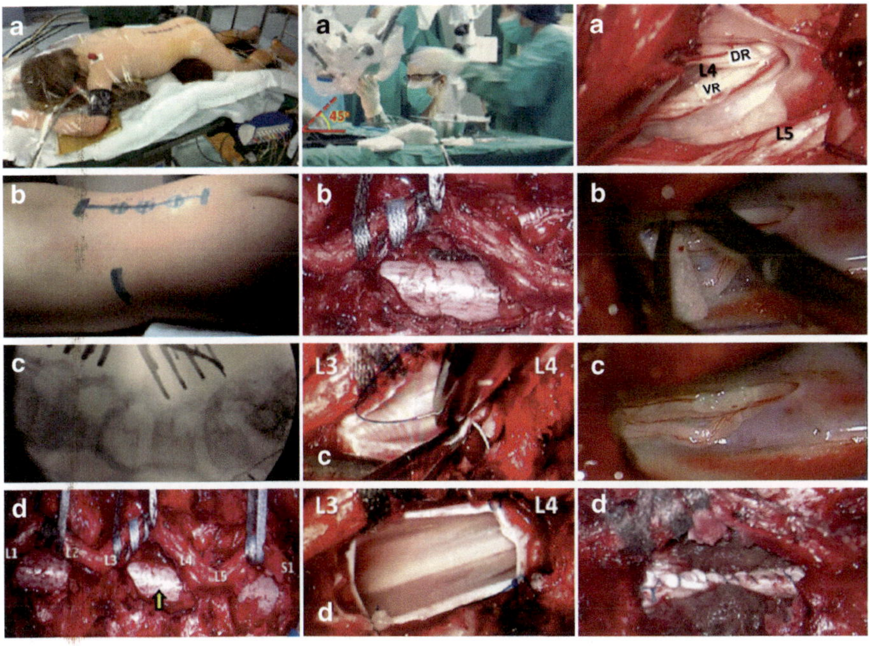

Fig. 11.2 Organization and microsurgical steps of the KIDr method. Left column: (**a**) The patient is in the prone position, with the head 10 cm lower than the body to minimize loss of cerebrospinal fluid. (**b**) Cutaneous landmarks of the lumbosacral spinous processes for skin incision (from Th12 to S2) with the three selected interlaminar spaces to approach. (**c**) Intraoperative X-ray to check the lumbosacral levels (from L1 to S2) to count from the sacrum. (**d**) View of the interlaminar (enlarged) spaces at the L1–L2, L3–L4, and L5–S1 levels, with preservation of the spinous processes and interspinous ligaments. At each "window" level, the lower two-thirds of the superior lamina and the upper three-quarters of the inferior lamina are dissected in the midline, and the ligamentum flavum is removed so that the dura and arachnoid can be exposed (in the midline) at a height of more than 20 mm. The L3–L4 space to approach the *L4* and *L5* roots—as an example—is indicated by the yellow arrow. **Central column:** (**a**) The surgeon is positioned with the axis of the surgical microscope at a 45 degrees angle so that the contralateral roots are accessible passing diagonally under the interspinous ligaments. (**b**) Exposure of the L3–L4 interlaminar space as an example. Note the preservation of the interspinous ligaments. (**c**) Opening and suspension of the dura. (**d**) Dura completely open and suspended, with the arachnoid membrane still intact. **Right column:** (**a**) View of the intradural space, diagonally below the interspinous ligaments, from the left side for contralateral access to the pair of right L4 and L5 roots: L4 upward proximally to the foramen and L5 downward. At this point, the L4 root is clearly separated into dorsal (DR) and ventral root (VR). (**b**) Partial rhizotomy of the dorsal L4 root with microscissors. (**c**) Final result of L4 dorsal rootlets sectioned (two-thirds). (**d**) Tight suturing of the dura under the interspinous ligament bridge

i.e., the intensity and diffusion of the muscle responses to dorsal root stimulation (Table 11.1).

At the end, the dural incision is tightly sutured at each of the openings. The paravertebral muscles are repositioned and attached at the interspinous ligament line and the skin closed. A compression draping and a soft lumbar corset are placed for

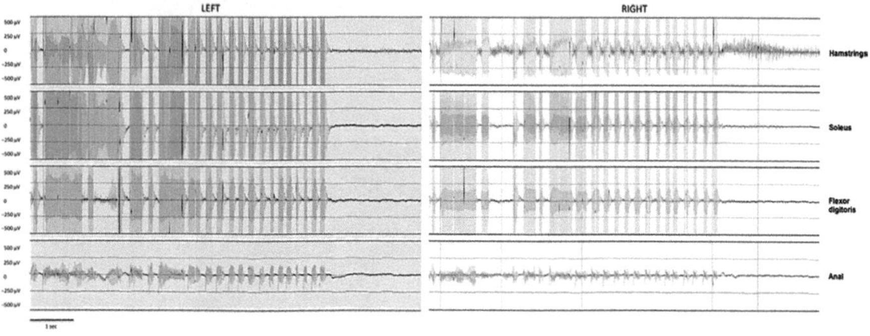

Fig. 11.3 Intraoperative electromyographic recordings obtained after stimulation (1 second train at 50 Hz, at intensity of 1 mA) of the left S1 dorsal root in a diplegic child. Recordings show diffusion of response in the contralateral right lower limb. An abnormality score of 4 was assigned to this electromyographic response pattern characterized by sustained, polyphasic response

Table 11.1 Scoring of muscle responses to dorsal root stimulation for decision regarding incision and extent, according to Fasano's classification

Grade	Muscular response to dorsal root stimulation with a 50 Hz stimulus train for 1 s
0	Unsustained motor response in muscles innervated by the segmental level of the stimulated dorsal nerve root or rootlets
1	Sustained motor response in myotome of stimulated nerve root
2	Contraction of muscles in myotomes of adjacent segmental level(s)
3	Contraction of muscles in myotomes at a distance from that of stimulated nerve root
4	Contraction of muscles in contralateral leg or upper limbs

a couple of weeks so that the may start standing and ambulating in the next following days and physical therapy be continued.

11.1.2 Anesthesia Protocol and Early Postoperative Care

11.1.2.1 Anesthesia Protocol

Dorsal rhizotomy necessitates general anesthesia with endotracheal intubation. It is advisable to insert a urinary catheter, which will remain in place for several days postsurgery until the patient achieves bladder control. The patient is positioned on the operating table in a prone position, supported by flexible devices to minimize thoracic and abdominal pressure. The head is positioned approximately 10 cm lower than the trunk to reduce the cerebrospinal fluid loss.

When administering muscle relaxants of the curare type, it is imperative that they have a short duration to preserve muscle responses to stimulation.

Anesthesia involves a combination of inhaled sevoflurane (or 50–70% nitrous oxide) and intravenous sufentanil (or remifentanil). In older children, the protocol may incorporate propofol alongside sevoflurane, although propofol may attenuate activities recorded by the EMG.

11.1.2.2 Early Postoperative Care

Following the procedure, the child spends the night in the intensive care unit before transitioning to the ward, where hospitalization typically lasts for a week. Subsequently, the child is transferred to the pediatric rehabilitation center for approximately 1 month. Postoperative pain management involves the use of low-dose opioids for wound discomfort and clonazepam for potential lower extremity paresthesias/dysesthesias until discharge.

Physical therapy, including sitting, standing, and walking (adjusted according to the child's degree of disability), commences on the second postoperative day and gradually intensifies.

11.2 Intraoperative Neurophysiology (ION)

Children diagnosed with spastic diplegia commonly exhibit Little's abnormal postural pattern [19]. For those capable of standing and movement, maintaining sufficient tone and strength in muscles contributing to antigravity function, particularly the quadriceps and gluteus, is imperative to preserve their function. The multidisciplinary preoperative chart should delineate the muscle groups to be targeted, specifying the desired reduction or preservation of tone.

Our experience led us to use and advise the necessity of intraoperative neurophysiological guidance to confirm and/or adjust the program preoperatively established [20].

Two distinct methodologies have been associated with different principles. The first, advocated by Gros, emphasizes anatomy. It involves identifying the motor innervation of exposed ventral (and corresponding dorsal) roots through electrical stimulation to determine which dorsal roots should be sectioned or preserved [21]. The second, introduced by Fasano, centers on physiology. It entails identifying abnormal (i.e., excessive) muscle responses to electrical stimulation of dorsal roots, indicative of involvement in dysfunctional spinal cord circuits [15].

The necessity and extent of intraoperative neurophysiology remains subject of debate [10–12]. On our side, we strongly advocate for neurophysiological guidance to ensure the maximal accuracy and safety of the procedure [16–18, 20], given the significant variations in myotome distribution between patient [14] and different degrees of excitability among segmental levels [16].

11.2.1 The Anatomical Mapping

Segmental identification, under anatomical mapping, involves ventral root (VR) electrical stimulation (preferably utilizing a bipolar stimulator) of the ventral roots at a rather low intensity to avoid diffusion (200 μA in our usual practice) and at a frequency of 2 Hz.

In Summary

- Stimulation of the L2 root elicits responses principally in the iliopsoas and adductor muscles of the hips.
- Stimulation of the L3 root elicits responses principally in the adductors and quadriceps.
- Responses to stimulation of the L4 root are observed predominantly in the quadriceps and tibialis anterior;
- Responses to stimulation of the L5 root are observed predominantly in the extensors of the toes and the gluteal muscles.
- Stimulation of the S1 root primarily elicits responses in the soleus and gastrocnemius group and the hamstrings. This triceps surae response can be confirmed by repeated testing of the Achilles reflex before, during, and after the rhizotomy. Noteworthy, in fact, the hamstrings response depends on the L5–S1–S2 roots.
- Stimulation of the S2 root produces muscle responses in the toes' flexors.
- The bladder and/or rectal response to stimulation of S2–S4 roots can be assessed using cystomanometry and rectomanometry, and/or by electromyographic recordings of the external anal sphincter [22], or more simply by gloved finger examination at the level of the sphincter.

All these responses can be palpated by examining the muscle groups in the lower extremities and/or monitored using electromyographic recordings.

Table 11.2 provides a comprehensive summary of the relevant features of this anatomical and topographic mapping.

Table 11.2 Predominant or specific motor response produced by stimulation of selected roots

Stimulated root	Predominantly responding muscle(s) (myotome)
L2	Iliopsoas, adductors of hips
L3	Adductors of hips, quadriceps
L4	Quadriceps, dorsal flexor of ankle (tibialis anterior)
L5	Extensors of toes, hamstrings
S1	Achilles ankle deep tendon reflex, gastrocnemius–soleus group, hamstrings, tibialis posterior
S2	Flexors of toes, hamstrings, bladder
S3	Anal sphincter, bladder
S4	Anal sphincter

11.2.2 The Physiological Testing

The objective of the physiological testing is to evaluate the excitability of the various lumbosacral segmental spinal circuitries by stimulating the dorsal roots/rootlets, according to Fasano's methodology [15], later modified by Philips and Park [23, 24] (Table 11.1).

This stimulation consists of a 1-second duration train at a frequency of 50 Hz with observation and quantification of the elicited muscle responses.

In its complete modality, the protocol proceeds as follows: First, the stimulation threshold is determined using 1-millisecond current pulses, starting at an intensity of 0.1 mA and gradually increasing until muscle contraction occurs. Once the threshold is established, a stimulus comprising a 50-Hz train of two to three times threshold intensity is applied to recruit a maximum of motor units. The resulting motor responses are then quantified using the grading scale system ranging from 0 to 4. Initially, a test is conducted on the entire dorsal root, followed by a potential second test at the level of the dissected rootlets if this modality is the one chosen by the surgical team. Although the latter may offer increased precision, it is time-consuming and carries a higher risk of trauma to the roots, potentially leading to nerve conduction disorders.

In our current practice, we employ a simplified protocol, which involves the estimation of the dorsal root as a whole, encompassing all its constituting rootlets globally, at an intensity of 1 mA. The choice of this intensity was based on our experience that this intensity is (slightly) above the threshold for the lumbosacral dorsal roots. This 1 mA intensity was used equally in all roots for testing and comparing excitability between the different segments of the lumbosacral spinal cord [16].

Determining the degree of response most indicative of which roots/rootlets should be sectioned remains a topic of debate [10–12]. Studies have demonstrated that in nonspastic individuals, a low-threshold and sustained dorsal root/rootlet response to a 50-Hz train lasting 1 s can occur. In many centers, determination is rather based on the diffusion of the response beyond the stimulated segmental level (Grade 3), extending even to the contralateral side or even more suprasegmentally to the upper extremities (Grade 4) (Fig. 11.3).

11.2.3 The Combined Anatomical and Physiological Intraoperative Evaluation

In our strategy, the integrated anatomical and physiological evaluation plays a pivotal role in confirming or adjusting the predetermined planning outlined in the preoperative chart mainly guided by the child's clinical presentation.

The preoperative diagram encompasses several key components: (a) description of all disabling aspects of spasticity; (b) enumeration of affected muscle groups bearing hypertonia; (c) identification of corresponding roots presumed to carry harmful afferent pathways based on classical anatomical knowledge; (d) determination of the number of dorsal rootlets to be sectioned for each selected and targeted root, proportional to hypertonia affecting specific muscle group(s); and (e) specification of muscles requiring tone preservation, thereby sparing corresponding dorsal roots/rootlets.

The following is our currently used protocol, as illustrated in an illustrative case in Figs. 11.4, 11.5, 11.6, 11.7, 11.8, 11.9, 11.10, 11.11, 11.12, and 11.13:

1. Initially, each root is electrically stimulated to identify its myotomal innervation region and confirm its topographical level. Anatomical mapping involves stimulation of the ventral root at 2 Hz and 200 μA (in our experience, just above threshold) and, subsequently, stimulation of the dorsal element of the root. If the "believed dorsal" root responds at this low intensity, it suggests inadequate anatomical differentiation between dorsal and ventral roots, necessitating continued microsurgical dissection until no response occurs from dorsal root stimulation at 2 Hz and 200 μA (Fig. 11.14).
2. Next, the dorsal root is meticulously dissected and isolated from the ventral root over 5–10 millimeters and then stimulated to assess its involvement in spinal cord excitability—globally with all its constituting rootlets together. Stimulation is with a train at a frequency of 50 Hz for 1 second and at 1 mA. Duration and spreading of the muscle responses are precisely noted.
3. Excessive excitability is defined by Fasano's calibration, manifested as a sustained, diffuse response to dorsal root stimulation. The amount of rootlets cut per selected dorsal root varies between one-third and four-fifths of the root, three-thirds on average as in most literature series.

11.2.4 Discussion on Quantification of Dorsal Rhizotomy

11.2.4.1 Radicular Resection Strategy

Across various dorsal rhizotomy methodologies, surgical teams typically report resection levels ranging from one-third to four-fifths of the targeted dorsal roots, averaging two-thirds of all dorsal roots. Temporary paresthesias may also manifest particularly after S1/S2 root cutting and predominantly affecting the plantar area,

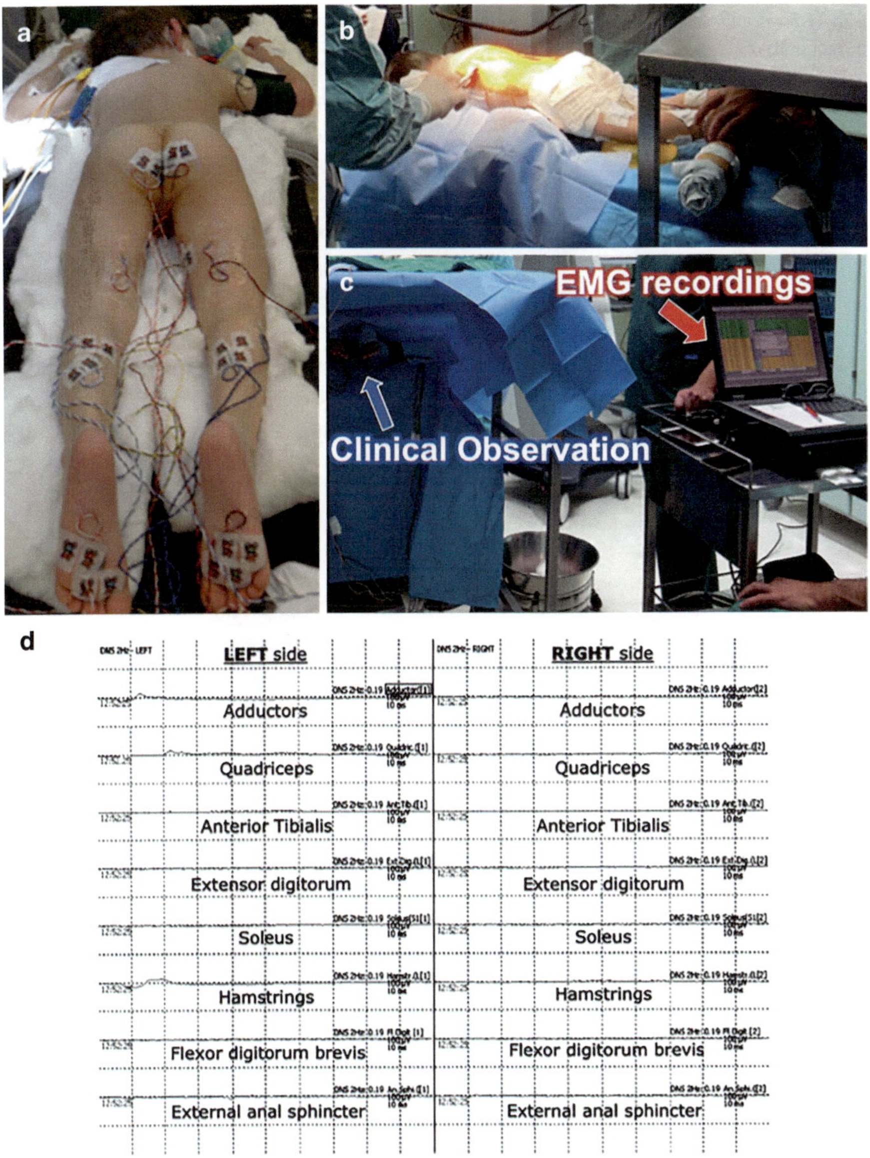

Fig. 11.4 Operating room, installation, and setup. (**a**) Needle electrodes inserted in the seven main muscular groups of both the lower limbs and in the external anal sphincter. (**b**) The child is in prone position. (**c**) The physical therapist should have optimal access to the patient's legs for clinical observation of the muscle responses. Neurophysiologist examines independently EMG responses. (**d**) EMG responses recorded from bipolar needle—electrodes implanted in adductors (for L2–L3 roots), quadriceps (for L3–L4), tibialis anterioris (for L4), extensor digitorum (for L5), soleus (for S1), biceps femoris (for S1–S2), flexor digitorum (for S2), and external anal sphincter (for S2–S3–S4)

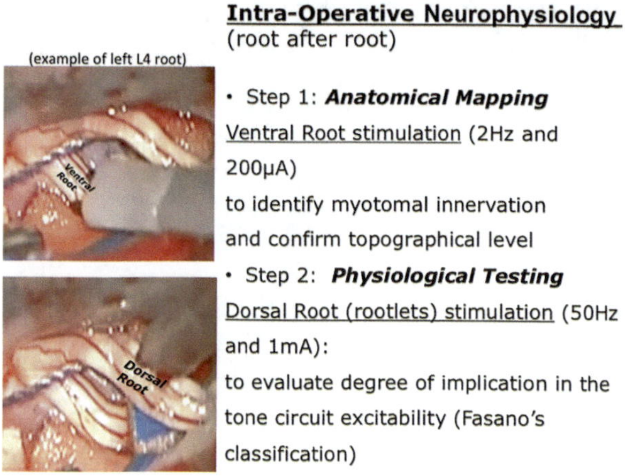

Fig. 11.5 Principles of intraoperative neurophysiology for dorsal rhizotomy (root after root) in two steps. Example of left L4 root

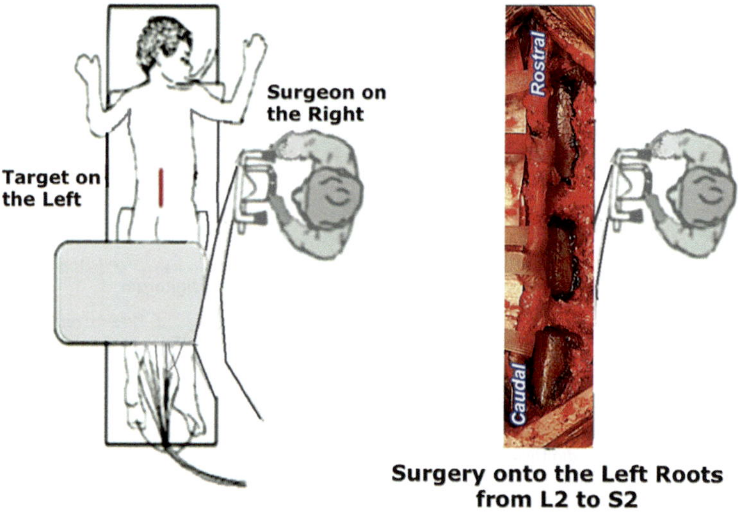

Fig. 11.6 Surgeon is located so that roots be accessed contralaterally, passing obliquely underneath the interspinous ligament. Surgeon with microscope on the right targets the left roots from L2 to S2

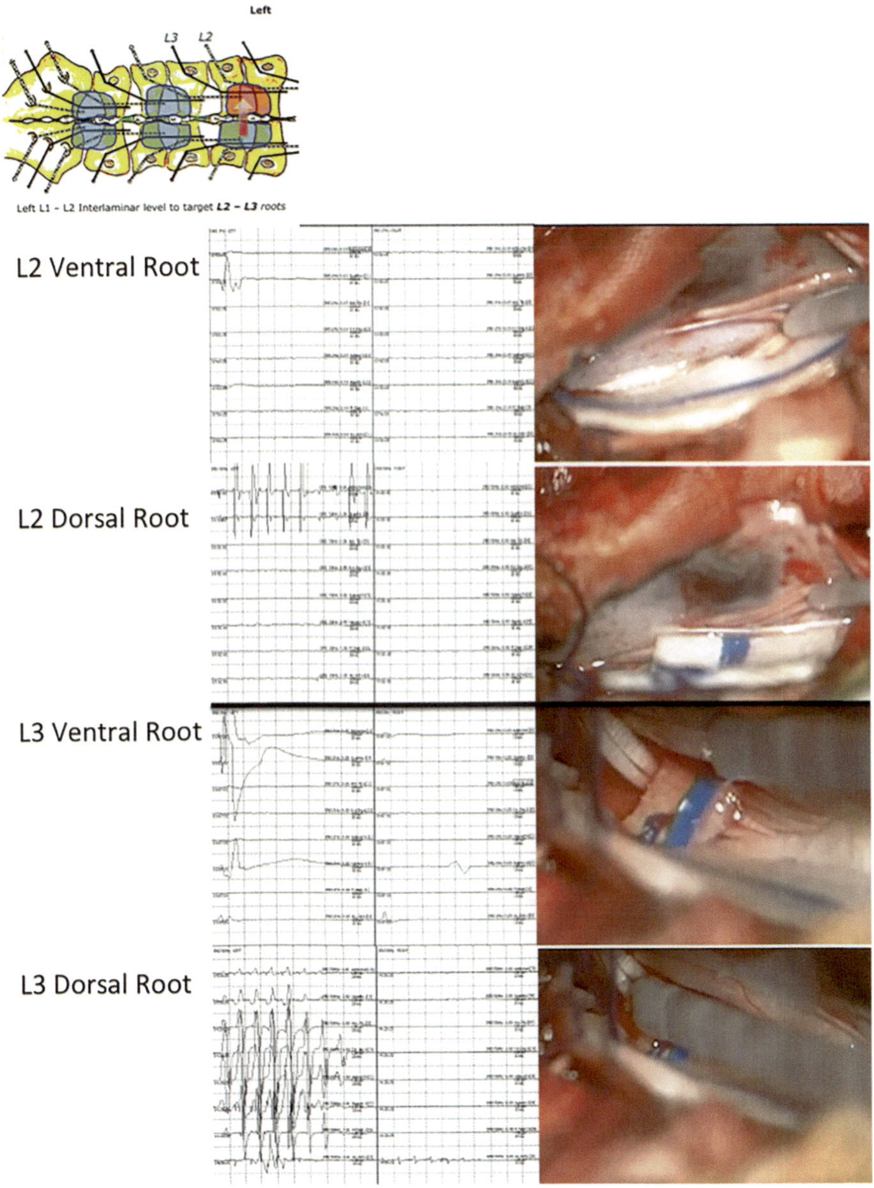

Fig. 11.7 Left L1–L2 interlaminar-level window to target left L2 and L3 roots. EMG recordings: L2 dorsal root Grade 2, sustained squared waveform; L3 dorsal root Grade 3, sustained multiphasic waveform

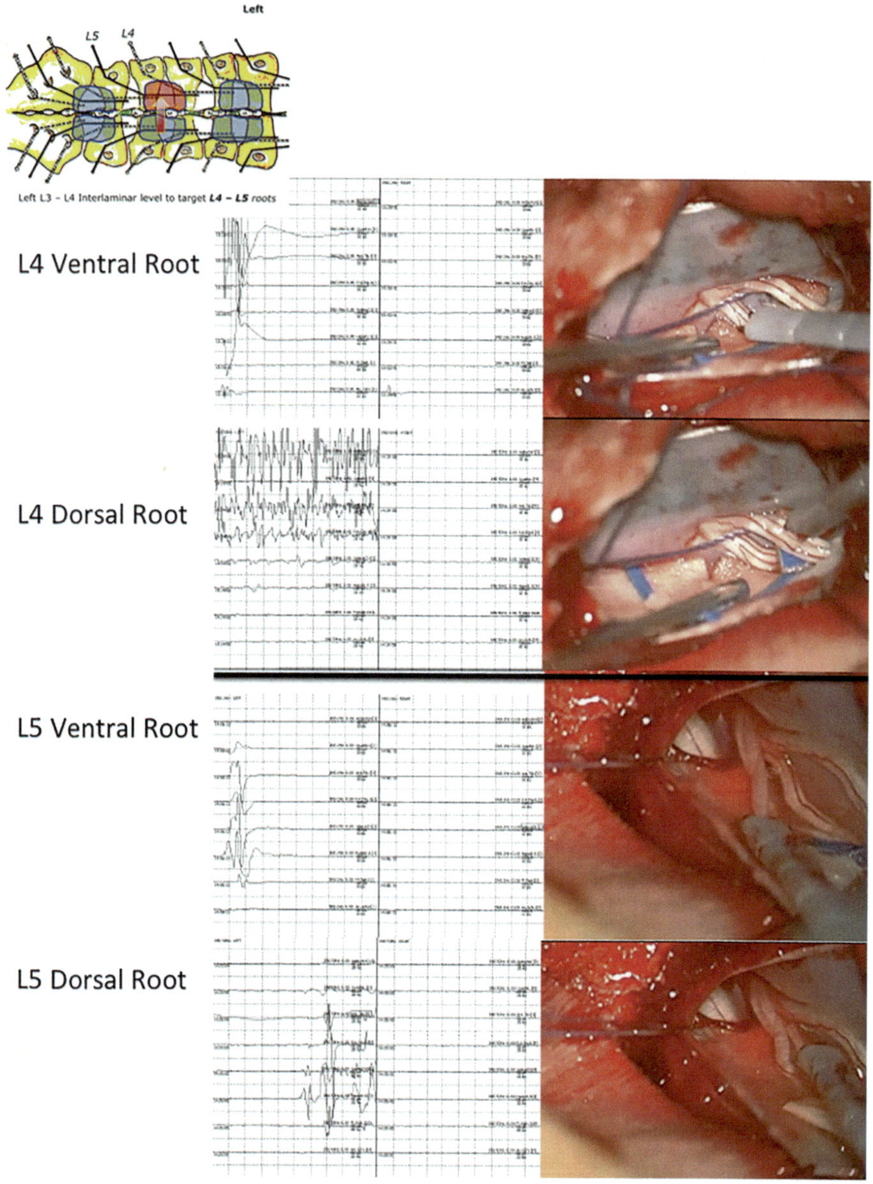

Fig. 11.8 Left L3–L4 interlaminar-level window to target left L4 and L5 roots. EMG recordings: L3 dorsal root Grade 3, sustained multiphasic waveform; L4 dorsal root Grade 3, sustained decremental waveform

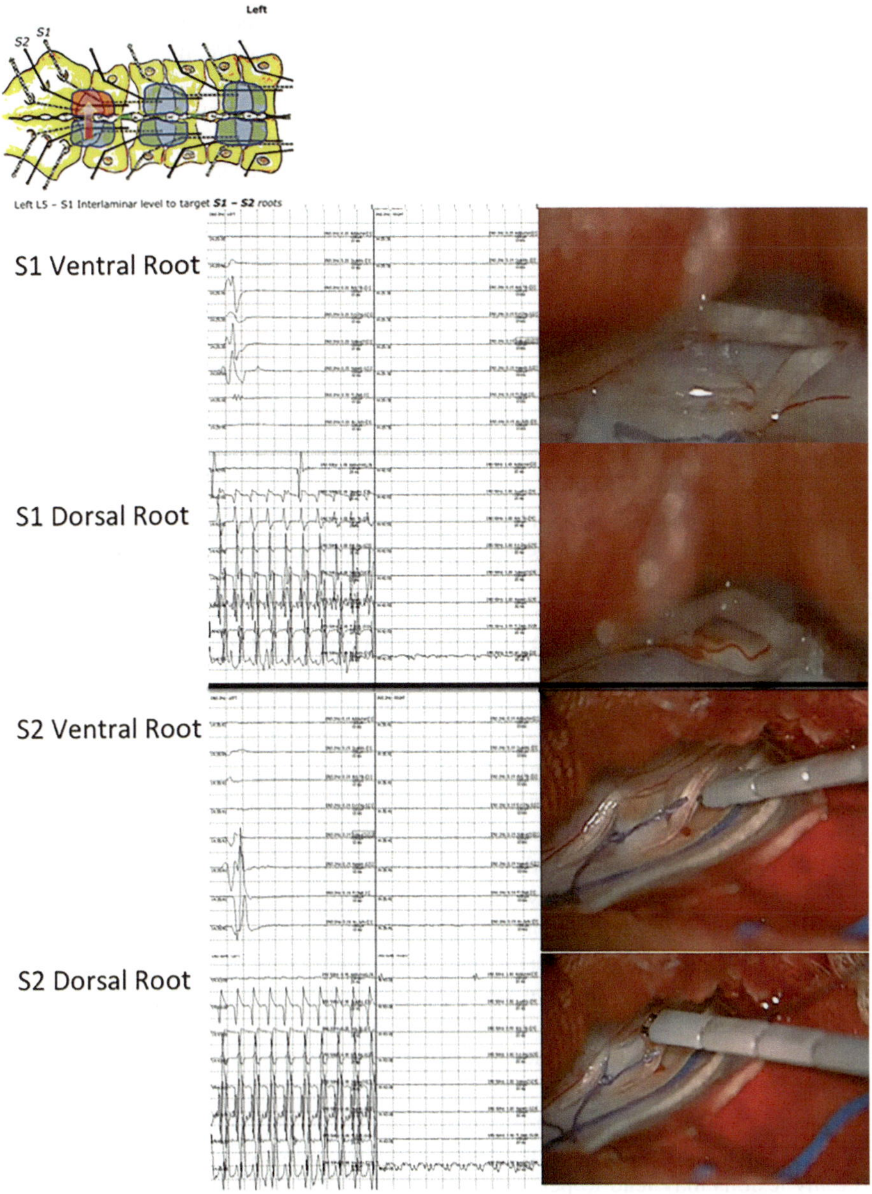

Fig. 11.9 Left L5–S1 interlaminar-level window to target left S1 and S2 roots. EMG recordings: S1 dorsal root Grade 3, sustained squared waveform; S2 dorsal root Grade 3, sustained squared waveform

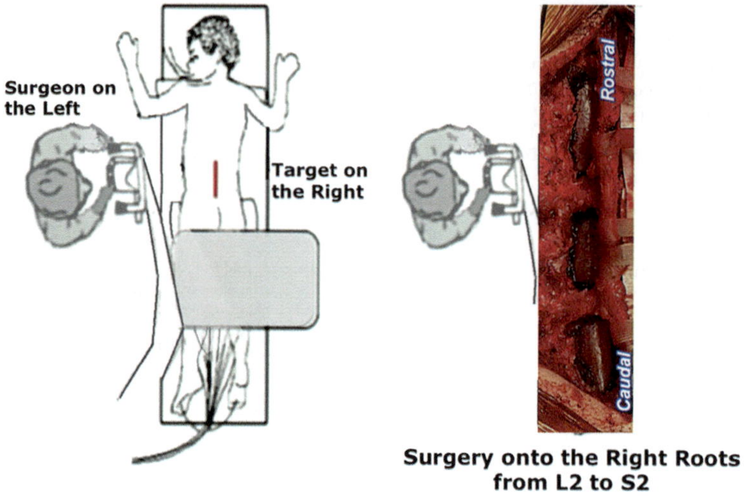

Fig. 11.10 Surgeon is located so that roots be accessed contralaterally, passing obliquely underneath the interspinous ligament. Surgeon with microscope on the left targets the right roots from L2 to S2

most often transient for a couple of weeks. When important, they can be controlled by anticonvulsants, principally clonazepam or pregabalin. Significant sensory pathway resection seldom results in appreciable long-term hypoesthesia [25]. However, neuropathic pain may occur in rare cases due to deafferentation mechanisms.

Empirical root cutting strategies based on segmental myotomal distribution are commonly employed by a majority of surgical teams. Most preoperative planning typically involves reducing L2 and L3 roots (by two-thirds cutting) to address hip and thigh flexion, adduction, and internal rotation. The L4 root, crucial for quadriceps innervation and antigravity function, is usually reduced by no more than a third. Preservation of the L5 root is prioritized to maintain gluteal muscle integrity essential for hip and thigh extension and pelvic stability during standing and walking. S1 root cutting is often set at three-quarters to four-fifths to address gait issues especially equinism. Regarding hamstrings' spasticity, theoretical targets include L5, S1, and S2 roots, although the latter is often spared to avoid compromising bladder and sexual functions.

Studies by Abbott and Deletis et al. underscore the importance of S2 root management [26–28]. Abbott's findings suggest that excluding S2 root from dorsal rhizotomy lesions may lead to persistent spasticity, while inclusion may increase the risk of postoperative genitourinary disorders, mitigated by intraoperative neuromonitoring techniques. Our policy is to involve S2 in the rhizotomy program, when intraoperative neurophysiology confirms involvement, providing cutting does not exceed 50% of rootlets [22].

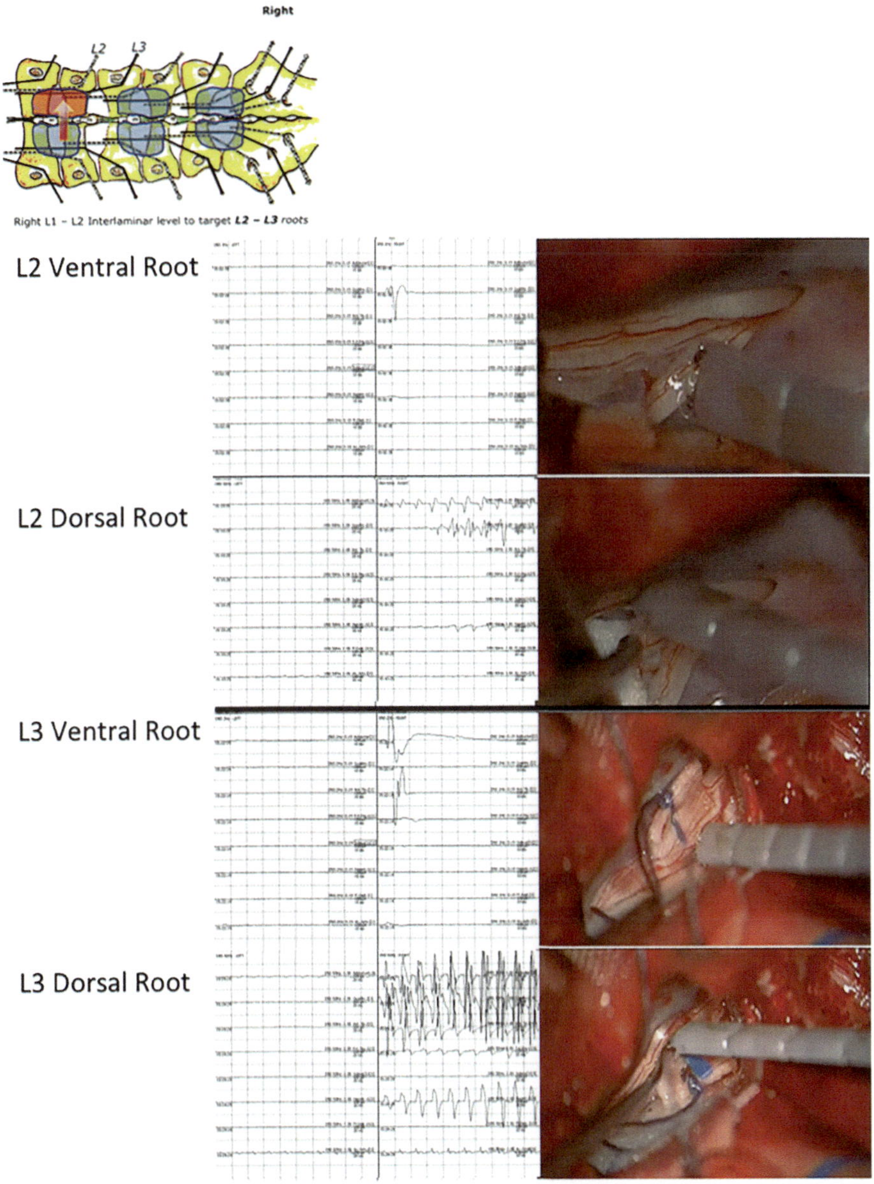

Fig. 11.11 Right L1–L2 interlaminar-level window to target right L2 and L3 roots. EMG recordings: L2 dorsal root Grade 1, sustained waveform; L3 dorsal root Grade 3, sustained incremental waveform

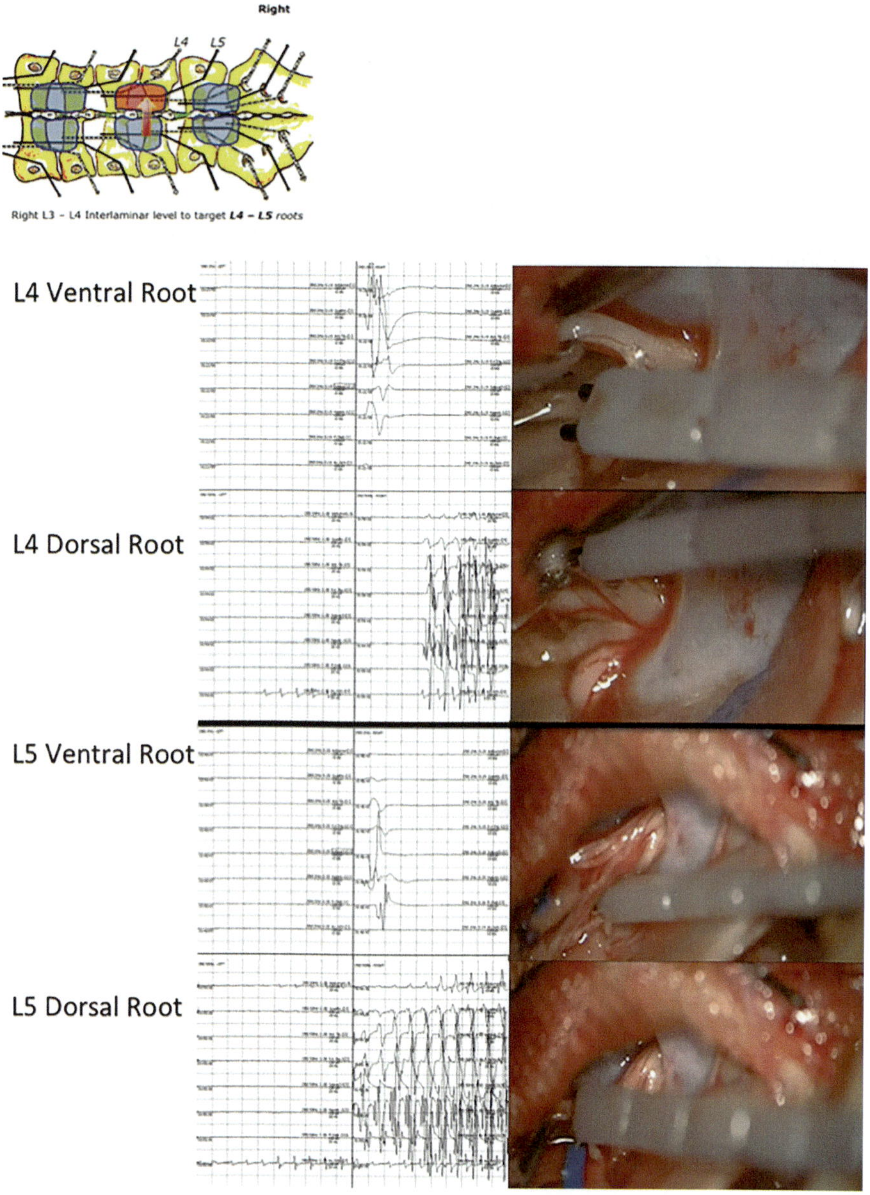

Fig. 11.12 Right L3–L4 interlaminar-level window to target right L4 and L5 roots. EMG recordings: L4 dorsal root Grade 3, sustained multiphasic waveform; L5 dorsal root Grade 3, incremental waveform

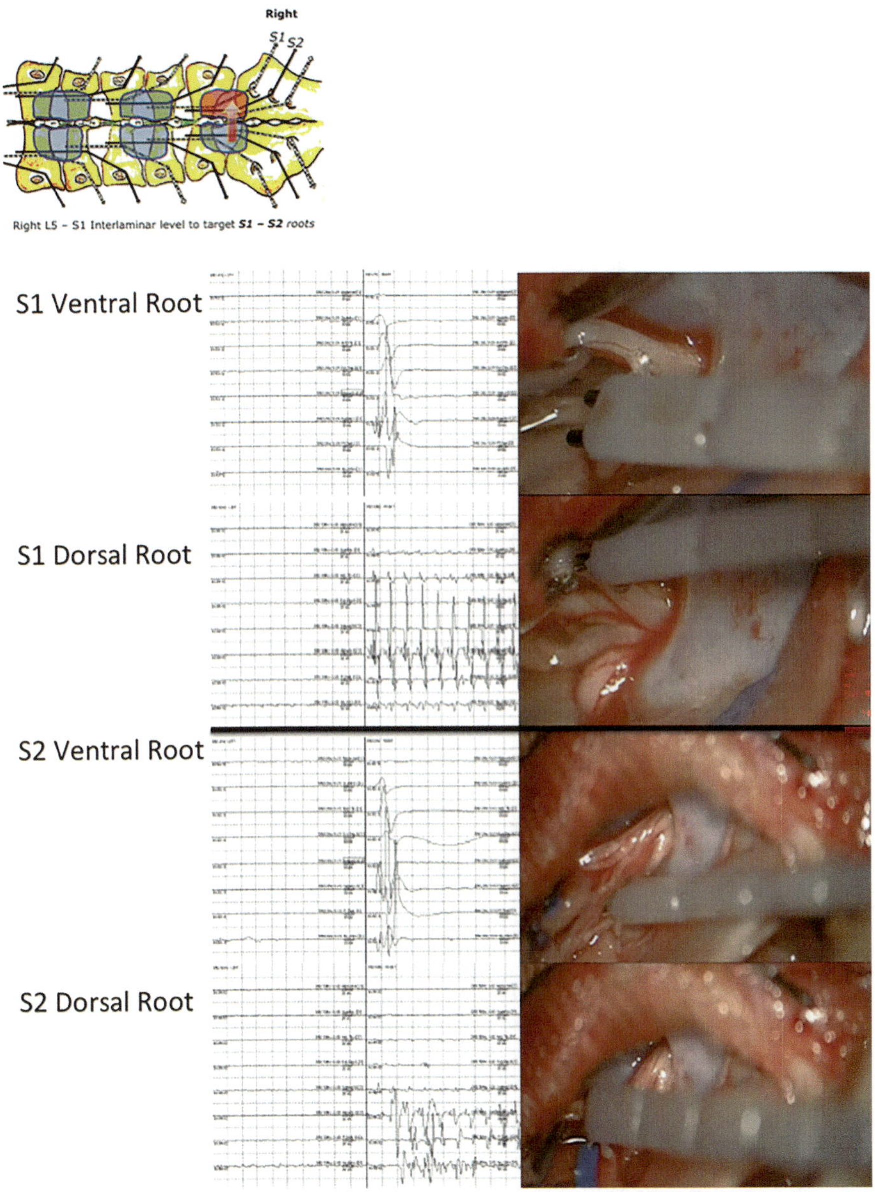

Fig. 11.13 Right L5–S1 interlaminar-level window to target right S1 and S2 roots. EMG recordings: S1 dorsal root Grade 3, decremental waveform; S2 dorsal root Grade 3, irregular waveform

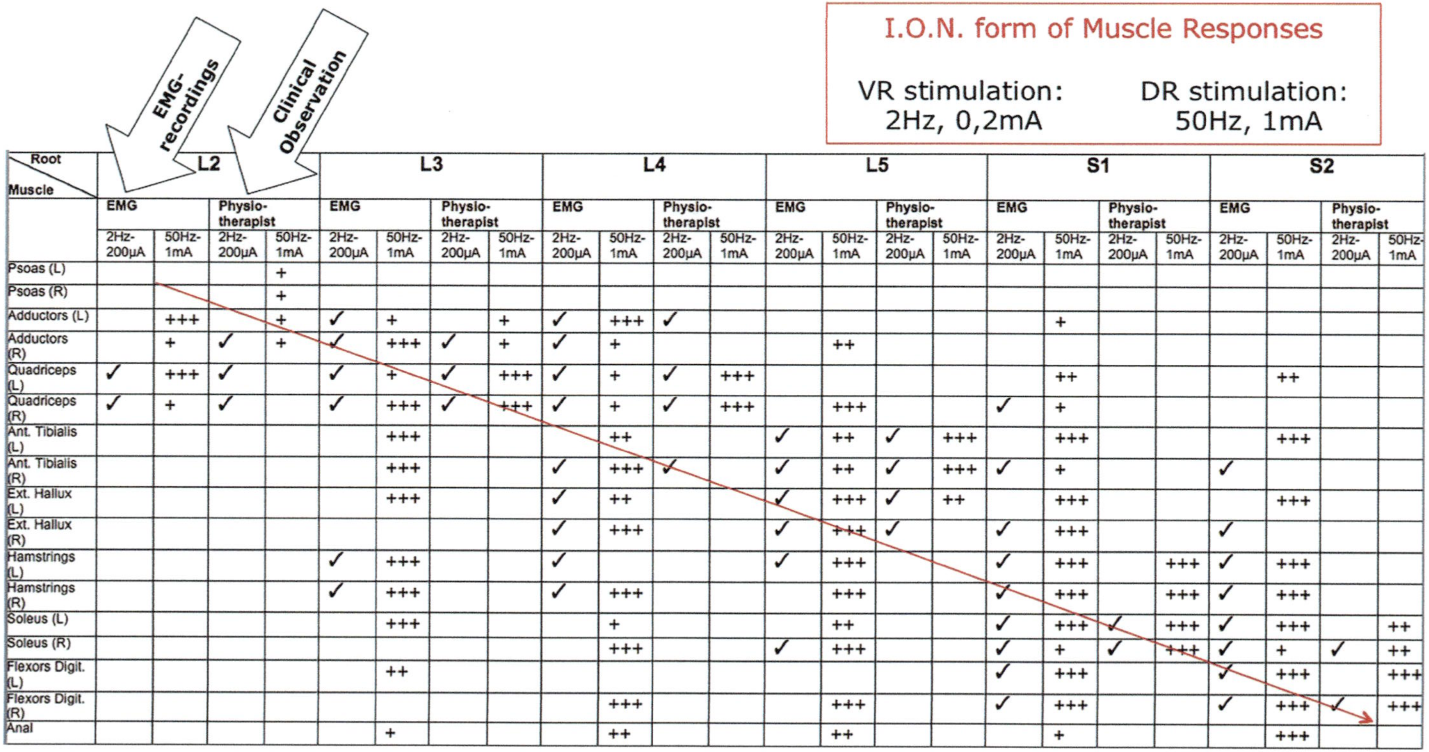

Root / Muscle	L2				L3				L4				L5				S1				S2			
	EMG		Physio-therapist		EMG		Physio-therapist		EMG		Physio-therapist		EMG		Physio-therapist		EMG		Physio-therapist		EMG		Physio-therapist	
	2Hz-200μA	50Hz-1mA	2Hz-200μA	50Hz-1mA	2Hz-200μA	50Hz-1mA	2Hz-200μA	50Hz-1mA	2Hz-200μA	50Hz-1mA	2Hz-200μA	50Hz-1mA	2Hz-200μA	50Hz-1mA	2Hz-200μA	50Hz-1mA	2Hz-200μA	50Hz-1mA	2Hz-200μA	50Hz-1mA	2Hz-200μA	50Hz-1mA	2Hz-200μA	50Hz-1mA
Psoas (L)				+																				
Psoas (R)				+																				
Adductors (L)		+++		+	✓	+		+	✓	+++	✓							+						
Adductors (R)		+	✓	+	✓	+++	✓	+	✓	+				++										
Quadriceps (L)	✓	+++	✓		✓	+	✓	+++	✓	+	✓	+++						++				++		
Quadriceps (R)	✓	+	✓		✓	+++	✓	+++	✓	+	✓	+++		+++			✓	+						
Ant. Tibialis (L)						+++				++			✓	++	✓	+++		+++				+++		
Ant. Tibialis (R)						+++			✓	+++	✓		✓	++	✓	+++	✓	+			✓			
Ext. Hallux (L)						+++			✓	++			✓	+++	✓	++		+++				+++		
Ext. Hallux (R)									✓	+++			✓	+++	✓		✓	+++			✓			
Hamstrings (L)					✓	+++			✓				✓	+++			✓	+++		+++	✓	+++		
Hamstrings (R)					✓	+++			✓	+++				+++			✓	+++		+++	✓	+++		
Soleus (L)						+++				+				++			✓	+++	✓	+++	✓	+++		++
Soleus (R)										+++			✓	+++			✓	+	✓	+++	✓	+	✓	++
Flexors Digit. (L)						++											✓	+++			✓	+++		+++
Flexors Digit. (R)										+++				+++			✓	+++			✓	+++	✓	+++
Anal						+				++				++				+				+++		

Fig. 11.14 Example of a form completed during intraoperative neurophysiologic assessment with muscle responses noted from clinical observation by physiotherapist and from electromyographic recordings. The red oblique arrow indicates the distribution of myotomes, classically aligned with the function of roots

11.2.4.2 Recent Insights and Neurophysiological Studies

Recent neurophysiological studies examining all roots from L2 to S2 during dorsal rhizotomy have yielded valuable insights. Muscle response studies to ventral (and dorsal as well) root stimulation have highlighted multiradicular innervation and interindividual variability in myotomal distribution, supporting intraoperative mapping [14]. Excitability studies in spastic diplegic/tetraplegic patients underscored significant differences in excitability levels across radicular levels, necessitating comprehensive investigation of L2–S2 roots for optimal sectioning ratios [16].

However, the threshold for defining an abnormal response justifying rhizotomy lacks strict physiological standards. Some neurosurgeons advocate for division if a grade 3 or 4 response is elicited, while others adhere strictly to grade 4. Hence, we advocate for both and combined anatomical/topographic mapping of roots based on the preoperative diagram and subsequent electrophysiological testing to quantify rootlet sectioning.

11.2.4.3 Unresolved Issues and Considerations

Currently, the empirical consensus suggests cutting approximately 60% ± 10% of dorsal roots; yet, the precise amount remains contentious. Morota's proposed formula, based on preoperative motor function assessed by GMFM-88 score, offers a reference point for estimating rhizotomy rates, subject to modification based on clinical severity and intraoperative neurophysiology [29]. The ratio of rootlets to be cut per root remains controversial, with some teams basing decisions on clinical spasticity severity and motor distribution, while others rely on muscle response diffusion to dorsal root stimulation.

In summary, the combination of anatomical mapping and physiological control remains our preferred approach, enabling a root-by-root strategy in dorsal rhizotomy planning and execution.

11.3 Indications and Timing

11.3.1 Selection

Before embarking on the selection process, it is essential for all stakeholders involved, from the child's family to caregivers, to align on the therapy's objectives and limitations. These are not the same according to the degree of handicap, categorized in a simplistic form by the Gross Motor Function Classification System (GMFCS). In ambulatory diplegic children, therapy aims to enhance functional status, mobility, and autonomy while preventing or halting deformities. Conversely, for nonambulatory diplegic or quadriplegic children, goals may be more modest, focusing on improving ease of care and comfort and reducing chronic pain. Steinbok emphasizes that reduced hypertonicity or improved range of motion are not the primary goals but rather means to achieve broader objectives [30].

The first step in the selection process is to identify whether hypertonia is the primary impediment to functional status and care or if other issues such as weakness, dystonia, dyskinesia, ataxia, or severe contractures are dominant. When contractures are evident, orthopedic surgery may take precedence or serve as a valuable adjunct to neurosurgery. Significant hypertonia prompts consideration for neurosurgery, particularly dorsal rhizotomy, in children with severe spasticity limiting function and/or complicating care.

11.3.2 Realistic Goals Setting

Realistic goals are pivotal for satisfaction and should be tailored to the child's functional status. For diplegic children capable of walking, surgery aims to enhance the quality of movement and independence, with objectives varying based on the Gross Motor Function Measure (GMFM) level. In severely disabled children, any reduction in spasticity can aid in care, pain reduction, comfort improvement, and prevention of deformities. Lumbosacral dorsal rhizotomies—thanks to its "distant effects"—can significantly ameliorate global and neck-cephalic posture, reduce parasitic movements in the upper limbs, decrease swallowing, and mitigate emotional hyperreactivity, so that it can be indicated in quadriplegic patients.

Objectives shall be clearly explained to the patient and caregivers written down under the form of a "Gain Attainment" project. The Goal Attainment Scale (GAS) assesses functional performance in rehabilitation by focusing on personalized patient goals. It quantifies objectives set by the patient, family, caregivers, and surgeon, prioritizing therapy impact evaluation.

11.3.3 Timing of Surgery

Determining the optimal timing for surgery is challenging, balancing the risk of negatively impacting central nervous system maturation with the potential for irreversible contractures and deformities if delayed. Early intervention may impede

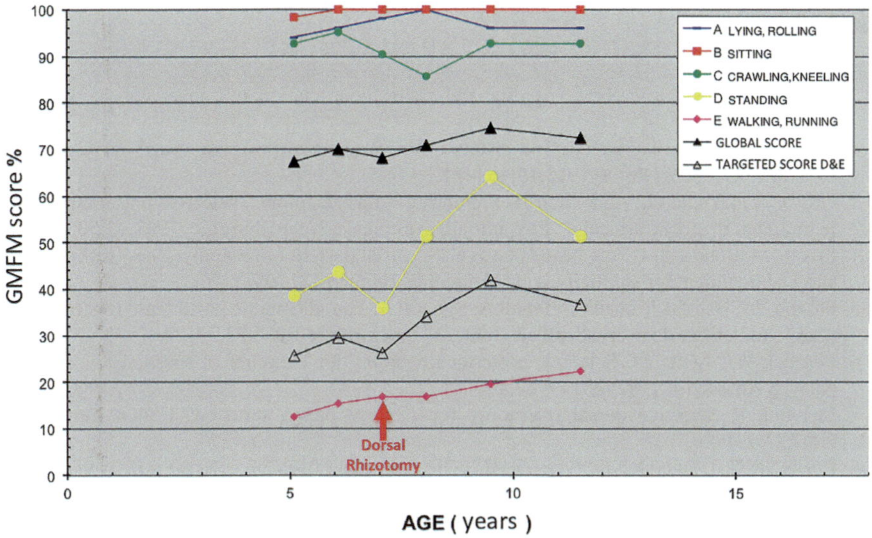

Fig. 11.15 Illustrative example for timing of dorsal rhizotomy. Decision for surgery according to the evolution of the Gross Motor Function Measure (GMFM) score (figure with global and walking scores). Decision for dorsal rhizotomy corresponded to functional "plateau" in GMFM, in spite of conservative treatment. Note that after surgery the GMFM curve shows improvement in targeted and global scores at least 4 years postoperatively

CNS maturation, while delayed intervention will be ineffective on irreversible deformities. Decisions and timing should be multidisciplinary and informed by regular, objective evaluations using tools like the GMFM score, offering insights into motor function ability and progression. The establishment of the GMFM curve does help to indicate, under the form of decrease or even a plateau, the appropriate time for surgery (Fig. 11.15).

11.4 Conclusion

Dorsal rhizotomy emerges as a viable treatment option for children with cerebral palsy, offering significant improvements in spasticity and motor function. Dorsal rhizotomy demands careful patient selection and thorough preoperative evaluation to optimize outcomes and mitigate risks. Long-term follow-up studies underscore its sustained benefits and potential to enhance quality of life for patients with cerebral palsy. As research evolves, collaborative efforts among healthcare professionals, researchers, and patients contribute to a deeper understanding of dorsal rhizotomy's role in the comprehensive management of cerebral palsy. Keyhole Interlaminar Dorsal rhizotomy (KIDr) modality, focusing intradurally to juxtaforaminal zone, allows accurate and selective control of excess tone, with minimal harm to the posterior spine structures.

References

1. Sherrington CS. Decerebrate rigidity and reflex coordination of movements. J Physiol. 1898;22:319–32.
2. Foerster O. On the indications and results of the excision of posterior spinal nerve roots in men. Surg Gynecol Obstet. 1913;16:463–74.
3. Gros C, Ouaknine G, Vlahovitch B, Frèrebeau P. La radicotomie sélective postérieure dans le traitment neurochirurgical de l'hypertonie pyramidale. Neurochirurgie. 1967;13:505–18.
4. Privat JM, Benezech J, Frerebeau P, Gros C. Sectorial posterior rhizotomy, a new technique of surgical treatment for spasticity. Acta Neurochir. 1976;35:181–95.
5. Fasano VA, Barolat-Romana G, Ivaldi A, Sguazzi A. La radicotomie postérieure fonctionnelle dans le traitement de la spasticité cérébrale. Neurochirurgie. 1976;22:23–34.
6. Peacock WJ, Arens LJ. Selective posterior rhizotomy for the relief of spasticity in cerebral palsy. S Afr Med J. 1982;62:119–24.
7. Steinbok P. Selective dorsal rhizotomy for cerebral palsy: a review. Childs Nerv Syst. 2007;23:981–90.
8. Enslin JMN, Langerak NG, Fieggen AG. The evolution of selective dorsal rhizotomy for the management of spasticity. Neurotherapeutics. 2019;16(1):3–8.
9. Warsi NM, Tailor J, Coulter IC, Shakil H, Workewych A, Haldenby R, Breitbart S, Strantzas S, Vandenberk M, Dewan MC, Ibrahim GM. Selective dorsal rhizotomy: an illustrated review of operative techniques. J Neurosurg Pediatr. 2020;7:1–8.
10. Warf BC, Nelson KR. The electromyographic responses to dorsal rootlet stimulation during partial dorsal rhizotomy are inconsistent. Pediatr Neurosurg. 1996;25(1):13–9.
11. Pollack MA. Limited benefit of electrophysiological studies during dorsal rhizotomy. Muscle Nerve. 1994;17(5):553–5.
12. Steinbok P, Keyes R, Langill L, Cochrane DD. The validity of electrophysiological criteria used in selective functional posterior rhizotomy for treatment of spastic cerebral palsy. J Neurosurg. 1994;81(3):354–61.
13. Sindou M, Duraffourg M, Georgoulis G. Neurosurgery for spasticity – a practical guide for treating children and adults. In: Dorsal rhizotomy for children with cerebral palsy. 2nd ed. Springer Nature; 2022. p. 255–84.
14. Georgoulis G, Sindou M. Muscle responses to radicular stimulation during lumbo-sacral dorsal rhizotomy for spastic diplegia: insights to myotome innervation. Clin Neurophysiol. 2020;131(5):1075–86.
15. Fasano VA, Barolat-Romana G, Zeme S, Squazzi A. Electrophysiological assessment of spinal circuits in spasticity by direct dorsal root stimulation. Neurosurgery. 1979;4(2):146–51.
16. Sindou M, Georgoulis G, Joud A, Neromyliotis E, Dinopoulos A. Excitability of the radiculo-medullary circuitry in spastic cerebral palsy: an intraoperative neurophysiological study in children undergoing selective dorsal rhizotomy. Dev Med Child Neurol. 2023;65(1):78–85.
17. Sindou M, Georgoulis G. Keyhole interlaminar dorsal rhizotomy for spastic diplegia in cerebral palsy. Acta Neurochir. 2015;157(7):1187–96.
18. Sindou M, Joud A, Georgoulis G. How I do it: selective dorsal rhizotomy, using interlaminar approaches, for spastic diplegia/quadriplegia in children with cerebral palsy. Acta Neurochir. 2021;163(10):2845–51.
19. Little WJ. On the influence of abnormal parturition, difficult labours, premature birth and asphyxia neonatorum on the mental and physical condition of the child, especially in relation to deformities. Trans Obstet Soc Lond. 1861;3:293–344.
20. Georgoulis G, Brînzeu A, Sindou M. Dorsal rhizotomy for children with spastic diplegia of cerebral palsy origin: usefulness of intraoperative monitoring. J Neurosurg Pediatr. 2018;22(1):89–101.
21. Gros C. Spasticity – clinical classification and surgical treatment. In: Advances and technical standards in neurosurgery. Wien: Springer; 1979.

22. Sindou M, Joud A, Georgoulis G. Usefulness of external anal sphincter EMG recording for intraoperative neuromonitoring of the sacral roots – a prospective study in dorsal rhizotomy. Acta Neurochir. 2021;163(2):479–87.
23. Phillips LH 2nd, Park TS. Electrophysiologic mapping of the segmental anatomy of the muscles of the lower extremity. Muscle Nerve. 1991;14(12):1213–8.
24. Phillips LH, Park TS. Electrophysiologic studies of selective posterior rhizotomy patients. In: Park TS, Phillips LH, Peacock WJ, editors. Management of spasticity in cerebral palsy and spinal cord injury. Neurosurgery: state of the art reviews, vol. 4. Philadelphia: Hanley & Belfus; 1989. p. 459–70.
25. Parise M, Sindou M, Mertens P, Mauguière F. Somatosensory evoked potentials following functional posterior rhizotomy in spastic children. Stereotact Funct Neurosurg. 1997;69(1–4 Pt 2):268–73.
26. Abbott R. Indications for surgery to treat children with spasticity due to cerebral palsy. In: Sindou M, Abbott R, Keravel Y, editors. Neurosurgery for spasticity: a multidisciplinary approach; 1991.
27. Lang FF, Deletis V, Cohen HW, Velasquez L, Abbott R. Inclusion of the S2 dorsal rootlets in functional posterior rhizotomy for spasticity in children with cerebral palsy. Neurosurgery. 1994;34(5):847–53.
28. Deletis V, Vodusek DB, Abbott R, Epstein FJ, Turndorf H. Intraoperative monitoring of the dorsal sacral roots: minimizing the risk of iatrogenic micturition disorders. Neurosurgery. 1992;30:72–5.
29. Morota N. Clinically practical formula for preoperatively estimating the cutting rate of the spinal nerve root in a functional posterior rhizotomy. Childs Nerv Syst. 2019;35(4):665–72.
30. Ailon T, Beauchamp R, Miller S, Mortenson P, Kerr JM, Hengel AR, Steinbok P. Long-term outcome after selective dorsal rhizotomy in children with spastic cerebral palsy. Childs Nerv Syst. 2015;31(3):415–23.

Chapter 12
Selective Dorsal Rhizotomy: What, When, and Why to Cut

Federico Bianchi, Giuliano Di Monaco, and Gianpiero Tamburrini

12.1 Introduction

Since its advent and application in the early 1900s, the surgical technique of selective dorsal rhizotomy (SDR) has undergone a nuanced evolution. Several refinements mark the continuous enhancement in methodology as well as a substantial reduction in postoperative complications. In particular, the aforementioned evolution involves the selection criteria for root or rootlet cut. In this context, the incorporation of intraoperative neurophysiological monitoring (IONM) represents the major innovation, allowing for real-time assessment and adjustments during the surgical procedure.

Nonetheless, there remains a lack of consensus on a standardized procedure secondary to the very multifaceted nature of spasticity and patients' individual variability. In this chapter, the authors aim to discuss root and rootlet selection criteria and technique for SDR.

F. Bianchi (✉)
Pediatric Neurosurgery, Fondazione Policlinico Agostino Gemelli IRCCS, Rome, Italy
e-mail: federico.bianchi@policlinicogemelli.it

G. Di Monaco
Università Cattolica del Sacro Cuore, Rome, Italy

G. Tamburrini
Pediatric Neurosurgery, Fondazione Policlinico Agostino Gemelli IRCCS, Rome, Italy

Università Cattolica del Sacro Cuore, Milan, Italy
e-mail: gianpiero.tamburrini@unicatt.it

N. Morota, P. Steinbok (eds.), *Dorsal Rhizotomy: Neurosurgery for Childhood Spasticity*, Advances and Technical Standards in Neurosurgery 51,
https://doi.org/10.1007/978-3-031-86441-4_12

12.2 Electrophysiological Background

To understand how to choose the proportion of rootlets to cut, gaining insight into the electrophysiological background of spasticity and intraoperative stimulation is paramount.

Whenever there is CNS damage, nerve cell membranes tend to remain in a more depolarized state, and the normal inhibitory network is impaired, favoring excitation and consequently increasing nerve excitability. This combination decreases action potential thresholds, leading to increased activity of structures innervated by the affected nerves. The described imbalance between excitatory and inhibitory input to α motor neurons results in increased muscle excitability, causing spasticity [1–3].

In light of these notions, SDR aims to interrupt this short circuit, restoring lost balance. Pivotal to the diffusion of SDR is the 1976 report by Fasano and colleagues, wherein they postulated the possibility of evaluating the loss of suprasegmental inhibition on the alpha-gamma muscle loop through stimulation using a train of stimuli [1]. This discovery led to the definition of several surgical techniques that evolved over the years. The more commonly used techniques are those proposed by Peacock in 1982, which center on the cauda equina (L2–L5 laminectomy), and Park's method, which focuses on the conus (single-level laminectomy) [4, 5].

Furthermore, the previously described techniques slowly evolved toward less invasive surgeries, further complicating anatomical-only rootlet differentiation and stressing the importance of IONM.

12.3 Root Selection

Transitioning to the selection of rootlets, IONM now stands as the gold standard for defining surgical targets. There are two major areas of interest here: discharge pattern and percentage of resected rootlets.

Discharge pattern represents the more commonly employed method of selecting surgical targets. In fact, both Peacock's and Park's approaches substantially align on the criteria for selecting roots/rootlets for severance, primarily grounded in the electrophysiological studies conducted by Fasano. To identify pathological rootlets, the surgeon has to test their elicitability one by one. For this reason, it is common to divide roots into three to ten rootlets and probe them using single stimuli lasting 0.1 ms at a rate of 0.5 Hz. Such stimulation facilitates the identification of each rootlet's muscular contraction threshold. Subsequently, the surgeon administers 50 Hz trains of stimuli through a bipolar electrode to the rootlet for 1 s, gradually increasing intensity until a response is obtained.

Pathological rootlets might present the following abnormal patterns:

1. Abnormalities in threshold response to the single stimulus.
2. Presence of sustained discharges during stimulus train.

3. Presence of pathological spread of the response to ipsilateral or contralateral muscle groups distant from the stimulated segment.

SDR Reflex Grading Criteria regroup those considerations, facilitating the differentiation of stimulation responses into five grades, ranging from 0 to 4+ (Table 12.1) [4, 6].

Rootlets graded as 0 exhibit either a nonsustained or a single discharge to the train of stimuli and are considered healthy and unaffected. Rootlets graded as 3+ and 4+ respond to stimuli with sustained discharges from ipsilateral muscles distant from the stimulated segment or contralateral muscles, suggesting pathology and warranting excision. Rootlets with intermediate responses, specifically 1+ and 2+, respond with sustained discharges but from muscles directly innervated by the stimulated segment or directly adjacent to it and are typically unaffected unless there are rootlets for that segment with a response grade of 3+ or 4+ (Fig. 12.1) [4, 6].

Another notable parameter to consider is the H-reflex study, specifically the H-reflex recovery curve. Under normal conditions, stimulation of sensitive dorsal fibers elicits a motor response through the H-reflex. However, this response tends to diminish due to descending inhibitory control on the interneurons governing it. In pathological conditions, this inhibitory response is absent. Consequently, the refractory period of the H-reflex's interneurons is shorter. By studying the ratio between the second and first H-reflex obtained (H2/H1 ratio), it is possible to identify pathological roots where this ratio exceeds 50% at all stimulation frequencies [7, 8].

As previously mentioned, an alternative method for selecting rootlets for excision involves determining the actual percentage of rootlets to be resected at each level. Despite the possibility of defining a cutting percentage, there is no unanimous consensus in the literature on the matter, with cutting percentages varying widely from 15% to 85%. Most authors concur that a preoperative multidisciplinary approach is imperative to set realistic treatment goals and tailor the procedure to each patient's unique characteristics [9, 10].

Several authors have posited a correlation between cutting percentage and preoperative motor function, as well as spasticity degree. The underlying principle suggests that children with severe spasticity and limited motor function may require a higher cutting percentage compared to those with mild spasticity and more

Table 12.1 SDR Reflex Grading Criteria

Grade	EMG response
0	Unsustained or single discharge to a train of stimuli
1+	Sustained discharges from muscles innervated trough the segment stimulated in the ipsilateral lower extremity
2+	Sustained discharges from muscles innervated trough the segment stimulated and immediately adjacent segments
3+	Sustained discharges from segmentally innervated muscles and muscles innervated trough segments distant to the segment stimulated
4+	Sustained discharges from contralateral muscles with or without sustained discharges from the ipsilateral muscles

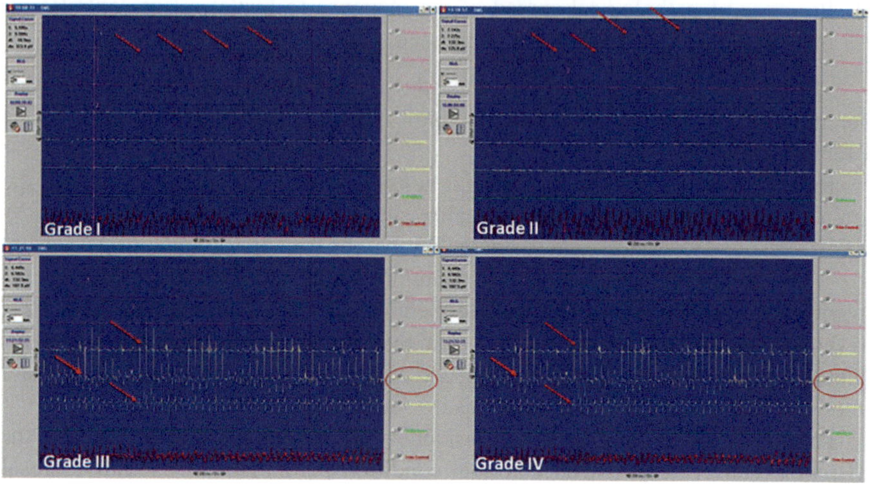

Fig. 12.1 EMG response grading according to single rootlet bipolar stimulation. Grades I and II show an example of quadriceps response in both legs highlighting the difference depending from rootlet anomaly. Grades III and IV show the same kind of difference in the hamstring bilaterally depicting aberrant stimulus diffusion

preserved preoperative motor function. Thus, the need for a standardized method for assessing spasticity and motor function has led to the definition and use of grading scales such as the Gross Motor Function Measure (GMFM) score and the Gross Motor Function Classification System (GMFCS) [11, 12].

One of the more interesting papers analyzing the relation between cutting percentage and spasticity degree is the one from Morota et al. In this study, the authors reviewed a personal series of 137 children with cerebral palsy treated with SDR, demonstrating a negative correlation between the cutting rate of the posterior root and preoperative motor function assessed by the GMFM. Additionally, the study derived a formula for calculating cutting percentage based on preoperative GMFM scores: $y = -0.5539x + 73.896$ (where x = GMFM score; = overall cutting percentage). Consistent with previous studies, Morota et al. confirmed that the percentage of cut rootlets increased in tandem with the GMFCS level, ranging from 17% to 30% in children with GMFCS level I to 49–83% in cases with GMFCS level V [12]. Interestingly, other studies highlighted the impact of additional, non-electrophysiological factors such as gender, body side (left- or right-biased asymmetry), and reference level, in influencing and predicting the degree of intraoperative EMG response. One study revealed a higher-graded EMG response being more frequent in boys and at lower segmental levels (L5 and S1), with a prevalence of left-biased asymmetry in higher-graded rootlets observed in the male population [13].

Even though IOM represents a gold standard adjuvant technique, these considerations might somehow lessen its significance. Indeed, several authors have cast doubt on the imperative necessity of IONM during surgery [14, 15]. Notably, a somewhat provocative study by Steinbok et al. in 2009, involving 22 children undergoing SDR, demonstrated that at a 1-year follow-up, no statistically significant differences persisted in terms of complications or outcome measures between the group undergoing SDR with intraoperative monitoring and the group treated without electrophysiological guidance. The study highlighted that the percentage of rootlet cutting was comparable between the two groups and the absence of IOM led to a reduction in operative time and associated complications. A closer look at this study shows that the author's intention wasn't to downplay the importance of intraoperative monitoring. Instead, they aimed to promote selective dorsal rhizotomy as a treatment for children with cerebral palsy, even in centers and regions where intraoperative monitoring is unavailable. This study, in fact, demonstrated that with meticulous preoperative study and the acquisition of substantial neurosurgical experience, the technique could yield favorable clinical results even in the absence of electrophysiological guidance [15].

Analyzing the whole literature on the subject, it is evident that a combination of IONM usage and anatomical cutting percentage could present the most effective method for achieving optimal surgical outcomes. Notably, a paper by Georgoulis, Brînzeu, and Sindou highlighted that the use of IONM resulted in differences in the final percentage of root sectioning for all root levels. According to the authors, it led to a decrease in the percentage of dorsal root sectioning for roots L2 and L3 and an increase for roots L4 and L5, compared to predictions based on the preoperative study, highlighting that IONM significantly contributed to adapting SDR to the clinical presentation and therapeutic goals of each patient [16].

Having defined how preoperative planning and IOM might affect the variability of dorsal root sectioning, it is worth mentioning that it is possible to underline level-specific consideration (Table 12.1). L2–L3 roots, innervating iliopsoas muscles, abductors, and part of the quadriceps femoris, are responsible for controlling hip and thigh flexion, adduction, internal rotation, and knee extension. These roots are often excised up to about two-thirds due to their crucial role in determining spasticity. L4 rootlet excision encloses up to a maximum of one-third of the rootlet, unless there is patella ascension, given their key role in innervating the femoral quadriceps and, consequently, maintaining upright posture and ambulation. Similarly, the L5 root, crucial for hip stability and its antigravity function, is often excised up to a maximum of one-third. Finally, the S1 root is excised up to three- to four-fifths, especially in cases of equinus or varus foot [17] (Table 12.2).

The case is different for the S2 root, historically unaffected by Peacock's approach due to its role in controlling urinary function. However, the S2 root is also involved in the reflex arcs of the plantar flexors (PFs), prompting consideration of its rhizotomy in the presence of claw toes. S2 rootlet lesioning again relies on IONM, particularly on a technique known as the "pudendal neurogram," previously employed to avoid bladder dysfunction during the sectioning of sacral roots. The technique involves testing the cutaneous branches of the pudendal nerve that innervate the dorsal surface of the penis or the clitoris (the dorsal penile or clitoral nerve). The surgeon can divide the rootlets further if stimulating a pathological one activates pudendal dorsal root action potentials while ensuring roots essential for

Table 12.2 Cutting percentage for each root level

Rootlets	Innervated muscles	Function	Cutting percentage
L2–L3	Iliopsoas muscles, abductors, and part of the quadriceps femoris	Hip and thigh flexion, adduction, internal rotation, and knee extension	Up to two-thirds
L4	Femoral quadriceps	Maintaining upright posture and ambulation	Up to one-thirds
L5	Tibialis anterior, extensor hallucis longus, extensor digitorum brevis, and the lateral head of gastrocnemius	Hip stability and its antigravity function	Up to one-thirds
S1	Biceps femoris, semimembranosus, semitendinosus, and the ischial portion of the adductor magnus	Knee flexion and hip adduction	Three- to four-fifths
S2	Plantar flexors	Genitourinary function and plantar flexion	Variable depending from IONM

vegetative functions are preserved. This modification significantly reduces long-term bowel or bladder complications and safeguards fibers crucial for sexual function, translating into a 71% reduction in the number of patients with residual PF spasticity [18, 19].

12.4 Conclusion

SRD represents a powerful tool in spasticity treatment. Identifying surgical targets to cut is the crucial step in procedures relying primarily on IONM. Nonetheless, careful preoperative planning can mitigate the need for IOM when it is unavailable.

Acknowledgement None.

Conflict of Interest None.

References

1. Fasano VA, Barolat-Romana G, Ivaldi A, Sguazzi A. Functional posterior radiculotomy, in the treatment of cerebral spasticity. peroperative electric stimulation of posterior roots and its use in the choice of the roots to be sectioned. Neurochirurgie. 1976;22(1):23–34.
2. Gros C, Ouaknine G, Vlahovitch B, Frèrebeau P. Selective posterior radicotomy in the neurosurgical treatment of pyramidal hypertension. Neurochirurgie. 1967;13(4):505–18.
3. Pasquali C, Deletis V, Sala F. Selective dorsal rhizotomy: functional anatomy of the conus-cauda and essentials of intraoperative neurophysiology. Childs Nerv Syst. 2020;36(9):1907–18.

4. Park TS, Johnston JM. Surgical techniques of selective dorsal rhizotomy for spastic cerebral palsy. Neurosurg Focus. 2006;21(2):e7.
5. Peacock WJ, Staudt LA. Selective posterior rhizotomy: evolution of theory and practice. Pediatr Neurosurg. 1991;17(3):128–34.
6. Phillips LH, Park TS. Electrophysiological studies of selective posterior rhizotomy patients. In: Neurosurgery: state of the art reviews 4. Management of spasticity in cerebral palsy and spinal cord injury. Philadelphia: Hanley and Belfus; 1989. p. 459–69.
7. Logigian EL, Wolinsky JS, Soriano SG, Madsen JR, Scott RM. H reflex studies in cerebral palsy patients undergoing partial dorsal rhizotomy. Muscle Nerve. 1994;17(5):539–49.
8. Storrs BB, Nishida T. Use of the "H" reflex recovery curve in selective posterior rhizotomy. Pediatr Neurosci. 1988;14(3):120–3.
9. McLaughlin J, Bjornson K, Temkin N, et al. Selective dorsal rhizotomy: meta-analysis of three randomized controlled trials. Dev Med Child Neurol. 2002;44(1):17–25.
10. Steinbok P. Selective dorsal rhizotomy for spastic cerebral palsy: a review. Childs Nerv Syst. 2007;23(9):981–90.
11. Graham D, Aquilina K, Mankad K, Wimalasundera N. Selective dorsal rhizotomy: current state of practice and the role of imaging. Quant Imaging Med Surg. 2018;8(2):209–18.
12. Morota N. Clinically practical formula for preoperatively estimating the cutting rate of the spinal nerve root in a functional posterior rhizotomy. Childs Nerv Syst. 2019;35(4):665–72.
13. Wolter S, Haberl H, Spies C, et al. Frequency distribution in intraoperative stimulation-evoked EMG responses during selective dorsal rhizotomy in children with cerebral palsy-part 2: gender differences and left-biased asymmetry. Childs Nerv Syst. 2020;36(9):1955–65.
14. Hays RM, McLaughlin JF, Bjornson KF, Stephens K, Roberts TS, Price R. Electrophysiological monitoring during selective dorsal rhizotomy, and spasticity and GMFM performance. Dev Med Child Neurol. 1998;40(4):233–8.
15. Steinbok P, Tidemann AJ, Miller S, Mortenson P, Bowen-Roberts T. Electrophysiologically guided versus non-electrophysiologically guided selective dorsal rhizotomy for spastic cerebral palsy: a comparison of outcomes. Childs Nerv Syst. 2009;25(9):1091–6.
16. Georgoulis G, Brînzeu A, Sindou M. Dorsal rhizotomy for children with spastic diplegia of cerebral palsy origin: usefulness of intraoperative monitoring. J Neurosurg Pediatr. 2018;22(1):89–101.
17. Sindou M. Surgery in the dorsal root entry zone for spasticity. In: Textbook of stereotactic and functional neurosurgery. Berlin: Springer; 2019. p. 1–26.
18. Huang MH, Mouradian WE, Cohen SR, Gruss JS. The differential diagnosis of abnormal head shapes: separating craniosynostosis from positional deformities and normal variants. Cleft Palate-Craniofacial J. 1998;35(3):204–11.
19. Lang FF, Deletis V, Cohen HW, Velasquez L, Abbott R. Inclusion of the S2 dorsal rootlets in functional posterior rhizotomy for spasticity in children with cerebral palsy. Neurosurgery. 1994;34(5):847–53.

Chapter 13
Functional Posterior Rhizotomy with the Use of Intraoperative Neurophysiology

Nobuhito Morota

Abbreviations

cMAP	Compound muscle action potential
DAP	Dorsal action potential
FPR	Functional posterior rhizotomy
GMFCS	Gross Motor Function Classification System
GMFM	Gross Motor Function Measurement
ION	Intraoperative neurophysiology

13.1 Introduction

Intraoperative neurophysiology (ION) plays critical role in dorsal rhizotomy as a surgery for spasticity. ION in general consists in intraoperative neurophysiological monitoring and mapping. ION mapping of the root/rootlet constitutes a major ION procedure during dorsal rhizotomy. Delivering electrical stimulation, surgeons evaluate the degree of abnormality in the root/rootlet, enabling informed decisions on which roots/rootlets to be cut selectively and functionally for spasticity reduction.

Reflecting on the history of dorsal rhizotomy, the first surgery took place over 130 years ago, as conducted by Abbe [1]. Foerster, in 1908, pioneered the application of dorsal rhizotomy for reducing spasticity. In his 1913 paper, he underscores key insights: [1] surgical outcomes were unfavorable in patients with athetosis; [2] surgery could reduce spasticity, and long-term rehabilitation was essential for motor

N. Morota (✉)
Department of Neurosurgery, Kitasato University Hospital, Minami-Ku, Sagamihara, Japan

N. Morota, P. Steinbok (eds.), *Dorsal Rhizotomy: Neurosurgery for Childhood Spasticity*, Advances and Technical Standards in Neurosurgery 51,
https://doi.org/10.1007/978-3-031-86441-4_13

improvement; and [3] preservation of the fourth lumbar root was recommended to maintain truncal support. Notably, Foerster advocated for the use of electrical stimulation to discern the spinal level of the root, acknowledging the wide variability among individuals [2]. It should be remembered that he had already incorporated ION monitoring into his dorsal rhizotomy procedure more than a century ago, ensuring the safety of the surgical process.

In the late 1970s, Fasano played a pivotal role in revitalizing dorsal rhizotomy [3–5]. He introduced what we call the modern ION procedure in dorsal rhizotomy, by incorporating tetanic 50 Hz electrical stimulation. He classified the electromyographic (EMG) response to assess the abnormality of root/rootlet, providing guidance to decide whether to cut or preserve the root/rootlet [3–5]. Subsequently, Peacock modified Fasano's surgical procedure in the 1980s by relocating the surgical field from the conus medullaris to the cauda equina [6, 7]. This modification significantly contributed to the widespread adoption of the procedure, as it ensured safety and facilitated the precise identification of the spinal level of the lumbar root, along with distinguishing between dorsal and ventral roots. In the early 1990s, Park reverted the surgical field to the conus medullaris with the use of the microscope [8, 9]. Phillips and Park further refined Fasano's EMG classification by introducing a grading system [10]. Concurrently, during this resurgence of dorsal rhizotomy, Deletis developed the pudendal mapping technique as an ION procedure to avoid urinary complications associated with dorsal rhizotomy [11].

The significant role of ION as an indispensable tool in dorsal rhizotomy for spasticity has been well-established and recognized [12–18]. The anticipated validity of ION in dorsal rhizotomy encompasses its ability to [1] identify the root/rootlet to be cut for spasticity reduction, [2] differentiate between dorsal and ventral roots, and [3] preserve urinary function. However, despite these recognized roles, there exist controversies, and a universally acknowledged standard for the application of ION in dorsal rhizotomy is lacking [19–23]. Furthermore, there is currently no ION procedure providing evidence of reduced spasticity following root/rootlet cutting during the surgery.

In this chapter, the author delineates his practice of dorsal rhizotomy and the application ION during the surgery. The emphasis is placed on elucidating the neurophysiological concept for distinguishing the root/rootlet to be cut to alleviate spasticity, in conjunction with the utilization of pudendal mapping to prevent urological complications after dorsal rhizotomy. Additionally, a novel concept validating the adequacy of root/rootlet cutting for spasticity reduction using the F-wave is discussed [24–28].

The author designated the dorsal rhizotomy incorporating full use of ION as functional posterior rhizotomy (FPR) in this chapter. This nomenclature is employed because the application of ION in dorsal rhizotomy extends beyond mere selection of roots/rootlets for excision; rather, it represents a functionally oriented rhizotomy guided by ION [29].

13.2 Surgical Procedure

Surgical procedures of FPR can be classified into two main categories [30] (Fig. 13.1). The first category involves surgery at the conus medullaris, originally described by Fasano and later modified by Park using a microscope [3–5, 8, 9]. The second category comprises surgery at the cauda equina, as introduced by Peacock [6, 7]. This category is further subdivided into the standard procedure, involving L2–L5 osteoplastic laminotomy and S1 (-S2) laminectomy, and the limited procedure, involving L4–L5 osteoplastic laminotomy and S1 (-S2) laminectomy [31]. Sindou added a less invasive procedure called interlaminal approach to the cauda equina [32], which is described in detail in Chap. 13.

The author employs FPR using Peacock's procedure because it offers direct visualization of the spinal level of the root and the dorsal root from the ventral one [14, 15]. The standard procedure is implemented for children exhibiting a moderate to severe degree of spasticity, extending to the hip joint (GMFCS levels 3–5). The limited procedure is applied for children with mild to moderate degree of spasticity, which usually affects predominantly the ankle joint (GMFCS levels 1–3). The rostral end of the lumbar spine level for the osteoplastic laminotomy is L2 and L4, respectively. It is one level caudal to the original procedures. The caudal end of the

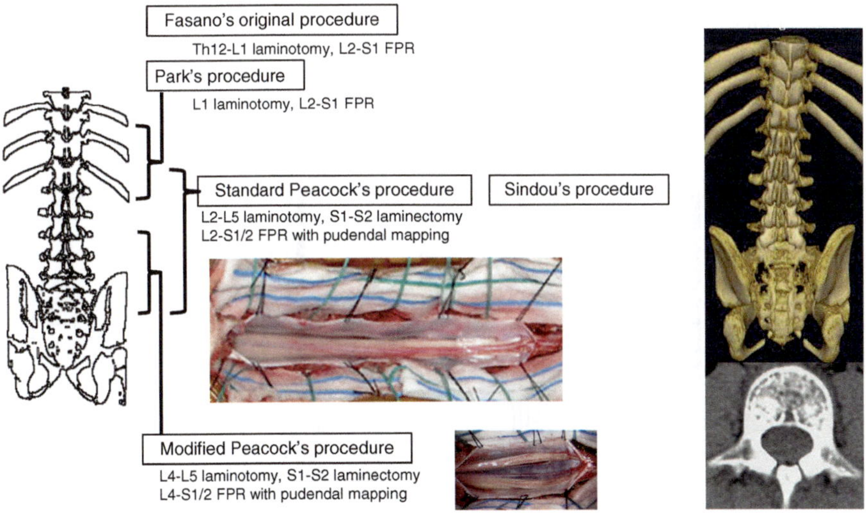

Fig. 13.1 Surgical procedures for dorsal rhizotomy. Left: Surgical procedures are classified into two main types. The first category involves surgery at the conus medullaris, originally described by Fasano and later modified by Park. The second category comprises surgery at the cauda equina, as introduced by Peacock. This category is further subdivided into the standard procedure, involving L2–L5 osteoplastic laminotomy and S1 (-S2) laminectomy, and the limited procedure, involving L4–L5 osteoplastic laminotomy and S1 (-S2) laminectomy. Sindou added a less invasive procedure called interlaminal approach to the cauda equina. Right: Postoperative CT scans after osteoplastic laminotomy for dorsal rhizotomy. It is essential to firmly fix the laminas unilaterally, and subsequently, ossification follows

dural exposure is determined based on the caudal end of the dural sac. The length of the skin incisions is about 12 cm and 5 cm, respectively.

Following the osteoplastic laminotomy and dural opening, bilateral dorsal roots ranging from L2 to S2 (standard procedure) or L4 to S2 (limited procedure) are separated from the ventral roots. Then, ION procedures are conducted for FPR. After completing dorsal rhizotomy, the dura is closed, the laminas are repositioned, and the skin is closed layer-by-layer. Correct application of osteoplastic laminotomy should minimize the likelihood of postoperative spinal deformity. It is essential to firmly fix the laminas unilaterally, and ossification follows subsequently as shown in Fig. 13.1.

13.3 Intraoperative Neurophysiological Procedures

ION procedures applied for FPR are classified into three groups. The first involves determining the root/rootlet to be cut and utilizes direct root/rootlet stimulation. The second group focuses on ION procedures aimed at preserving urinary function, incorporating pudendal mapping, and monitoring the bulbocavernosus reflex (BCR) [33]. The final ION procedure is employed to verify the reduction of spasticity following FPR, utilizing the F-wave for this purpose. Figure 13.2 demonstrates the comprehensive schema of ION applied for FPR.

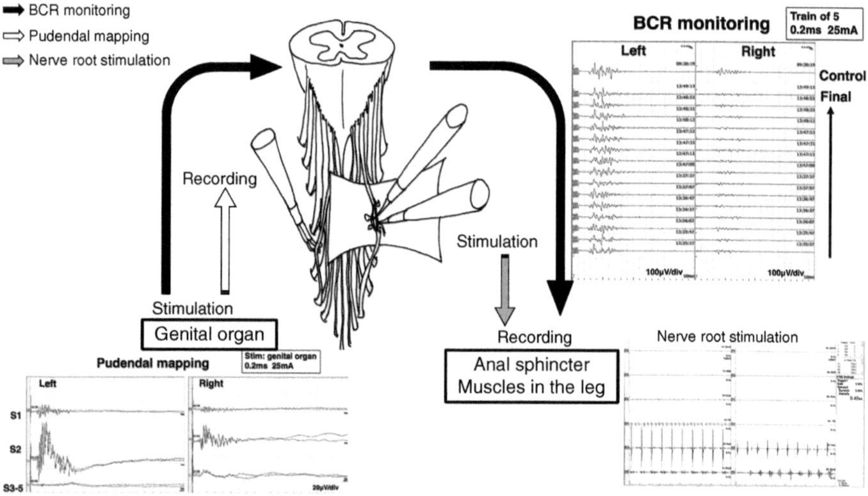

Fig. 13.2 Intraoperative neurophysiological procedures for dorsal rhizotomy. ION procedures applied for dorsal rhizotomy are classified into three groups. The first involves determining the root/rootlet to be cut and utilizes direct root/rootlet stimulation. The second group focuses on ION procedures aimed at preserving urinary function, incorporating pudendal mapping and the BCR monitoring. The last group, the F-wave, is employed to verify the degree of spasticity (the F-wave is not shown in the figure. Please see Fig. 13.6)

13.3.1 Dorsal Root/Rootlet Stimulation

The author applies a 10 Hz tetanic electrical stimulation for 1 s in order to test a root/rootlet. Following the dissection of the dorsal root from the ventral one, each dorsal root is secured using a pair of electrodes previously utilized for the root dissection. It is the bipolar stimulation with the cathode positioned on the rostral side. A 10 Hz electrical stimulation is delivered, and the resulting muscle contraction, evoked by suprathreshold intensity, is recorded by EMG. The electrical stimulation for testing the dorsal root initiates from a caudal root and progresses in the rostral direction. An example of EMG record and the parameters for root/rootlet stimulation are detailed in Figs. 13.3 and 13.4.

All dorsal roots in the range of lesioning undergo testing, and dorsal roots displaying highly abnormal EMG patterns are identified. These functionally selected dorsal roots are further divided into several rootlets depending on their diameter, typically ranging from three to six. Subsequently, the same electrical stimulation is delivered to the rootlet. Rootlets exhibiting markedly abnormal EMG patterns again are then cut after coagulation.

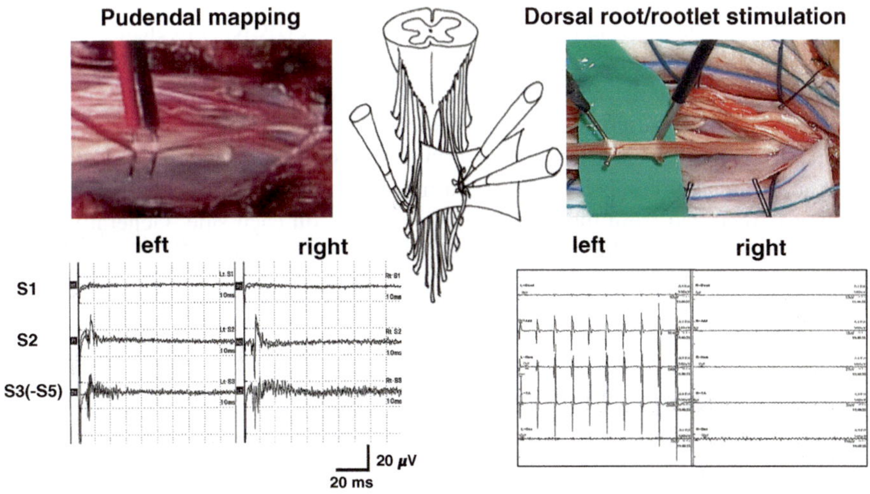

Fig. 13.3 Dorsal root/rootlet stimulation and pudendal mapping. A schema of both procedures and records: The results of pudendal mapping show a high DAP from bilateral S2 and S3 (-S5) roots (left). They are excluded from dorsal rhizotomy. The 10 Hz tetanic electrical stimulation to the left S1 root demonstrated highly abnormal EMG responses (right). It is further divided into several rootlets, and the same stimulation is repeated to judge the rootlet cutting

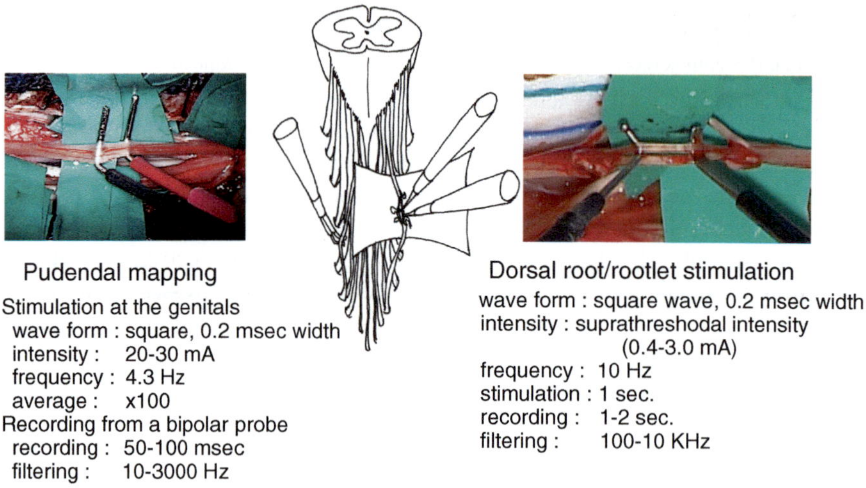

Fig. 13.4 Parameters for dorsal root/rootlet stimulation and pudendal mapping

13.3.2 The BCR Monitoring

The purpose of monitoring the bulbocavernosus reflex (BCR) is to ensure the preservation of urinary function during surgery, particularly when involving sacral roots. Technical details of the BCR monitoring have been documented elsewhere [33, 34]. The BCR parameters and EMG records for BCR monitoring are presented in Fig. 13.5. Briefly, electrical stimulation is applied to the genital organ at suprathreshold intensity but below the supra-maximum level, and the resulting EMG finding is recorded from the anal sphincter muscle on each side. Generally, BCR tends to be robust in children with spasticity. The preservation of BCR provides the surgeon with assurance that urinary function is maintained during the surgery [34].

13.3.3 Pudendal Mapping

Pudendal mapping was initially developed to prevent postoperative urinary complications following dorsal rhizotomy [11]. An example of the record and the parameters for pudendal mapping are shown in Figs. 13.3 and 13.4. The genital organ is electrically stimulated with suprathreshold intensity but below the supra-maximum level, and the dorsal action potential (DAP) of the pudendal nerve is recorded from a handheld bipolar electrode. Pudendal mapping is conducted across the S1–S3 (-S5) dorsal roots.

Stimulation	
Intensity	Submaximal intensity (20 ~ 40 mA, max. 45 mA)
Wave from	Biphasic rectangular
Peak duration	0.5m sec
Train	x5
ISI	2 msec (500 Hz)
Average	x2
Rate	2.3 ~ 4.3 Hz
Recording	
Average	x2
Filter	50 ~ 500 Hz
Epock time	100 msec

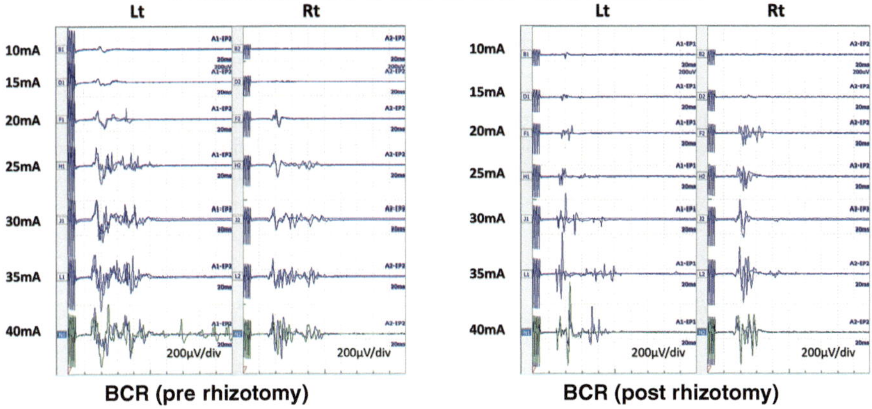

Fig. 13.5 BCR parameters and EMG records. Pre- and post-rhizotomy records are shown. There is change in the BCR waveform, but the EMG responses remain robust

13.3.4 The F-Wave Measuring

The F-wave serves as an indicator of the excitability of alpha motor neurons in the anterior horn of the spinal cord, thereby reflecting spasticity [24–26, 28]. To validate the reduction of spasticity in the ankle joint, the F-wave is measured by stimulating the tibial nerve at the ankle joint, and the compound muscle action potential (cMAP) of F-waves is recorded from the ipsilateral abductor hallucis muscle.

Following the completion of dorsal rhizotomy, the reduction of spasticity in the ankle joint is reflected in the F-wave. Generally, in children with spasticity, the F-wave exhibits consistently abnormal cMAP patterns, which tend to normalize by diminishing the amplitude or appearing disperse following FPR. As a result, surgeons can assess the outcome of dorsal rhizotomy even during the course of the surgery (Fig. 13.6).

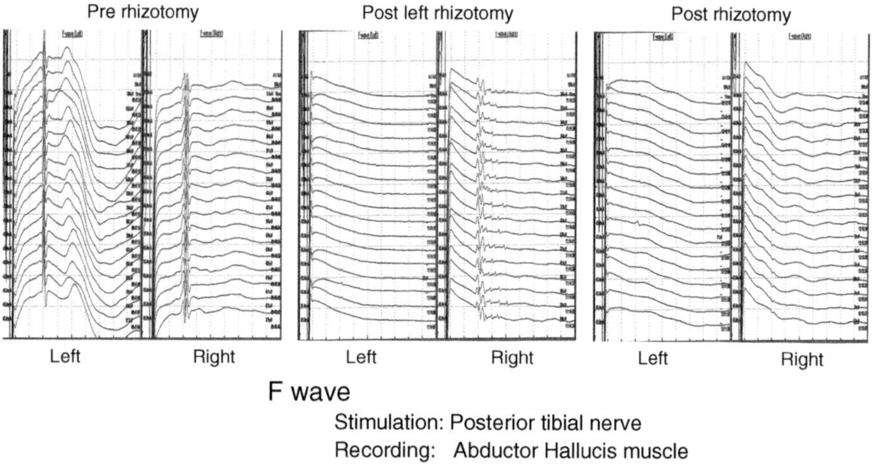

Fig. 13.6 F-waves during dorsal rhizotomy (stimulation intensity: 40 mA). Left: The F-wave showed a highly abnormal cMAP pattern before rhizotomy. Middle: After completing left dorsal rhizotomy, F-waves from the left side disappeared. Right: After completing right dorsal rhizotomy, bilateral F-waves disappeared. Reduction of spasticity at the bilateral ankle joints is expected from the result of the F-wave change

13.3.5 Application of Intraoperative Neurophysiology During Surgery

These ION procedures are systematically applied during FPR (Fig. 13.7).

1. After introduction of anesthesia, baseline recording of the BCR is monitored.
2. Following the dural opening, a baseline record of F-waves from each side is obtained before rhizotomy.
3. Following the dissecting of the dorsal root from the ventral one, pudendal mapping is conducted from the S1 dorsal root to S3 (-S5) roots to map the DAP of the pudendal afferent nerve. Dorsal roots exhibiting a high amplitude of DAP are excluded from rhizotomy, and the range for dorsal root lesioning is determined. The highest DAP of the pudendal nerve is typically recorded from the S2 or S3 dorsal root [35, 36].
4. Based on the pudendal mapping result, L2–S1 (S2) dorsal roots are included in the standard procedure, while L4–S1 are included in the limited procedure [15, 35]. Tetanic electrical stimulation is then delivered to each dorsal root to identify highly abnormal roots. Roots judged as highly abnormal from the EMG record are further divided into several (three to six) rootlets, and the same tetanic electrical stimulation is applied to each rootlet. Rootlets judged as highly abnormal again are cut after coagulation.
5. Finally, the F-wave is remeasured at the end of rootlet cutting to confirm the disappearance of abnormal patterns in the ipsilateral F-wave trends. If abnormal patterns persist, additional dorsal rhizotomy is performed.

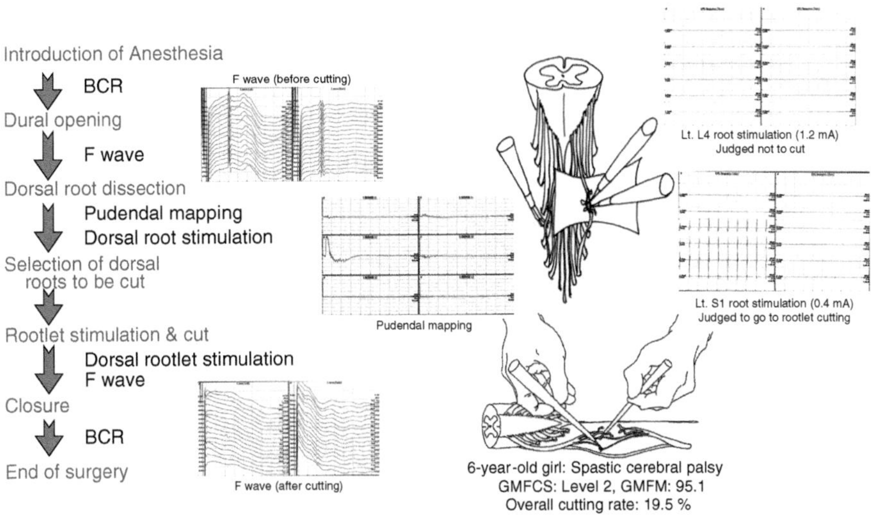

Fig. 13.7 Systemic application of ION procedures during dorsal rhizotomy. ION procedures are systematically applied from the introduction of anesthesia to the end of surgery

6. Steps 4 and 5 are repeated in a similar manner on the contralateral side.
7. After completing bilateral dorsal rhizotomy, meticulous hemostasis is confirmed before initiating dural closure. During closure, BCR is recorded to confirm the preserved urinary function during dorsal rhizotomy.

13.3.6 S1 Dorsal Root with High Pudendal Action Potentials

Cutting the S1 dorsal root is crucial for reducing spasticity at the ankle joint when the titanic electrical stimulation of the S1 dorsal root evoked highly abnormal EMG records from the gastrocnemius muscle. If a S1 dorsal root exhibits relatively high pudendal DAP, even though it is uncommon, special attention is required for S1 dorsal root rhizotomy [37]. Under such circumferences, additional pudendal mapping is performed for each S1 rootlet. The rootlet that demonstrated a relatively high DAP of the pudendal nerve should be preserved, irrespective of the EMG outcomes after rootlet electrical stimulation (Fig. 13.8).

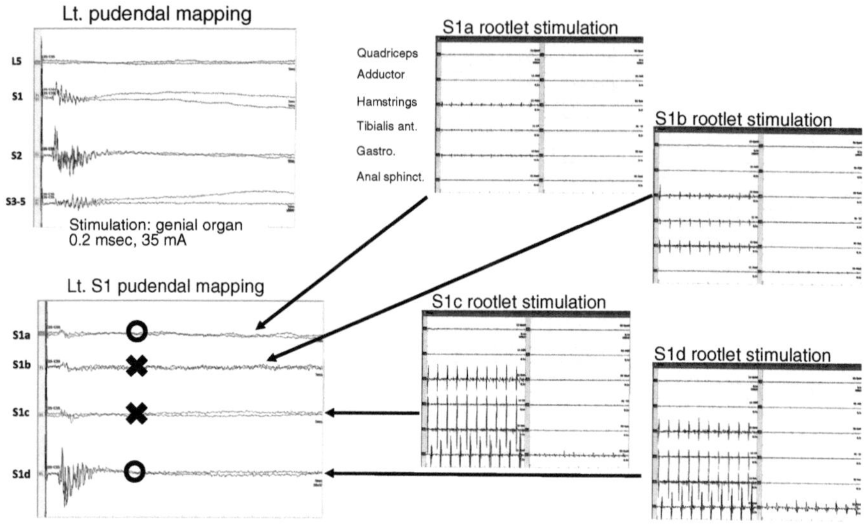

Fig. 13.8 S1 dorsal root with high pudendal action potentials. If an S1 dorsal root exhibits relatively high pudendal DAP, additional pudendal mapping is performed for each S1 rootlet. The rootlet that demonstrated a relatively high DAP of the pudendal nerve should be preserved, irrespective of the EMG outcomes after rootlet electrical stimulation. In the figure, left S1 pudendal mapping showed high DAP from a rootlet S1d. The rootlet stimulation demonstrated moderate to high abnormal EMG responses from rootlet S1b, S1c, and S1d. Based on the IOM results, S1b and S1c were cut, while S1d was preserved because of its high pudendal DAP

13.4 Tailor-Made Dorsal Rhizotomy Guided by Intraoperative Neurophysiology

Decision-making regarding whether to cut or preserve a root/rootlet is the highlight of FPR. Major causes influencing this decision are multifactorial (Fig. 13.9).

The primary and most crucial factor is the result of intraoperative neurophysiology. Two major principles are employed to assess abnormal muscle responses by EMG recordings. Firstly, the extent and distribution of muscle contraction based on the spinal dorsal root level are evaluated. If muscle contraction beyond segmental innervation is elicited following tetanic electrical stimulation of the dorsal root/rootlet, it is deemed abnormal. Another criterion for judging abnormality is measured by the loss or reduction of central inhibition, as defined by Futagi and Abe in 1985 using the H_2/H_1 ratio of H reflex [38, 39]. Accordingly, the H_2/H_1 ratio during 10 Hz tetanic stimulation should remain less than 0.5. Thus, EMG recordings with sustained or increased muscle contractions or contractions with an amplitude ration exceeding 0.5 are considered abnormal. The degree of abnormality of the tested dorsal root/rootlet is determined using the previously published grading system [10, 13]. These two major principles, abnormal segmental distribution of muscle contraction and the loss or decrease of central suppression, form the core of the ION evaluation for dorsal root/rootlet cutting.

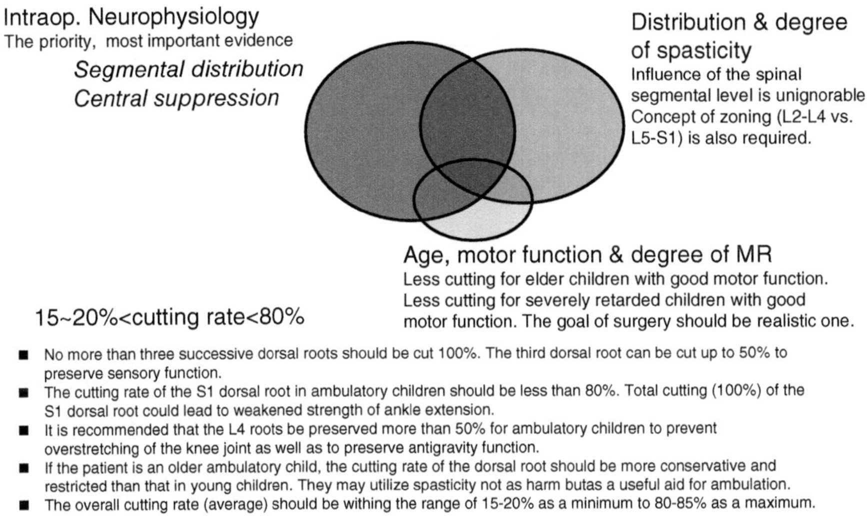

Fig. 13.9 Decision-making for root/rootlet cutting. Factors influencing the decision-making regarding whether to cut or preserve a root/rootlet are shown. The results of ION stand as the primary and most crucial factor. However, other factors need to be considered for the final decision of root/rootlet cutting

The second factor is the distribution and the degree of spasticity in the lower extremities, which should be evaluated preoperatively by a multidisciplinary spasticity team. The spinal segmental level of the spastic muscle is crucial and should be considered during decision-making. The presence of severe subluxation at the hip joint suggests more cutting at the levels of L2 and L3, while a gait with prominent pes equinus requires more weighted cutting at the level of S1. It should be noted that, in general, the degree of abnormal muscle contractions tends to be higher at the level of L5 and S1 dorsal root [40, 41] (Figs. 13.10 and 13.11). The concept of zoning of the dorsal root into the upper dorsal root (L2 and L3: correspond to the hip joint spasticity) and the lower one (L5 and S1: correspond to the ankle joint spasticity) can aid in estimating the cutting rate prior to surgery based on preoperative evaluation.

The third factor is the patient's age, preoperative motor function, and presence or degree of mental retardation. Some older children tend to utilize spasticity for gait as truncal support to compensate for muscle weakness. In such cases, a reduction in spasticity may lead to deteriorated motor function after surgery. The presence of severe mental retardation would hinder intensive postoperative neurorehabilitation. Thus, less cutting of the dorsal root/rootlet is rationalized under these conditions.

Apart from the above three factors, several criteria should be considered before reaching the final decision about rootlet cutting.

1. No more than three successive dorsal roots should be cut 100%. The third dorsal root can be cut up to 50% to preserve sensory function.

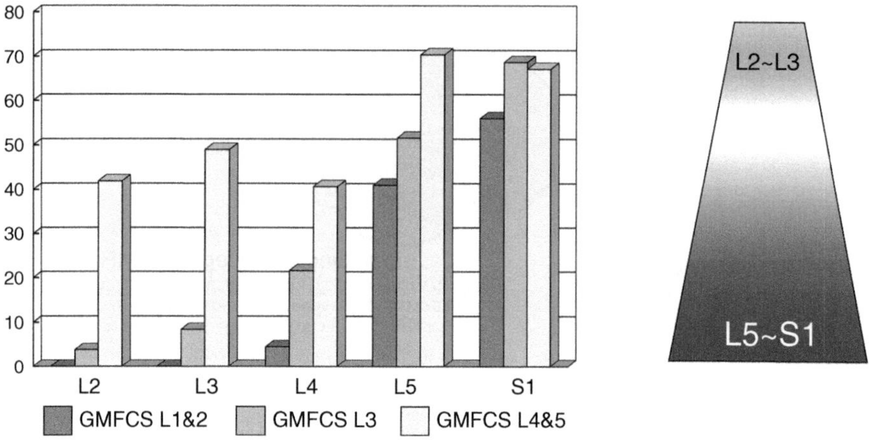

Fig. 13.10 Cutting rate of each root. The average cutting rate of each dorsal root in the last 43 cases is shown. The cutting rate correlates with GMFCS level. It should be noted that the degree of abnormal muscle contractions tends to be higher at the level of L5 and S1 dorsal root

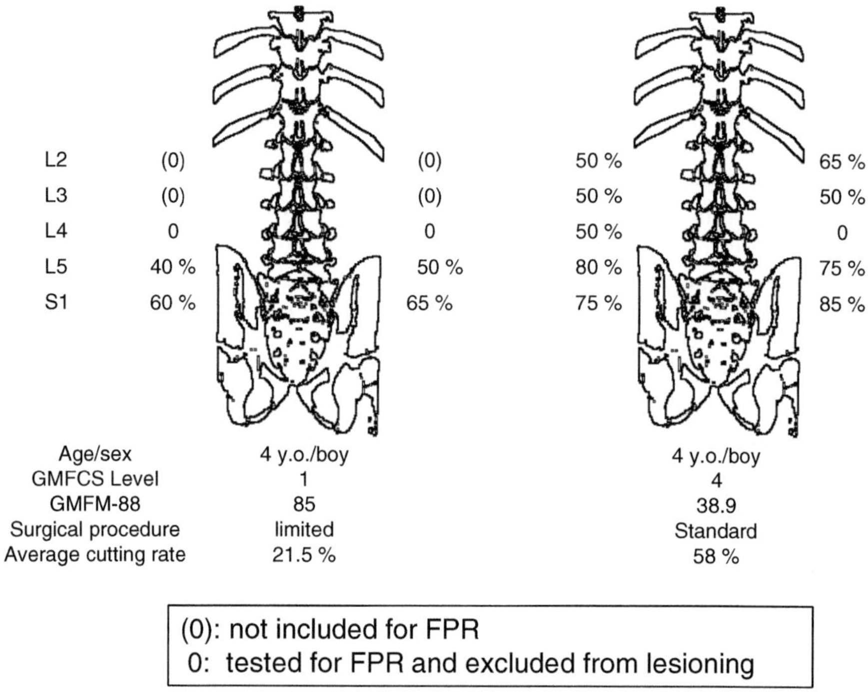

Fig. 13.11 Tailor-made dorsal rhizotomy guided by ION. ION introduces individualized dorsal rhizotomy, called functional posterior rhizotomy. GMFCS levels 1–2 (left) require less dorsal root cutting compared to those classified under levels 4–5 (right)

2. The cutting rate of the S1 dorsal root in ambulatory children should be less than 80%. Total cutting (100%) of the S1 dorsal root could lead to weakened strength of ankle extension.
3. It is recommended that the L4 roots be preserved more than 50% for ambulatory children to prevent overstretching of the knee joint as well as to preserve anti-gravity function [2].
4. If the patient is an older ambulatory child, the cutting rate of the dorsal root should be more conservative and restricted than that in young children. They may utilize spasticity not as harm but as a useful aid for ambulation.
5. The overall cutting rate (average) should be within the range of 15–20% as a minimum to 80–85% as a maximum.

13.5 Cutting Rate: Functional vs. Selective Dorsal Rhizotomy

It is reasonable to hypothesize that the severity of spasticity is inversely correlated with the cutting rate of the dorsal root (Fig. 13.11). This correlation should exhibit a negative association with preoperative motor function, suggesting that individuals classified under GMFCS levels 1–2 would require less dorsal root cutting compared to those classified under levels 4–5. Similarly, spastic children with high GMFM scores are expected to have a lower cutting rate, whereas those with lower GMFM scores may necessitate a higher cutting rate.

In 2019, the author proposed a practically useful formula for preoperatively estimating the cutting rate of the dorsal root during FPR [34]. The statistical analysis of the relationship between preoperative GMFM-88 and the cutting rate (overall) resulted in the following simple linear regression formula:

$$y = -0.5539x + 73.896$$

where x represents the GMFM-88 score and y represents the cutting rate, with a correlation coefficient of −0.89. The formula demonstrates a very high negative correlation between the cutting rate of the dorsal root and the GMFM-88 score. This statistical formula is approximated for practical use as:

$$y = 100 - x$$

The simple formula is useful to estimate the approximate cutting rate before the surgery. A similar simple regression was also presented by Xiao et al. using the GMFM-66 score with a correlation coefficient of −0.66 [17].

In the surgical practice of RPR, the formula is applied as follows. For instance, in a case of a spastic child with a GMFM-88 score of 72, the estimated cutting rate is 100–72 = 28. During the surgery, ION procedures are performed, and the dorsal rootlet to be cut is functionally determined. It is then expected to achieve a cutting

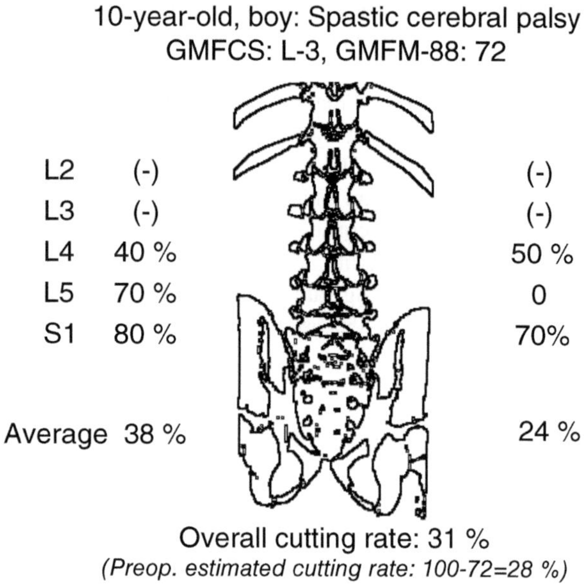

Fig. 13.12 Preoperative estimation of dorsal root cutting rate. The overall cutting rate of dorsal roots is estimated from the formula "Cutting rate = 100 – preoperative GMFM-88 score." In this case, the preoperative GMFM-88 score was 72, and the estimated cutting rate was 28. FPR with the use of limited procedure resulted in an overall cutting rate of 31, with satisfactory reduction of spasticity after surgery

rate of around 25–35% (Fig. 13.12). F-wave measurements confirm whether the cutting is sufficient. If the F-wave persists with highly abnormal pattern, additional dorsal rootlet cutting is performed. The surgical goal is to achieve functional improvement with minimum cutting of the dorsal root. In this sense, this approach is more functional than selective surgery [29].

Figure 13.12 illustrates a series of surgical and neurophysiological procedures of FPR in a case of a child with spastic diplegia.

13.6 Conclusions

ION plays a critical role in FPR, guiding the functional selection of dorsal root/rootlet for cutting while preserving urinary function. The implementation of ION procedures ensures that the cutting rate remains at a minimum while achieving maximum outcomes in spasticity reduction. This, in turn, can lead to improvements in functional performance and a decrease in the burden experienced by both patients and their families due to spasticity. Furthermore, the utilization of F-wave measurements allows for the prediction of FPR outcomes, specifically the reduction of spasticity, even during the surgery itself. In the context of functional surgery, ION serves as the key factor for the successful implementation of FPR.

References

1. Abbe R. Intradural section of the spinal nerves for neuralgia. Boston Med Surg J. 1896;135:329–44.
2. Foerster O. On the indications and results of the excision of posterior spinal nerve roots in men. Surg Gynecol Obstet. 1913;16:463–74.
3. Fasano VA, Broggi G, BArolat-Romana G, Sguazzi A. Surgical treatment of spasticity in cerebral palsy. Childs Brain. 1978;4:289–305.
4. Fasano VA, Barolat-Romana G, Zeme S, Sguazzi A. Electrophysiological assessment of spinal circuits by direct dorsal root stimulation. Neurosurgery. 1979;4:146–51.
5. Fasano VA, Broggi G, Zeme S. Intraoperative electrical stimulation for functional posterior rhizotomy. Scand J Rehab Med Suppl. 1988;17:149–54.
6. Peacock WJ, Arens LJ. Selective posterior rhizotomy for the relief of spasticity in cerebral palsy. S Afr Med J. 1982;62:119–24.
7. Peacock WJ, Arens LJ, Berman B. Cerebral palsy spasticity. Selective posterior rhizotomy. Pediatr Neurosci. 1987;13:61–6.
8. Park TS, Gaffney PE, Kaufman BA, Molleston MC. Selective lumbosacral dorsal rhizotomy immediately caudal to the conus medullaris for cerebral palsy spasticity. Neurosurgery. 1993;33:929–34.
9. Park TS, Johnston JM. Surgical techniques of selective dorsal rhizotomy for spastic cerebral palsy. Technical note. Neurosurg Focus. 2006;21:e7.
10. Phillips LH II, Park TS. Electrophysiologic studies of selective posteiror rhizotomy patients. In: Park TS, editor. Neurosurgery: state of the art reviews 4. Management of spasticity in cerebral palsy and spinal cord injury. Philadelphia: Hanley & Belfus; 1989. p. 459–69.
11. Deletis V, Vodusek D, Abbott R, Epstein F, Turndorff H. Intraoperative monitoring of the dorsal roots: minimizing the risk of iatrogenic micturition disorders. Neurosurgery. 1992;30:72–5.
12. Hays RM, McLaughlin JF, Bjornson KF, Stephens K, Roberts TS, Price R. Electrophysiological monitoring during rhizotomy, and spasticity and GMFM performance. Develop Med Child Neurol. 1998;40:233–8.
13. Mittal S, Farmer JP, Al-Atassi B, Montpetit K, Gervais N, Poulin C, Cantin MA, Benaroch TE. Impact of selective posterior rhizotomy on fine motor skills. Pediatr Neurosurg. 2002;36:133–41.
14. Morota N. Functional posterior rhizotomy: the Tokyo experience. Childs Nerv Syst. 2007;23:1007–14.
15. Morota N, Ihara S, Ogiwara H. Neurosurgical management of childhood spasticity: functional posterior rhizotomy and intrathecal baclofen infusion therapy. Neuro Med Chir (Tokyo). 2015;55:624–39.
16. Georgoulis G, Brinzeu A, Sindou M. Dorsal rhizotomy for children with spastic diplegia of cerebral palsy origin: usefulness of intraoperative monitoring. J Neurosurg Pediatr. 2018;22:89–101.
17. Xiao B, Constantini S, Browd SR, Zhan Q, Jiang W, Mei R. The role of intra-operative neuroelectrophysiological monitoring in single-level approach selective dorsal rhizotomy. Childs Nerv Syst. 2020;36:1925–33. https://doi.org/10.1007/s00381-019-04408-5.
18. De Vloo P, Huttunen TJ, Forte D, Jankovic I, Lee A, Hair M, Cawker S, Chugh D, Carr L, BHA C, Pitt M, Aquilina K. Intraoperative electrophysiology during single-level dorsal rhizotomy: technique, stimulation threshold, and response data in a series of 145 patients. J Neurosurg Pediatr. 2020;25:597–606. https://doi.org/10.3171/2019.12.PEDS19372.
19. Cohen AR, Webster HC. How selective is selective posterior rhizotomy? Surg Neurol. 1991;35:267–72.
20. Hays RM, McLaughli JF, Bjornson KF, Stephens K, Roberts TS, Price R. Electrophysiological monitoring during selective dorsal rhizotomy, and spasticity and GMFM performance. Dev Med Child Neurol. 1998;40:233–8.

21. Steinbok P, Kestle JR. Variation between centers in electrophysiological techniques used in lumbosacral selective dorsal rhizotomy for spastic cerebral palsy. Pediatr Neurosurg. 1996;25:233–9.
22. Steinbok P, Tidemann AJ, Miller S, Mortenson P, Bowen-Roberts T. Electrophysiologically guided versus non-electrophysiologically guided selective dorsal rhizotomy for spastic cerebral palsy: a comparison of outcomes. Childs Nerv Syst. 2009;25:1091–6.
23. Young K. Correlating nerve rootlet and spastic muscle activation intraoperatively during selective dorsal rhizotomy. Dev Med Child Neurol. 2023;65:9–10. https://doi.org/10.1111/dmcn.15341.
24. Eisen A, Odusote K. Amplitude of the F wave: a potential means of documenting spasticity. Neurology. 1979;29:1306–9. https://doi.org/10.1212/wnl.29.9_part_1.1306.
25. Fox JE, Hitchcock ER. F wave size as a monitor of motor neuron excitability: the effect of deafferentation. J Neurol Neurosurg Pshychiatr. 1987;50:453–9.
26. Bischoff C, Schoenle PW, Conrad B. Increased F-wave duration in patients with spasticity. Electromyogr Clin Neurophsiol. 1992;32:449–53. PMID: 1396297Ca
27. Kimura J. The F wave and the a wave. In: Kimura J, editor. Electrodiagnosis in diseases of nerve and muscle: principles and practice. 3rd ed. New York: Oxford University Press Inc.; 2001. p. 439–49.
28. Mesrati F, Vecchierini MF. F-waves: neurophysiology and clinical value. Neurophysiol Clin. 2004;34:217–43. https://doi.org/10.1016/j.neucli.2004.09.005.
29. Morota N. Clinically practical formula for preoperatively estimating the cutting rate of the spinal nerve root in a functional posterior rhizotomy. Childs Nerv Syst. 2019;35:665–72.
30. Warsi NM, Tailor J, Coulter IC, Shakil H, Workewych A, Haldenby R, Breitbart S, Strantzas S, Vandenberk M, Dewan M, Ibrahim GM. Selective dorsal rhizotomy: an illustrated review of operative techniques. J Neurosurg Pediatr. 2020;25:540–7. https://doi.org/10.3171/2019.12.PEDS19629.
31. Galarza M, Fowler EG, Chipps L, Padden TM, Lazareff JA. Functional assessment of children with cerebral palsy following limited (L4-S1) selective posterior rhizotomy –a preliminary report. Acta Neurochir. 2001;143:865–72.
32. Sindou M, Georgoulis G. Keyhole interlaminar dorsal rhizotomy for spastic diplegia in cerebral palsy. Acta Neurochir. 2015;157:1187–96.
33. Deletis V, Vodusek DB. Intraoperative recording of the bulbocavernosus reflex. Neurosurgery. 1997;40:88–93.
34. Morota N. Intraoperative neurophysiological monitoring of the bulbocavernosus reflex during surgery for conus spinal lipoma: what are the warning criteria? J Neurosurg Pediatr. 2019;23:639–47.
35. Deletis V, Vodusek DB, Abbott R, Epstein FJ, Turndorf H. Intraoperative monitoring of the dorsal sacral roots: minimizing the risk of iatrogenic micturition disorders. Neurosurgery. 1992;30:72–5.
36. Ogiwara H, Morota N. Pudendal afferents mapping in posterior sacral rhizotomies. Neurosurgery. 2014;74:171–5.
37. Morota N. Pudendal mapping of S1 rootlets in a functional posterior rhizotomy: when an S1 posterior root shows a high pudendal dorsal action potential—a technical note. Childs Nerv Syst. 2020;36:1971–5.
38. Futagi Y, Abe J. H-reflex study in normal children and patients with cerebral palsy. Brain Dev. 1985;7:414–20.
39. Nishida T, Storrs B. Electrophysiological monitoring in selective posterior rhizotomy for spasticity. Principles, techniques and interpretation of responses. In: Sindou M, Abbott R, Keravel Y, editors. Neurosurgery for spasticity. A multidisciplinary approach. New York: Springer-Verlag; 1991. p. 159–63.
40. Wolter S, Spies C, Martin JH, Schulz M, Sarpong-Bengelsdorf A, Unger J, Thomale UW, Michael T, Murphy JF, Haberl H. Frequency distribution in intraoperative stimulation-evoked EMG responses during selective dorsal rhizotomy in children with cerebral palsy-part 1: clini-

cal setting and neurophysiological procedure. Childs Nerv Syst. 2020;36:1945–54. https://doi.org/10.1007/s00381-020-04734-z.

41. Sindou M, Georgoulis G, Joud A, Neromyliotis E, Dinopoulos A. Excitability of the radiculo-medullary circuitry in spastic cerebral palsy: an intraoperative neurophysiological study in children undergoing selective dorsal rhizotomy. Dev Med Child Neurol. 2023;65(1):78–85. https://doi.org/10.1111/dmcn.15315.

Part IV
Postoperative Rehabilitation and Outcome of Dorsal Rhizotomy

Chapter 14
Postoperative Functional Recovery and Rehabilitation Following Selective Dorsal Rhizotomy

Neil Wimalasundera

14.1 Introduction

Due to the heterogeneity of cerebral palsy and the historical variation in selective dorsal rhizotomy (SDR) technique, it is difficult to prescribe a standardized postoperative rehabilitation programme which will suit all children undergoing SDR.

There is a strong body of evidence which supports the short- and long-term reduction in spasticity following SDR; however, longer functional outcomes have had varied reports with very few studies looking directly at activity and participation goals [1–3].

The current long-term data compares groups of children who may have had SDR many years ago with different selection criteria, different procedures and different rehabilitation programmes. Despite this, there is an emerging body of evidence regarding the short- and long-term safety and efficacy of SDR. There is an expanded understanding that this is not just in relation to gait but also other parameters important to patients and their families [4–6].

There is now data to show which children will show improvement and who will sustain those improvements following SDR. Algorithms to help identify these groups such as the PILAR score (predictive index for long-term ambulation after rhizotomy) from Dudley's group are discussed later in this chapter [6].

Most long-term studies report sustained Gross Motor Function Measurement (GMFM) gains in children with Gross Motor Function Classification System (GMFCS) levels 1 and 2 with maximum gains approximately up to 3–5 years following the procedure followed by plateauing. GMFCS level 3 make gains; however, there is loss of these gains with age but not to below baseline. Most children

N. Wimalasundera (✉)
Royal Children's Hospital, Melbourne, Australia
e-mail: Neil.wimalasundera@rch.org.au

N. Morota, P. Steinbok (eds.), *Dorsal Rhizotomy: Neurosurgery for Childhood Spasticity*, Advances and Technical Standards in Neurosurgery 51,
https://doi.org/10.1007/978-3-031-86441-4_14

undergoing SDR maintain the same GMFCS level or gain one level. They tend not to drop GMFCS levels. These factors need to be taken into consideration when deciding at which age to perform an SDR and the natural history of cerebral palsy.

Children who are physically more able with less impairment prior to SDR will have a better long-term outcome in relation to walking goals specifically. This is highlighted by the Oswestry experience where they had a very strict selection criteria and very good outcomes with many children improving their GMFCS level by 1 [7].

SDR in GMFCS levels 4–5 children despite not leading to sustained long-term motor gains can have its own benefits in terms of comfort and care goals and has been proposed as an alternative treatment to ITB implantation or ITB replacement [8, 9].

14.2 Presurgical Optimization

If mobility goals are the priority for SDR, as the evidence suggests a better GMFM score relates to a better outcome; then, a period of preoperative optimization is indicated. As well as ensuring standard selection criteria are considered, these other presurgical areas should be considered.

1. Physiotherapy programme prior to SDR to ensure the child and family are psychologically prepared for the intensive programme postoperatively.
2. Specific focus on a strengthening programme prior to SDR.
3. Orthotic prescription and increasing tolerance of wearing them.
4. Orthopaedic evaluation—will existing contracture or bony alignment issues interfere with postop rehabilitation?
5. Equipment evaluation—some children will need additional mobility aids including crutches, quad sticks, a walking frame or a wheelchair postoperatively. Consider or equipment for washing and toileting such as a commode.
6. Evaluation of community access (home and school).
7. Discussion (especially in GMFCS level 4) that some physical activity may initially be more difficult, especially if children are relying on spasticity for upright mobility with an aid.
8. Management of concurrent difficulties such as constipation—opiate analgesia and relative immobility can exacerbate these difficulties postoperatively.
9. Consider weaning of hypertonia medications such as baclofen prior to surgery.
10. It is now common practice to start children on gabapentin just prior to surgery or soon after SDR surgery to manage the expected dysesthesia following the procedure.

14.3 Postoperative Management

14.3.1 General Management

Specific postop precautions will be dependent on the procedure performed. Children with a single-level laminotomy usually have less postoperative needs and are often ready for transfer to a rehabilitation programme by day 5 [10].

If children have a larger laminectomy procedure, there is usually a longer period of spinal care, prior to formal transfer to a rehabilitation programme. There will be slower progress to increasing seating time and walking activities.

Postoperatively, consideration should be given to the management of pain, bladder and bowel function and general nutrition. Some children will be young and have limited understand of what is happening, so good family and social support is essential.

14.3.2 Early Symptom Management Following SDR

Postoperative pain is common, and each team will have their own preferred protocol depending on the procedure performed. Pain intervention may range from opioid infusions to epidural or even intrathecal treatments. These medications are usually quickly weaned to intravenous or oral medications including opiates, clonidine, nonsteroidal medications and paracetamol [11].

Postoperative dysesthesia is common, and many children are started prophylactically on gabapentin just prior to surgery to help manage this. Some advocate early weaning at 3–4 weeks, but it is often useful for 2–3 months to help manage sensory difficulties, so they don't interfere with the rehabilitation programme. Gabapentin can also be beneficial for managing pain and, in some cases, residual dystonia.

The urinary catheter is usually removed on day 1–2, and most children do not need NG tube feeding supplementation in this early period of rehabilitation.

Constipation can occur following surgery and is exacerbated by opiate use and immobilization. This can be managed with good fluid intake and aperients such as Movicol and Senna.

Spinal laminectomy restrictions are usually guided by the neurosurgeon and depend on the procedure performed.

Other immediate surgical and postsurgical adverse events were reported in one cases series of 150 SDR patients as intubation difficulty, urinary catheter-related difficulty, minor CSF leak, transient urinary retention, postoperative nausea, superficial infection, neuropathic pain, transient sensory disturbance in the legs, single case of temporary hypertonia, orthostatic headaches (self-resolving), drug reaction, urinary tract infection, lower respiratory tract infection, allergy to dressings, pressure sore, hallucinations and dystonia [10].

14.4 Early Rehabilitation Programmes and Duration of Admission

The overall duration of admission is dependent on the procedure the child receives and the rehabilitation protocol of the provider. Some children who are receiving an SDR for predominantly care and comfort goals (GMFCS levels 4–5) may be discharged as early as day 5 without a formal inpatient programme, whereas many children may remain inpatients for 6–8 weeks of rehab [9].

In some services following a single-level laminotomy SDR, children are medically ready for discharge by the end of the first week and can therefore receive their rehabilitation as a day rehabilitation programme, without requiring the use of an acute hospital bed. The family may stay in accommodation near the hospital (walking/manual wheelchair distance), and this can relieve the stress on acute hospital beds. These centres usually provide 2–3 weeks of intensive rehabilitation following SDR.

Therapy programmes are guided by the baseline functional level of the child. Children who are GMFCS level 2, especially following single-level laminotomy, will be able to engage upright activities faster than a child who is GMFCS 3 and has undergone a larger laminectomy procedure. Therapy often begins in the first few days after surgery, involving early in-bed mobilization with range of motion exercises and positioning strategies. Improving sitting tolerance in different positions and improving trunk control in conjunction with bed strengthening exercises are usually the priority. Specific focus is given to strengthening of quadriceps, hamstrings, hip abductors, and hip extensors. This is followed by increasing upright time, sometimes with the assistance of standing frame or gait aids. Facilitating early self mobilisation with a wheelchair or prone laying board will help with mood and motivation postoperatively.

Several studies have provided reviews of rehabilitation protocols following SDR [12, 13]. Physical therapies started anywhere between day 1 and day 5 following the SDR surgery, but generally, therapy is started in the first week following surgery.

Inpatient therapy then often ranges between 2 and 6 weeks. Therapy is daily and a combination of physiotherapy and occupational therapy, usually 2–3 sessions per day (3 hrs).

Some centres have recommended early muscle lengthening surgery following SDR (Limpaphayom et al., 2020) [14]; however, the general international consensus is to wait to see the effect of the SDR before lengthening muscles. This will help to avoid overlengthening muscles and exacerbating weakness, especially when other factors are affecting gait such as selective motor control, weakness and bony deformity. There are sometimes exceptions to this, such as when there is significant contracture interfering with orthotic tolerance and therefore effective rehabilitation cannot take place.

Some children following SDR can have residual muscle hypertonia. This can be either spasticity or dystonia. It may manifest in muscles such as posterior tibialis which can interfere with orthotic tolerance.

Table 14.1 Hypotheses of upper limb improvement following SDR

Hypotheses of upper limb improvement following SDR
Somatosensory cortex reorganization favouring the hand region of the leg region
Decrease in abnormal electrical transmission throughout the spinal cord
Indirect result of improved posture due to improved truncal and leg stability
Indirect consequence of occupational and physical therapy intensification
Maturation effect

Overweakening muscles in this early phase should be avoided, but sometimes, it is necessary to use focal botulinum toxin or medications such as baclofen, diazepam, or clonidine to help a child engage with the physical rehabilitation programme. Most children will already have been started on gabapentin perioperatively to help with dysesthesia. Higher doses of gabapentin can help with managing unwanted dystonia.

There is increasing evidence of upper limb functional improvement following SDR [15, 16]. It is therefore important not only to have physiotherapy as the main physical therapy but also occupational therapy. This can be focused functional hand use and development of independence of activities of daily living (see Table 14.1).

As the initial inpatient stay is often up to 6 weeks long, it is important to incorporate other therapies and teams which are important in the child's life and will contribute to improved engagement. This can include play therapy, music therapy, psychological support and education.

14.5 Early Equipment and Orthotics Following SDR

The early use of knee gaiters (leg wraps) is often recommended when there has been significant hamstring tightness prior to surgery. SDR is especially good at improving knee extension, so if there was mild contracture at the knee level preoperatively, knee gaiters are recommended for use in both laying and standing positions.

The early use of ankle foot orthosis (AFOs) is recommended. They are needed for all standing activities and can also be used while in bed intermittently to provide a long stretch. They are most effective when the knee is in extension with the gaiters on.

Most international service providers of SDR recommend the long-term use of AFOs rather than weaning their use in the months following SDR. The rationale for this is that the calf muscles can have residual spasticity and unmasked weakness will cause the feet to roll in to valgus, promoting a crouch gait pattern. This is the same reason for not promoting early calf muscle lengthening surgery unless absolutely necessary.

Many children will require equipment following SDR especially in the early rehabilitation phase and on return to home and school. There may be initial loss of motor function, especially in children who are GFMCS level 4. Some children may have relied on spasticity for upright function, and they may not be able to perform in the same way initially post-SDR. Weakness may be unmasked, and children will also fatigue faster initially. Equipment may include the following:

1. Walking aids—crutches, four-point sticks, walking frame
2. Wheelchair
3. Standing frame
4. Equipment for activities of daily living—shower chair, commode

14.6 Longer-Term Therapy

Intensive therapy is recommended for the first 6–12 months following SDR, with intensity ranging from 2 hrs per week to 5 hrs per week. After the first 6 months, the intensity drops to once or twice per week as it is hoped that some of the formal therapy sessions will be replaced with the child's usual physical activities such as sports and swimming. They will also be able to practice walking more independently at this stage [12, 13].

Formal rehabilitation programmes following SDR have been described, and rehabilitation will usually be a combination of physiotherapy and occupational therapy. Sessions can also be performed by allied health assistants or exercise physiologists. Some children may require psychological support due to the intensity and duration of rehabilitation therapy [15, 16].

Families should be counselled regarding the long-term commitment to physical therapy with many protocols extending for 1–2 years post-SDR [17].

The research shows that most children following SDR will need ongoing assessment and intervention, including gait analysis, hypertonia management and orthopaedic surgery [1–4, 6].

SDR is sometimes portrayed as a single curative procedure especially in popular media; however, in reality, the process will be over many years, extending into adolescence and full growth.

14.7 Post-SDR Follow-Up Protocols

SDR postoperative follow-up protocols are varied around the world. Standardized long-term follow-up is essential to ensure SDR safety and efficacy into adulthood. There is good evidence for the short-term improvement in GMFM score and spasticity reduction following SDR, with more recent studies also showing short-term improvement in quality of life measures [7, 18–20].

Timing of data collection for SDR-AUS registry study						
			Follow-up			
Assessment domains/study phase	**Baseline**	**Sx**	**12 months**	**2 years**	**5 years**	**10 years**
Personal and medical history	X					
CP assessment	X		X	X	X	X
Physical assessment	X		X			
Surgery and admission details		X				
Surgical complications		X				
Assessment of gross motor function and mobility	X		X	X	X	X
Instrumented gait analysis	X		X	X	X	X
Goal attainment	X		X	X		
Musculoskeletal interventions	X		X	X	X	X
Long-term adverse events			X	X	X	X
Assessment of pain	X		X	X	X	X

CP, cerebral palsy; SDR-AUS, Australian selective dorsal rhizotomy; Sx, surgical.

Fig. 14.1 Suggested timing of data collection following SDR—Australian protocol

Long-term evidence for the benefits of SDR is less robust and difficult to generalize from the available studies due to the different selection criteria and different surgical and rehabilitation protocols. Outcome is also influenced by growth and subsequent orthopaedic intervention. Despite some conflicting reports, the evidence does suggest long-term reduction in spasticity, longer-term gains in motor function especially in GMFCS level 2 children, the need for fewer orthopaedic operations and that SDR is safe in terms of long-term complications [1–4, 6, 21, 22].

Data collection should include the following areas:

1. Attainment of pre-SDR family-focused goal setting
2. GMFM and other motor measures
3. Radiographic measures—hip and spine
4. Gait analysis
5. Clinical assessment—spasticity levels and musculoskeletal joint range assessment
6. Quality of life measures—independence and participation
7. Continence (bowel and bladder)
8. Sensory change
9. Pain

Lewis in 2019 proposed a protocol for a national registry of multidimensional outcomes following SDR in Australia [23]. See Figs. 14.1 and 14.2.

They have suggested the timing and battery of assessments which should be performed when considering SDR.

The primary and secondary outcome measures	
Gross motor function and mobility (activity)	Gross motor function measure-66 Functional Mobility Scale Gillette Functional Assessment Questionnaire Six min walk test Timed up-and-go
Gait (body structure and functions)	Gait Profile Score and Gait Variable Scores from 3DGA (barefoot)
Goal attainment (activity and participation)	Canadian Occupational Performance Measure
Musculoskeletal interventions (body structure and functions)	Botulinum toxin A injections Musculoskeletal surgeries
Pain (body structure and functions)	Faces Pain Scale-Revised Checklist of pain location PROMIS Paediatric Pain Interference Scale
Quality of life (personal factors)	Cerebral Palsy Quality of Life Questionnaires

3DGA: three-dimensional gait analysis.

Fig. 14.2 Suggested primary and secondary outcome measures following SDR—Australian protocol

14.8 Factors Influencing Functional Outcome Following SDR

Despite using different surgical protocols, most data shows the benefit of SDR in the short term (2 years) on spasticity reduction and improvement in GMFM. Recent evidence highlighting this, is from the United Kingdom, and the benefit of these studies is that they are larger cohorts of children undergoing SDR with similar selection, surgical and postoperative protocols. They used a single-level laminotomy procedure and have been focused on children with cerebral palsy GMFCS levels 2 and 3 [10, 20]. One study reported on 150 patients from a single centre including patients GFMCS 2–4 and the other was a national study, following up 137 GMFCS 2–3 patients.

Several studies have looked at the factors influencing outcome following SDR as part of long-term follow-up studies. There is a developing consensus that SDR has long-term benefits, but there continues to be some conflicting evidence, which is understandable. For example, most studies report long-term reduction in spasticity many years following SDR. Tedroff reported on 17 years post-SDR follow-up and concluded that the spasticity reducing effect did not however improve long-term functioning nor prevent contractures but may reduce pain [24]. Tedroff's 2020 systematic review on the long-term effects of SDR felt the evidence available was low level, and at 10 years post-SDR, there wasn't convincing evidence of functional improvement with SDR over conventional treatment [2]. It is possible that this is due to the heterogeneity of the studies at the time and highlights why national and even international standardization of procedures is necessary.

Munger and MacWilliams have published data which may be contrary to much of the published data on long-term outcome following SDR [1, 3]. Munger concluded that both SDR and non-SDR patients improved in their gait 10 years after surgery. Patients without SDR had larger improvements in gait but underwent significantly more interventions. MacWilliams published a multicentre trial which showed that spasticity was effectively reduced in the long term following SDR; however, this SDR group underwent more orthopaedic surgery and antispasmodic injections to the legs. They had a control group and concluded that untreated spasticity doesn't cause meaningful impairment in young adult hood at the level of pathophysiology, function or quality of life.

The more recent larger cohorts of patients going through the same selection criteria and the same procedure for SDR will hopefully provide more consistent data on long-term outcome [10, 20].

It is important to acknowledge the influence of parental and child expectations regarding perceived outcome following SDR. Some measures are more subjective than others, and it may be that parents who actively pursued SDR will report better outcomes or conversely be disappointed if overly optimistic outcomes are not achieved [25, 26].

Children who are GMFCS levels 2 and 3 will do better in their mobility scores in the long term compared with GMFCS levels 4 and 5. Within the GMFCS levels 2 and 3, a further subset of children with higher GMFMs preoperatively will have the additional and sustained benefit. Several studies report the motor gains seen in GMFCS level 4 are lost at longer-term follow-up [6].

If a service, however, has very strict selection criteria based on GMFM score, this may be prohibitive in providing the procedure to the wider population of children who may benefit from it.

For the GMFCS level 4–5 group, it has been proposed that different outcome measures are needed such as the PEDI score (Paediatric Evaluation of Disability Inventory), which some earlier studies have not used. Comfort and caregiver satisfaction may be more important for this group, so proposed SDR is still indicated [9, 27]. Some studies have proposed SDR instead of intrathecal baclofen pump replacement in this population, as they report it confers similar efficacy. In children who had SDR instead of ITB pump replacement, only those with mixed tone and high levels of dystonia had ongoing difficulties following the SDR [9, 27].

Dudley's study in 2013 suggested a PILAR score (predictive index for long-term ambulation after rhizotomy) to help identify which children will do better with regard to long-term mobility following SDR. Their follow-up was at 10 years and the index was largely based on the GMFM-88 [6].

Components of the PILAR Score

1. Preop GMFCS SCORE—Better outcome the lower the GMFCS level (1 vs. 4)
2. Preop GMFM-88 score—Better outcome with GMFM-88 over 60 compared to under 60
3. Spasticity distribution—Better outcome with diplegia compared to triplegia or quadriplegia
4. Hip adductor tone (Ashworth score)—Better outcome under 3 compared to over 3

Several studies have followed children up for many years following SDR. Tedroff published outcomes at 17 years post-SDR, and in 2022, Langerak published 26–35 years post-SDR gait status from their original cohort operated on by Peacock [21, 24].

Some studies have demonstrated that the natural history of spasticity in spastic cerebral palsy is to decline with age [30]. This is another reason why timing of SDR is crucial with better gains seen when it is not delayed into late childhood or early adolescence.

A few centres believe that spasticity is the main cause of motor difficulties in spastic cerebral palsy and hence advocate early SDR, even as young as 2 years old. In most international centres, however, the consensus is to wait until the child is older, usually around 4 years old to identify what are the main issues affecting mobility, such as motor control, weakness, dystonia and even cognition. Children will also naturally make rapid gains in motor function between the ages of 2 years and 4 years in milder forms of cerebral palsy, and gains from very early SDR may be confounded by these expected gains. It is important not to delay SDR too long to help avoid fixed contracture formation, and it should be considered when there is plateauing of motor skills with conventional spasticity treatments. The evidence suggests that contracture development in cerebral palsy is not related to spasticity alone, but interventions for spasticity may alter the musculoskeletal trajectory if done early enough [28, 29].

14.9 What the Evidence Suggests Regarding Long-Term Outcome of SDR

As time goes on and as protocols become more standardized, it will be easier to assess the effect of SDR, but looking at the key long-term studies of outcome following SDR, a few themes have become evident [1–6, 15].

1. SDR causes the long-term reduction in spasticity.
2. Children who are GMFCS levels 2 and 3, with better GMFM scores and milder levels of spasticity, will do better in terms of mobility outcomes in the short and long term following SDR.
3. Most children who undergo SDR will remain or improve in one level on the GMFCS scale. Most children do not deteriorate on the GMFCS scale following SDR surgery.
4. Most of the motor gains in the GMFCS levels 2 and 3 are in the first 3–5 years following SDR with then plateau or decline, but usually, levels of function remain above baseline. The nadir is around 10–14 years of age.
5. SDR may delay the functional peak and protect against the decline somewhat in GMFCS 3.
6. Motor gains in GMFCS levels 4 and 5 are often lost at longer-term follow-up, but other gains following the reduction in spasticity may be evident.

7. SDR is best performed before the onset of fixed musculoskeletal deformity and prior to the plateau or reduction in function due to the natural history of cerebral palsy. This is commonly around the age of 5 in most children with bilateral spastic CP. The mobility outcomes are worse if SDR is performed after the age of 10.
8. Most studies identified that there is no reduction in strength or strength has increased post-SDR.
9. Several studies show long-term improvement in areas such as GMFM score, ambulator status, range of movement and gait quality, but this may not be consistent with improvements in participation or quality of life. In very long-term studies, the gait improved or stayed the same in approximately 80% at 18 years post-SDR.
10. Most children need ongoing orthopaedic follow-up and intervention to maintain mobility gains following SDR. A systematic review in 2020 showed 60% required orthopaedic post-SDR (51% soft tissue and 22% bony surgery) [4]. Earlier age of SDR tends to indicate less need for orthopaedic surgery with O'Brien showing 34% of patients requiring orthopaedic surgery if SDR was performed before 6 years old compared to 70% requiring orthopaedic surgery if SDR was performed after 6 years old [31].
11. Children who have had SDR have the same gait outcomes as children receiving conventional cerebral palsy treatment in the long term but have significantly less procedures to achieve this (spasticity treatments and orthopaedic interventions).
12. More studies are identifying dystonia as part of the spastic cerebral palsy classification phenotype. Dystonia associated with PVL appears to be less of an issue post-SDR compared to dystonia due to primary hypoxic basal ganglia injury or congenital brain malformation. GMFCS levels 4–5 will have higher incidence of mixed muscle tone, and uncontrolled dystonia following SDR in this population can be problematic [9].
13. Some children with cerebral palsy (especially GMFCS level 4) rely on hypertonia to maintain upright postures. Unmasked weakness following SDR can be an issue in these children, and they may find some upright (standing) function harder.
14. Weight gain is common following SDR and this can affect the long-term mobility outcome.
15. It is important to set realistic goals with families when counselling for SDR. Parental expectation and acceptance will be an important factor interpreting some outcome measures following SDR.
16. There evidence to support that there is short- and long-term upper limb functional improvement following SDR.
17. SDR does not reduce the long-term energy consumption in children with ambulant cerebral palsy compared to controls. Some studies have shown an energy consumption reduction post-SDR, but they didn't have control groups. The natural history is for energy consumption and spasticity to reduce with age in cerebral palsy [30].

18. Some papers quote long-term high levels of independence in self-care tasks post-SDR, with GMFCS level 1 doing better than GMFCS level 3 [21]. When measured on the PEDI, there are increases to 3 years post-SDR then stabilization. It is hard to ascertain the effect of SDR on actual independence.

14.10 Potential Long-Term Complications Following SDR

Mishra et al. performed a systematic review of complications following SDR both long and short term in 2023 [32]. Overall, they categorized the complications into two distinct groups, structural and neurological. They concluded that the majority of complications following SDR are managed conservatively, but there will still be a physical, psychological and financial burden which should be taken into account. Tu, also provided a systematic review of long-term complications following SDR and concluded very low levels of long-term complications [4].

14.10.1 Hip Subluxation

Despite anecdotal and case reports of accelerated hip subluxation following SDR, Miller concluded that the incidence of hip displacement post-SDR is consistent with population-based studies when evaluated by GMFCS. Their study had neither a positive nor negative effect on hip displacement when assessed at least 5 years post-SDR [33]. This supports that children still need orthopaedic follow and specifically hip surveillance following SDR.

14.11 Spinal Deformity

The natural history of spinal deformity in cerebral palsy is 20–25%. Tu's systematic review showed that the rate of spinal deformity following SDR is 29.5% with only 3% requiring spinal deformity surgery [4]. This study concluded that SDR doesn't seem to change the rates of spinal deformity significantly, but ongoing surveillance is recommended. Mishra's 2022 systematic review of complications reported 5–7% of patients across 15 studies had scoliosis with the greatest risk in quadriplegia and young children [32]. High Cobb angle of more than 30 degrees preop was associated with increased progression. Hyperlordosis was noted in eight studies with a prevalence of 18.4% with the highest risk being in female gender, younger age at surgery, quadriplegia, scoliosis and intellectual delay. Kyphosis was reported across ten studies with a prevalence of 8.4%. Scoliosis and lower kyphosis preoperatively are highly indicative of abnormal kyphosis postoperatively.

Spondylolysis and spondylolisthesis were noted across nine studies with a prevalence of 9.6%. Spondylosis and spondylolisthesis are associated with higher levels of mobility, greater lumbar lordosis and loading across the posterior lower spine, so are more common in GMFCS levels 1–3.

14.12 Pain

Daunter et al. looked at a cohort of patients averaging 22 years post-SDR [34]. This was a case control study, and they reported that SDR was not related to lower levels of pain interference, pain intensity or fatigue compared to controls. Lower back and lower extremity pain was the most common reported areas. The group with SDR did report higher levels of function, had fewer complaints of gross motor decline and needed less assistance compared to those who didn't have SDR. Tu's 2020 systematic review of long-term outcome in SDR identified that 50% complained of back pain at least once per week and 42% complained of leg discomfort, but it was generally minor, and it isn't clear if chronic pain is a long-term problem post-SDR [4]. In a study of patients 25–35 years post-SDR, 28% had lower back pain, but 80% reported no or minimal disability in relation to this [35].

14.13 Weight Gain

Weight gain is a common feature following SDR. The Oswestry team published on 19 children undergoing SDR [7]. They reported excessive weight gain in 18 of the 19 patients and advised specific counselling regarding this. Excessive weight gain in children with existing motor difficulty may counter the gains of spasticity reduction during initial rehabilitation and later during transition into adolescence.

14.14 Bowel and Bladder Dysfunction

Bowel and bladder continence issues are common in cerebral palsy and are related to age of the child, physical ability and cognition. New bowel and bladder problems were seen in 8.9% of patients post-SDR, with 2% having transient dysfunction for a few weeks following the procedure. In a report of follow-up at over 18 years post-SDR, 7.3% had bladder dysfunction, but there was no baseline data to link this to the SDR procedure. None of these patients required catheterization suggesting the difficulty was non-neurogenic. Overall bladder dysfunction is not a common problem in the long term, and bowel dysfunction appears to be mainly an issue in the perioperative period.

14.15 Conclusion

Despite differing SDR protocols, there is now good evidence to show short- and long-term efficacy, associated with good long-term safety data. It is easier to identify which cohorts of children will have sustained benefit in mobility and which children will benefit from improvements in care and comfort goals.

Post-SDR rehabilitation protocols are dependent on the procedure performed and do not necessarily need to be as an inpatient, as in the case of single-level laminotomy procedures. Many of these children are medically stable to be discharged at 1 week postop and can then continue their rehabilitation in an outpatient day rehabilitation programme. This has significant benefits for services with limited inpatient hospital resources. Family counselling regarding the long-term commitment to therapy is very important if long-term motor gains following SDR are to be sustained.

References

1. Munger ME, Aldahondo N, Krach LE, Novacheck TF, Schwartz MH. Long-term outcomes after selective dorsal rhizotomy: a retrospective matched cohort study. Dev Med Child Neurol. 2017;59:1196–203.
2. Tedroff K, Hägglund G, Miller F. Long-term effects of selective dorsal rhizotomy in children with cerebral palsy: a systematic review. Dev Med Child Neurol. 2020;62:554–62.
3. McMulkin ML, MacWilliams BA, Nelson EA, et al. The long-term effects of aggressive spasticity reducing treatment, including selective dorsal rhizotomy, on joint kinematic outcomes of persons with cerebral palsy. Gait Posture. 2023;105:139–48.
4. Tu A, Steinbok P. Long term outcome of selective dorsal Rhizotomy for the management of childhood spasticity-functional improvement and complications. Childs Nerv Syst. 2020;36:1985–94.
5. Ailon T, Beauchamp R, Miller S, Mortenson P, Kerr JM, Hengel AR, Steinbok P. Long-term outcome after selective dorsal rhizotomy in children with spastic cerebral palsy. Childs Nerv Syst. 2015;31:415–23.
6. Dudley RWR, Parolin M, Gagnon B, et al. Long-term functional benefits of selective dorsal rhizotomy for spastic cerebral palsy: clinical article. J Neurosurg Pediatr. 2013;12:142–50.
7. Cole GF, Farmer SE, Roberts A, Stewart C, Patrick JH. Selective dorsal rhizotomy for children with cerebral palsy: the Oswestry experience. Arch Dis Child. 2007;92:781–5.
8. Gillespie CS, Hall BJ, George AM, Hennigan D, Sneade C, Cawker S, Silva AHD, Vloeberghs M, Aquilina K, Pettorini B. Selective dorsal rhizotomy in non-ambulant children with cerebral palsy: a multi-center prospective study. Childs Nerv Syst. 2024;40:171–80.
9. D'Aquino D, Moussa AA, Ammar A, Ingale H, Vloeberghs M. Selective dorsal rhizotomy for the treatment of severe spastic cerebral palsy: efficacy and therapeutic durability in GMFCS grade IV and V children. Acta Neurochir. 2018;160:811–21.
10. Jeffery SMT, Markia B, Pople IK, et al. Surgical outcomes of single-level bilateral selective dorsal Rhizotomy for spastic Diplegia in 150 consecutive patients. World Neurosurg. 2019;125:e60–6.
11. Hesselgard K, Reinstrup P, Stromblad LG, Undén J, Romner B. Selective dorsal rhizotomy and postoperative pain management. A worldwide survey. Pediatr Neurosurg. 2007;43:107–12.

12. Shahid J, Kashif A, Shahid MK. Enhancing post-operative recovery in spastic Diplegia through physical therapy rehabilitation following selective dorsal Rhizotomy: a case report and thorough literature analysis. Children (Basel). 2023; https://doi.org/10.3390/children10050842.
13. Nicolini-Panisson RD, Tedesco AP, Folle MR, Donadio MVF. Selective dorsal rhizotomy in cerebral palsy: selection criteria and postoperative physical therapy protocols. Rev Paul Pediatr. 2018;36:9.
14. Limpaphayom N, Stewart S, Wang L, Liu J, Park TS, Dobbs MB. Functional outcomes after selective dorsal rhizotomy followed by minimally invasive tendon lengthening procedures in children with spastic cerebral palsy. J Pediatr Orthop B. 2020;29:1–8.
15. Mortenson P, Sadashiva N, Tamber MS, Steinbok P. Long-term upper extremity performance in children with cerebral palsy following selective dorsal rhizotomy. Childs Nerv Syst. 2021;37:1983–9.
16. Merckx L, Poncelet F, De Houwer H, Laumen A, Peeters L, Nuttin B, Pauwels P, Van Campenhout A, Ortibus E, De Vloo P. Upper-extremity spasticity and functionality after selective dorsal rhizotomy for cerebral palsy: a systematic review. J Neurosurg Pediatr. 2023;32:673–85.
17. Blatt K, Lewis J, Bican R, Leonard J. Selective dorsal Rhizotomy: patient demographics and postoperative physical therapy. Pediatr Neurol. 2023;147:56–62.
18. McLaughlin J, Bjornson K, Temkin N, et al. Selective dorsal rhizotomy: meta-analysis of three randomized controlled trials. Dev Med Child Neurol. 2002;44:17–25.
19. Sargut TA, Haberl H, Wolter S, Tafelski S, van Riesen A, Linhard M, Kaindl AM, Thomale U-W, Schulz M. Motor and functional outcome of selective dorsal rhizotomy in children with spastic diplegia at 12 and 24 months of follow-up. Acta Neurochir. 2021;163:2837–44.
20. Summers J, Coker B, Eddy S, et al. Selective dorsal rhizotomy in ambulant children with cerebral palsy: an observational cohort study. Lancet Child Adolesc Health. 2019;3:455–62.
21. Langerak NG, Veerbeek BE, Fieggen AG, Lamberts RP. Gait status 26–35 years after selective dorsal rhizotomy: a 9 year follow up study. Gait Posture. 2022;91:284–9.
22. Josenby AL, Wagner P, Jarnlo GB, Westbom L, Nordmark E. Functional performance in self-care and mobility after selective dorsal rhizotomy: a 10-year practice-based follow-up study. Dev Med Child Neurol. 2015;57:286–93.
23. Lewis J, Bear N, Baker F, et al. Australian children undergoing selective dorsal rhizotomy: protocol for a national registry of multidimensional outcomes. BMJ Open. 2019;9:e025093.
24. Tedroff K, Löwing K, Åström E. A prospective cohort study investigating gross motor function, pain, and health-related quality of life 17 years after selective dorsal rhizotomy in cerebral palsy. Dev Med Child Neurol. 2015;57:484–90.
25. Paget SP, Campbell L, Blaxland A, Lewis J, Morrow AM, Wimalasundera N. "Life-changing surgery": English-language news media representation of selective dorsal rhizotomy. Child Care Health Dev. 2021;47:844–50.
26. Waite G, Chugh D, Cawker S, Oulton K, Wray J, Harniess P. "Wanting no regrets": parental decision making around selective dorsal rhizotomy. Child Care Health Dev. 2023;49:382–91.
27. Buizer AI, van Schie PEM, Bolster EAM, van Ouwerkerk WJ, Strijers RL, van de Pol LA, Stadhouder A, Becher JG, Vermeulen RJ. Effect of selective dorsal rhizotomy on daily care and comfort in non-walking children and adolescents with severe spasticity. Eur J Paediatr Neurol. 2017;21:350–7.
28. Tedroff K, Löwing K, Jacobson DNO, Åström E. Does loss of spasticity matter? A 10-year follow-up after selective dorsal rhizotomy in cerebral palsy. Dev Med Child Neurol. 2011;53:724–9.
29. Nordmark E, Hägglund G, Lauge-Pedersen H, Wagner P, Westbom L. Development of lower limb range of motion from early childhood to adolescence in cerebral palsy: a population-based study. BMC Med. 2009;7:65.
30. Zaino NL, Steele KM, Donelan JM, Schwartz MH. Energy consumption does not change after selective dorsal rhizotomy in children with spastic cerebral palsy. Dev Med Child Neurol. 2020;62:1047–53.

31. O'Brien DF, Park TS, Puglisi JA, Collins DR, Leuthardt EC. Effect of selective dorsal rhizotomy on need for orthopedic surgery for spastic quadriplegic cerebral palsy: long-term outcome analysis in relation to age. J Neurosurg. 2004;101:59–63.
32. Mishra D, Barik S, Raj V, Kandwal P. A systematic review of complications following selective dorsal rhizotomy in cerebral palsy. Neurochirurgie. 2023;69:101425.
33. Miller SD, Juricic M, Bone JN, Steinbok P, Mulpuri K. The effect of selective dorsal Rhizotomy on hip displacement in children with cerebral palsy: a long-term follow-up study. J Pediatr Orthop. 2023;43:e701–6.
34. Daunter AK, Kratz AL, Hurvitz EA. Long-term impact of childhood selective dorsal rhizotomy on pain, fatigue, and function: a case-control study. Dev Med Child Neurol. 2017;59:1089–95.
35. Veerbeek BE, Lamberts RP, Fieggen AG, Mankahla N, de Villiers RVP, Botha E, Langerak NG. A long-term follow-up study of spinal abnormalities and pain in adults with cerebral palsy and spastic diplegia more than 25 years after selective dorsal rhizotomy. J Neurosurg Spine. 2020;34:228–35.

Chapter 15
Long-Term Outcome of Selective Dorsal Rhizotomy for Spastic Children

Nelleke G. Langerak, Berendina E. Veerbeek, and Robert P. Lamberts

Abbreviations

CP	Cerebral palsy
FMS	Functional Mobility Scale
GDI	Gait Deviation Index
GMFCS	Gross Motor Function Classification System
GPS	Gait Profile Score
HRQoL	Health-Related Quality of Life
ICF	International Classification of Functioning, Disability and Health
LIFE-H	Life Habits questionnaire
MACS	Manual Ability Classification System
ROM	Range of motion
SF-36v2	The Health-Related Quality of Life Health Survey Version 2
TUG	Timed Up and Go
SDR	Selective dorsal rhizotomy
2DGA	2-Dimensional Gait Analysis
3DGA	3-Dimensional Gait Analysis

N. G. Langerak (✉)
Division of Neurosurgery and Neuroscience Institute, Faculty of Health Sciences, University of Cape Town, Cape Town, South Africa

Departement of Research, Sint Maartenskliniek, Nijmegen, The Netherlands

B. E. Veerbeek
Division of Neurosurgery and Neuroscience Institute, Faculty of Health Sciences, University of Cape Town, Cape Town, South Africa

R. P. Lamberts
Department of Human Movement Sciences, University Medical Center Groningen & University of Groningen, Groningen, The Netherlands

N. Morota, P. Steinbok (eds.), *Dorsal Rhizotomy: Neurosurgery for Childhood Spasticity*, Advances and Technical Standards in Neurosurgery 51,
https://doi.org/10.1007/978-3-031-86441-4_15

15.1 Aging with Spastic Cerebral Palsy

Owing to advancements in medical care and interventions, the lifespan of individuals with cerebral palsy (CP) has significantly extended [1]. A remarkable outcome of these improvements is the survival of almost all higher-functioning children with CP into adulthood. The life expectancy of individuals with CP is close to that of typically developing adults [2]. Consequently, a pivotal challenge in the current era revolves around understanding the life trajectory of adults who have undergone maturation with a 'pediatric condition' such as CP [3].

The demographic landscape has evolved to the extent that there are now more adults living with CP than children, accentuating the importance of addressing the challenges associated with healthy aging [1]. Effective intervention during childhood is crucial to prevent secondary complications. Treatment is often primarily focused on the musculoskeletal system to enhance overall functional status and quality of life across the lifespan [3, 4].

Given that approximately 80% of individuals with CP exhibit spasticity [5], it becomes imperative to specifically address spasticity to avert secondary abnormalities such as lower extremity deformities, contractures, joint dysplasia, and pain. Managing spasticity is integral to facilitating optimal physical development [6, 7].

Selective dorsal rhizotomy (SDR) is endorsed as an irreversible intervention for spasticity treatment in children with spastic CP [8, 9]. Despite numerous studies investigating the impact of this neurosurgical procedure, the majority are characterized by relatively short-term follow-up assessments in children and adolescents with CP. The most extensive follow-up studies on adults who underwent SDR during childhood have been conducted by the research group in Cape Town [10–13]. These follow-up studies conducted more than 25 years post-SDR are crucial for comprehensively assessing the long-term implications of SDR on various aspects of functioning and quality of life in adults with CP.

15.2 ICF Model Framework to Describe Outcomes of SDR

A common framework for evaluating the outcomes of management in CP is the International Classification of Functioning, Disability and Health (ICF) model from the World Health Organization [14]. This framework adopts a biopsychosocial perspective, emphasizing functioning, disability, and health [14]. It provides a conceptual framework for delineating functioning, disability, and health through the interplay of 'body structure and function', 'activities' and 'participation', 'personal factors', and 'environmental factors'. Change in any of these domains are postulated to exert an impact on other domains, influencing the individual's overall health. Quality of life is not being explicitly encompassed within the ICF model; however, there is a proposal for an expanded ICF model. This proposed model incorporates an overarching dimension of 'quality of life' since it is considered an indispensable concept that encapsulates and synthesizes various dimensions within the ICF model [15].

In the following paragraphs, the post-SDR outcomes are summarized using the ICF model domains and quality of life. This is a description of the literature focusing on studies conducted between 5 and 15 years and between 15 and 25 years post-SDR. Since SDR was first reintroduced by Warwick Peacock in Cape Town, South Africa [16], the Cape Town research group has the longest track record of research in this field. Their experiences, more than 25 years post-SDR, are also described below [10–13].

The Cape Town research group examined adults with bilateral spastic CP over a span of 25–35 years post-SDR. These results were compared to a previous follow-up study conducted with the same cohort 9 years ago and a cohort of typically developing adults [10, 11, 13]. The CP cohort participated in these studies underwent SDR following the 'Peacock' method (laminectomies L2–S1) [16, 17] at Red Cross War Memorial Children's Hospital in Cape Town, South Africa, between 1981 and 1991. These children were selected adhering strict SDR selection criteria [18, 19]. In addition, it is noteworthy to mention that the majority of the CP cohort had no other diagnosis influencing their medical status. As presented in Table 15.1, additional orthopedic surgical interventions were common, with 14 participants (54%) receiving surgery before SDR and 15 (58%) after SDR. However, none of the participants ever received other interventions such as intramuscular botulinum toxin or intrathecal baclofen. At time of the follow-up studies more than 25 years post-SDR, the median age of the participants was 35 years, and 60% were male. Preoperatively, 18 (69%) adults were classified as Gross Motor Function Classification System (GMFCS) level II and 8 (31%) as level III. This distribution changed with the majority (65%) of adults with CP showed improved gross motor

Table 15.1 Overview of orthopedic surgeries received by adults with CP who participated in the studies conducted >25 year after SDR (n = 26)

	Number of participants (%)	
Interventions	Pre-SDR	Post-SDR
Soft-tissue surgery		
Plantar flexors	12 (46)	12 (46)
Rectus femoris	3 (12)	2 (8)
Hamstrings	7 (27)	13 (50)
Adductors	7 (27)	2 (8)
Iliopsoas	1 (4)	1 (4)
At least one soft-tissue surgery	14 (54)	14 (54)
Bony surgery		
Femoral derotation	2 (8)	1 (4)
Tibial derotation	0 (0)	0 (0)
Ankle/foot	0 (0)	4 (15)
Toe	0 (0)	4 (15)
At least one bony surgery	2 (8)	7 (27)

function compared to preoperative levels (lower GMFCS level) and none showed deterioration. More than 25 years after SDR, half of the cohort were classified as GMFCS level I, 38% as level II, and 12% as level III [12].

15.3 Body Function and Structure

15.3.1 5–15 Years After SDR

Grunt et al. conducted a systematic review, analysing 21 articles encompassing a cohort of 966 children with a minimum follow-up duration of 5 years. The study showed that SDR exhibited a poor to moderately positive long-term effect on the ICF domain 'body function and structure', attributable to reductions in spasticity, increased range of motion (ROM), and improvements in gait [20]. Consistent with these findings, other studies also affirmed the enduring spasticity reduction effect of SDR [21–25]. Divergent results were observed concerning passive ROM, with some studies reporting improvements [21], others noting no change [22, 24], and some indicating deterioration [22, 23]. Muscle strength outcomes also varied, with some studies reporting no differences [21] and others observing sustained increases, particularly in quadriceps muscles [23]. In addition, selective motor control remained unchanged [21]. Regarding gait patterns, 3-Dimensional Gait Analysis (3DGA) demonstrated sustained improvements in Gait Profile Score (GPS) and Gait Deviation Index (GDI) [21, 26].

A potential association between SDR and spinal deformities in children and adolescents was reported by Grunt et al., acknowledging the inherent challenge of distinguishing such associations from the natural progression of deformities in CP [20]. Wheelwright et al. also noted that spinal deformities could be a potential complication of SDR [27]; however, a notable prevalence of spinal deformities is evident in the general CP population. The absence of control groups, representing individuals who did not undergo SDR, in the conducted studies introduces uncertainty regarding the causative relationship of these spinal deformities [20]. This uncertainty is further underscored by the findings of Van Schie et al. [25], who reported a minimal occurrence of spinal deformities, including scoliosis and spondylolysis, 6 years post-SDR.

An association between spinal deformities and back pain has been noted in the 5–15 years following SDR [28, 29]. Grunt et al. reported that between 5% and 29% of individuals who underwent SDR experienced back pain during long-term follow-up [20]. However, it is essential to consider that, in addition to spinal deformities, various factors can contribute to pain in adolescents and young adults with CP, such as comorbidities and persistent muscle spasticity [22, 30]. Moreover, the prevalence of pain in adults with CP is acknowledged to be higher than in the general population [31, 32]. Tedroff et al.'s study reported low pain severity and minimal interference with daily tasks based on the Brief Pain Inventory, suggesting a potential influence of SDR on pain outcomes [22]. Munger et al. similarly reported comparable results, emphasizing that pain caused minimal interference with activities [21]. Notably, while they did not attribute these results solely to SDR, they concluded that both SDR and alternative treatment regimens equally contribute to preventing the onset of pain through early adulthood.

15.3.2 15–25 Years After SDR

The reduction of spasticity following SDR appears to be widely accepted without significant controversy. However, there is a scarcity of literature available on (young) adults with CP with a follow-up period exceeding 15 years after surgery. Noteworthy studies by Dudley et al. (15 years post-SDR) and Langerak et al. (17–25 years post-SDR) have corroborated sustained reductions in muscle tone during early adulthood [33, 34]. This reduction in muscle tone was also evident in the gait pattern, as demonstrated by Langerak et al. (17–25 years post-SDR) in their 3DGA study [35]. Despite the presence of a mild crouch gait pattern in young adults, relatively good active joint ROM was observed. A 2DGA follow-up study conducted by the same research group over 1, 3, 10, and 20 years post-SDR affirmed this finding [36]. Additionally, another study by Langerak et al. (1 and 20 years post-SDR) reported sustained improvements in passive ROM, muscle strength, and voluntary movement (combination selectivity and muscle strength) across these parameters [37].

Regarding spinal abnormalities, only one study has reported on these issues in young adults with CP between 15 and 25 years after SDR. Conducted by the Cape Town research group, this study observed instances of scoliosis, hyperkyphosis, hyperlordosis, spondylolysis, and spondylolisthesis. The findings indicated that only the incidence of relatively mild scoliosis increased over time. However, it remained unclear to what extent these abnormalities were attributed to SDR versus the natural course of CP [34].

Chronic back pain was documented in (young) adults with CP at 19 years post-SDR, based on the Pain Numerical Rating Scale [38], and at 22 years post-SDR, utilizing the Patient-Reported Outcome Measurement Information System and pain assessment tools [39]. However, the incidence, interference, and location of pain in these adults were reported to be similar to what has been previously documented in the literature for adults with CP [38]. Additionally, the pain experiences of these individuals were comparable to those of an age-matched control group (adults with CP who did not undergo SDR) [39]. The long-term SDR follow-up study conducted by Langerak et al. [34], which primarily focused on spinal abnormalities, also reported on the occurrences of pain in the upper and lower extremities, as well as at the spinal level, more than 17 years after SDR. Notably, this pain had either minimal or no discernible influence on daily activities, as indicated by the Oswestry Disability Index.

15.3.3 Experience from Cape Town >25 Years After SDR

The Cape Town research group reported normalized muscle tone in adults with CP more than 25 years after SDR [12]. The reduction in muscle tone resulting from SDR had also long-lasting positive effects on the gait pattern of adults with CP [13]. Beyond 25 years after SDR, adults with CP and spastic diplegia demonstrated a mild crouch gait pattern with minimal signs of spasticity. Importantly, their walking pattern remained stable over a 9-year follow-up period and was associated with the GMFCS levels assessed concurrently [13]. Lower scores were identified for passive ROM, muscle strength, and selective motor control in comparison to the cohort with typically developing adults aligning with the anticipated characteristics in adults with CP [12]. These differences may be attributed to variances in the neurophysiology of muscles between individuals with CP and their peers [33, 37, 40].

In the follow-up examination conducted more than 25 years after SDR, spinal abnormalities, including scoliosis, hyperkyphosis, and hyperlordosis, were identified. However, these abnormalities did not appear to manifest more frequently than what has been reported in adults with CP. Notably, this observation was not found for spondylolysis and spondylolisthesis, which seemed to occur more frequently than reported in adolescents with CP. In addition, over a 9-year follow-up period, the overall prevalence of spinal abnormalities did not exhibit significant changes [10]. As also noted in shorter follow-up studies [20], it is essential to acknowledge the limited available data on the natural history of CP and its impact on spinal abnormalities, making it challenging to independently attribute effects solely to SDR. Furthermore, the identified spinal abnormalities showed no correlation with contextual factors, except for hyperkyphosis in females, abnormality in sensation, or the level of disability due to back pain. Participants reported minimal disability, which did not progress over time and did not impede their engagement in activities of daily living [10] (Table 15.2).

Table 15.2 Experiences of participants at certain time periods after SDR

5–15 years post-SDR	15–25 years post-SDR	> 25 years post-SDR Experience from Cape Town	
Body structure and function			
Spasticity	Reduced	Sustained reduced muscle tone	No change after 9 years follow-up
ROM	Mixed; increased, no change, decreased	Sustained improved passive ROM	No change after 9 years follow-up
Muscle strength	Mixed; increased, no change	Sustained improved muscle strength	No change after 9 years follow-up
Selective motor control	No change	Sustained improved voluntary movements	No change after 9 years follow-up
Gait	Improved gait pattern	Sustained mild crouch gait	No change after 9 years follow-up
Spinal deformity	Not deteriorated[a]	Sustained, only increase of mild scoliosis[a]	No change after 9 years follow-up
Pain	Not increased[a]	Sustained (back) pain[a]	No change after 9 years follow-up
Activity and participation			
Function	Mixed: Increased, no change, decreased	Sustained improved functional level	No change after 9 years follow-up
Participation	No change	Good; similar to typically developing peers, except for lower mobility and recreation levels	No change after 9 years follow-up
Quality of life			
Mental and physical status	Good	High levels of satisfaction	Good; similar to typically developing adults, except for lower physical functioning

[a]*Difficult to interpret the data with no control group of individuals with CP, who did not undergo SDR*

15.4 Activity and Participation

15.4.1 5–15 Years After SDR

The systematic review conducted by Grunt et al. [20] failed to discover compelling evidence supporting the positive impact of SDR on the 'activity' and 'participation' domains of the ICF model. Subsequent to this review, a spectrum of studies has been published, presenting distinct findings. Van Schie et al. [25], Bolster et al. [41], and Josenby et al. [24] reported sustained improvements in the Gross Motor Function Measurement (GMFM) 6–10 years post-SDR. In contrast, Tedroff et al. documented a decline in GMFM 10 years post-SDR [22], and Munger et al. found no discernible difference in function, as assessed by the Median Gillette Functional Assessment Questionnaire and Functional Mobility Scale (FMS), between the SDR and control groups 10–17 years post-SDR [21].

There is a scarcity of long-term outcome studies examining the level of participation among children and adolescents in the community, particularly within the context of a SDR follow-up study. Grunt et al. reported the absence of such studies [20], and to the best of our knowledge, only Munger et al. incorporated this domain in their 13-year SDR follow-up study. Utilizing the Frequency of Participation Questionnaire, Munger et al. concluded that there were no differences in participation levels between a group that underwent SDR and a group that did not undergo SDR [21].

15.4.2 15–25 Years After SDR

Favourable outcomes in terms of functioning were documented for young adults more than 15 years after SDR. Dudley et al. [33] reported sustained improvement in GMFM 15 years post-SDR. Langerak et al. [37] similarly noted sustained improvement in functioning, utilizing the Berman scale, 20 years after SDR, and observed high levels of functioning based on the FMS 17–25 years post-SDR [42]. Additionally, Hurvitz et al. showed self-reported higher functional levels and a lower incidence of motor function decline (based on GMFCS) and Manual Ability Classification System (MACS) in comparison to a control group 19 years after SDR [38].

Only one research group has contributed to the body of literature by publishing a study on outcomes related to participation more than 15 years after SDR. This study demonstrated that adults with CP experience elevated levels of accomplishment and satisfaction in their daily activities and participation in the community, as assessed through the Life Habits questionnaire (LIFE-H) [42]. This questionnaire encompassed domains such as nutrition, fitness, personal care, communication, housing, and mobility. Notably, the majority of adults with CP exhibited independence in the execution of life habits, encompassing personal care, engagement in community life, and employment. However, challenges were identified in the domains of mobility and recreation [42].

15.4.3 Experience from Cape Town >25 Years After SDR

The concern regarding a decline in walking ability associated with aging in individuals with CP, which typically begins in their 20 s and 30 s [43, 44], did not align with the findings from the Cape Town cohort observed more than 25 years after SDR. The majority of the cohort did not demonstrate an increased risk for falls based on the Timed Up and Go (TUG) test [12]. In fact, 54% of adults with CP in the cohort were able to walk independently without the need for walking aids, and no decline in FMS scores was identified over a 9-year period [11] (Table 15.2).

These encouraging outcomes were mirrored in the consistently high levels of functioning observed in the accomplishment of daily activities, as assessed by the LIFE-H questionnaire [11]. Despite facing greater dependency and challenges in fitness, personal care, and mobility compared to adults of the typically developing cohort, adults with CP reported similar levels of satisfaction, except for the domain of mobility. The correlation identified between accomplishment levels and functional mobility underscores the crucial role of preserving walking function during aging to facilitate daily activities [11].

Regarding participation in the community, in the follow-up conducted at more than 25 years after SDR, a greater number of adults with CP were either married or living with partners. Additionally, more adults had children compared to 9 years prior, while there were fewer observable changes in education and employment over this extended time period. The proportion of these adults with CP who were in a relationship was comparable to adults of the typically developing cohort (61%). Nevertheless, adults of the typically developing cohort with a similar age were more likely to be parents (77% vs. 42%) and not residing with (grand)parents (89% vs. 62%). Additionally, a higher percentage of TD adults were employed (89%) compared to adults with CP in both studies (73%) [11] (Table 15.2).

15.5 Quality of Life

15.5.1 5–15 Years After SDR

More than 10 years after SDR, adolescents with CP were found to perceive their health-related quality of life favourably, as concluded by Tedroff et al. This assessment was based on the Health-Related Quality of Life Health Survey (SF-36v2), a questionnaire that covers eight health concepts and results into a physical and mental summary score [22]. Notably, adolescents who underwent SDR perceived their mental health (based on SF-36v2) to be even better than the age norm. Furthermore, their overall satisfaction with life, as measured by the Diener Satisfaction with Life Scale, was reported to be good and comparable to peers who did not undergo SDR in childhood [21].

15.5.2 15–25 Years After SDR

Limited information is available regarding the quality of life of adults with CP who have undergone SDR. In a study by Hurvitz et al. [38], satisfaction with life, as assessed by the Diener Satisfaction with Life Scale, was reported for adults with CP more than 15 years after SDR. The findings indicated that these adults perceived a high level of satisfaction with life, even 19 years after SDR. Similarly, Langerak et al. observed elevated satisfaction levels concerning the accomplishment of daily life activities and participation 17–25 years post-SDR [42].

15.5.3 *Cape Town Experience >25 Years After SDR*

The adults with CP who took part in the Cape Town studies more than 25 years after SDR reported a relatively positive health-related quality of life (HRQoL). In the SF-36v2 assessment, seven out of eight health concepts, including physical role functioning, bodily pain, general health, vitality, social functioning, emotional role functioning, and mental health, did not exhibit significant differences between adults with CP and adults of the typically developing cohort [12]. This finding contrasts with other studies where challenges in most of these areas were reported for adults with CP [45–48]. The only health concept where adults with CP in this study perceived a lower HRQoL compared to their peers was related to physical functioning [12].

The HRQoL mental score and the levels of anxiety and depression were comparable between adults with CP and typically developing adults. This suggests that, despite ongoing physical challenges faced by adults with CP, their mental health may not be directly impacted. Furthermore, the levels of anxiety and depression identified in the long-term Cape Town follow-up studies were lower than those reported in other studies. Only mild to moderate levels of anxiety were observed in 15% of the CP cohort, and no increased levels of depression were noted [12] (Table 15.2).

15.6 Personal Feedback from Adults >25 Years Post-SDR

Based on semistructured interviews, adults with CP who underwent SDR over 25 years ago, and were actively involved in the studies conducted by the Cape Town research team (as detailed in previous paragraphs), shared their perspectives and offered insights into their individual experiences with SDR [10].

In response to the question ‘Do you feel that SDR has been worthwhile?’, some participants (28% of the CP cohort) expressed difficulty answering, citing reasons such as being too young at the time of the operation (making it challenging to recall their condition before the operation) or finding it difficult to judge the potential outcomes of alternative treatment options. Among the adults capable of responding, 94% of the cohort provided positive feedback, expressing that they found SDR worthwhile, primarily attributing it to improvements in mobility and/or quality of life. However, one participant expressed the view that the operation was not worthwhile, citing the experience of pain as a determining factor [10].

Regarding the question 'What would you have done differently if you look back?', the most prevalent response, answered by 20% of the participants, was the wish to have engaged in more exercise in previous years. They expressed the feeling that they should have focused on improving the maintenance of their fitness levels [10].

Responding to the third question, 'If you had to decide by yourself now, would you make the same decision as your parents to undergo SDR?', some participants (16%) found it challenging to answer, citing difficulty in judging the potential outcomes of other treatment options. Among the remaining adults interviewed, 90% of the cohort expressed that they would undergo this neurosurgical operation based on the mobility and functional walking benefits they experienced more than 25 years post-SDR. However, the other 10% of the cohort stated that they would not choose to undergo the operation due to the pain they had experienced [10].

15.7 Complications Following SDR

Complications associated with SDR may arise directly as a consequence of the surgical procedure [49]. In addition, adverse outcomes may arise due to factors such as poor patient selection. Additionally, the variables of the percentage of cut rootlets and the involved spinal levels are also identified as contributing factors that can lead to suboptimal outcomes [50].

Acute complications linked to the operation may encompass infection, haemorrhage, and cerebrospinal fluid leakage [51]. Perioperative complications, such as sensory changes, neurogenic bladder, or bowel issues, have also been documented [49]. It is noteworthy, however, that major complications are relatively rare, and protocols implemented by neurosurgeons have been adjusted to mitigate and reduce the occurrence of such events [51].

Potential long-term suboptimal outcomes, as delineated in earlier studies, encompass hypotonia, weakness, sensory changes, spinal instability, hip subluxation, constipation, and urinary incontinence [49, 52–54]. The systematic review of Mishra et al. [54] on complications following SDR reported structural complications, scoliosis, and hyperlordosis as the commonest, while a review of Tu et al. [55] identified that the incidence of spinal deformity was not observed to be substantially elevated over that of natural history, as also mentioned by the Cape Town research group [10] and Grunt et al. [20].

15.8 Conclusion

This comprehensive literature overview presented both short- and long-term outcomes related to the ICF domains and quality of life. Besides the impact of SDR surgery, it is crucial to consider the inevitable interaction of the aging process with the motor disorder associated with CP. Continuous follow-up remains important for monitoring development and addressing challenges throughout the entire lifespan of adults with CP after SDR. These valuable clinical insights will help to develop the right management programs to support healthy aging in adults with CP and are anticipated to support parents, caregivers, and clinicians in their decision-making processes concerning children with CP.

References

1. Dan B. Is there early ageing in cerebral palsy? Dev Med Child Neurol. 2024;66(1):4–5.
2. Graham HK, Rosenbaum P, Paneth N, Dan B, Lin JP, Damiano DL, et al. Cerebral palsy. Nat Rev Dis Primers. 2016;2:15082.
3. Colver A, Fairhurst C, Pharoah PO. Cerebral palsy. Lancet (London, England). 2014;383(9924):1240–9.
4. Colver A. Quality of life and participation. Dev Med Child Neurol. 2009;51(8):656–9.
5. Blair E, Watson L. Epidemiology of cerebral palsy. Semin Fetal Neonatal Med. 2006;11(2):117–25.
6. Rosenbaum P. Cerebral palsy: what parents and doctors want to know. BMJ (Clinical Research ed). 2003;326(7396):970–4.
7. Stanley EBE, Alberman E. How common are the cerebral palsies? In: Stanley E, editor. Cerebral palsies: epidemiology and causal pathways. London: MacKeith Press; 2000. p. 14–21.
8. Novak I, Morgan C, Fahey M, Finch-Edmondson M, Galea C, Hines A, et al. State of the evidence traffic lights 2019: systematic review of interventions for preventing and treating children with cerebral palsy. Curr Neurol Neurosci Rep. 2020;20(2):3.
9. Ward AB. A summary of spasticity management--a treatment algorithm. Eur J Neurol 2002;9 Suppl 1:48–52. Discussion 3–61.
10. Veerbeek BE, Lamberts RP, Fieggen AG, Mankahla N, de Villiers RVP, Botha E, et al. A long-term follow-up study of spinal abnormalities and pain in adults with cerebral palsy and spastic diplegia more than 25 years after selective dorsal rhizotomy. J Neurosurg Spine. 2020:1–8.
11. Veerbeek BE, Lamberts RP, Fieggen AG, Verkoeijen PPJL, Langerak NG. Daily activities, participation, satisfaction, and functional mobility of adults with cerebral palsy more than 25 years after selective dorsal rhizotomy: a long-term follow-up during adulthood. Disabil Rehabil. 2019:1–9.
12. Veerbeek BE, Lamberts RP, Kosel E, Fieggen AG, Langerak NG. More than 25 years after selective dorsal rhizotomy: physical status, quality of life, and levels of anxiety and depression in adults with cerebral palsy. J Neurosurg. 2022;136(3):689–98.
13. Langerak NG, Veerbeek BE, Fieggen AG, Lamberts RP. Gait status 26-35 years after selective dorsal rhizotomy: a 9 year follow up study. Gait Posture. 2022;91:284–9.
14. Organization WH. International classification of functioning, disability and health. ICF: World Health Organization; 2001.
15. McDougall J, Wright V, Rosenbaum P. The ICF model of functioning and disability: incorporating quality of life and human development. Dev Neurorehabil. 2010;13(3):204–11.
16. Peacock WJ, Eastman RW. The neurosurgical management of spasticity. South African Med J Suid-Afrikaanse tydskrif vir geneeskunde. 1981;60(22):849–50.
17. Peacock WJ, Arens LJ. Selective posterior rhizotomy for the relief of spasticity in cerebral palsy. South African Med J Suid-Afrikaanse tydskrif vir geneeskunde. 1982;62(4):119–24.
18. Peacock WJ, Arens LJ, Berman B. Cerebral palsy spasticity. Selective posterior rhizotomy. Pediatr Neurosci. 1987;13(2):61–6.

19. Arens LJ, Peacock WJ, Peter J. Selective posterior rhizotomy: a long-term follow-up study. Childs Nerv Syst. 1989;5(3):148–52.
20. Grunt S, Becher JG, Vermeulen RJ. Long-term outcome and adverse effects of selective dorsal rhizotomy in children with cerebral palsy: a systematic review. Dev Med Child Neurol. 2011;53(6):490–8.
21. Munger ME, Aldahondo N, Krach LE, Novacheck TF, Schwartz MH. Long-term outcomes after selective dorsal rhizotomy: a retrospective matched cohort study. Dev Med Child Neurol. 2017;59(11):1196–203.
22. Tedroff K, Lowing K, Astrom E. A prospective cohort study investigating gross motor function, pain, and health-related quality of life 17 years after selective dorsal rhizotomy in cerebral palsy. Dev Med Child Neurol. 2015;57(5):484–90.
23. Ailon T, Beauchamp R, Miller S, Mortenson P, Kerr JM, Hengel AR, et al. Long-term outcome after selective dorsal rhizotomy in children with spastic cerebral palsy. Childs Nerv Syst. 2015;31(3):415–23.
24. Josenby AL, Wagner P, Jarnlo GB, Westbom L, Nordmark E. Motor function after selective dorsal rhizotomy: a 10-year practice-based follow-up study. Dev Med Child Neurol. 2012;54(5):429–35.
25. van Schie PE, Schothorst M, Dallmeijer AJ, Vermeulen RJ, van Ouwerkerk WJ, Strijers RL, et al. Short- and long-term effects of selective dorsal rhizotomy on gross motor function in ambulatory children with spastic diplegia. J Neurosurg Pediatr. 2011;7(5):557–62.
26. McFall J, Stewart C, Kidgell V, Postans N, Jarvis S, Freeman R, et al. Changes in gait which occur before and during the adolescent growth spurt in children treated by selective dorsal rhizotomy. Gait Posture. 2015;42(3):317–22.
27. Wheelwright M, Selvey PJ, Steinbok P, Singhal A, Ibrahim G, Fallah A, et al. Systematic review of spinal deformities following multi-level selective dorsal rhizotomy. Childs Nerv Syst. 2020;36(5):1025–35.
28. Johnson MB, Goldstein L, Thomas SS, Piatt J, Aiona M, Sussman M. Spinal deformity after selective dorsal rhizotomy in ambulatory patients with cerebral palsy. J Pediatr Orthop. 2004;24(5):529–36.
29. Turi M, Kalen V. The risk of spinal deformity after selective dorsal rhizotomy. J Pediatr Orthop. 2000;20(1):104–7.
30. Wang KK, Munger ME, Chen BP, Novacheck TF. Selective dorsal rhizotomy in ambulant children with cerebral palsy. J Child Orthop. 2018;12(5):413–27.
31. Hilberink SR, Roebroeck ME, Nieuwstraten W, Jalink L, Verheijden JM, Stam HJ. Health issues in young adults with cerebral palsy: towards a life-span perspective. J Rehabil Med. 2007;39(8):605–11.
32. Schwartz L, Engel JM, Jensen MP. Pain in persons with cerebral palsy. Arch Phys Med Rehabil. 1999;80(10):1243–6.
33. Dudley RW, Parolin M, Gagnon B, Saluja R, Yap R, Montpetit K, et al. Long-term functional benefits of selective dorsal rhizotomy for spastic cerebral palsy. J Neurosurg Pediatr. 2013;12(2):142–50.
34. Langerak NG, Vaughan CL, Hoffman EB, Figaji AA, Fieggen AG, Peter JC. Incidence of spinal abnormalities in patients with spastic diplegia 17 to 26 years after selective dorsal rhizotomy. Childs Nerv Syst. 2009;25(12):1593–603.
35. Langerak NG, Tam N, Vaughan CL, Fieggen AG, Schwartz MH. Gait status 17–26 years after selective dorsal rhizotomy. Gait Posture. 2012;35(2):244–9.
36. Langerak NG, Lamberts RP, Fieggen AG, Peter JC, van der Merwe L, Peacock WJ, et al. A prospective gait analysis study in patients with diplegic cerebral palsy 20 years after selective dorsal rhizotomy. J Neurosurg Pediatr. 2008;1(3):180–6.
37. Langerak NG, Lamberts RP, Fieggen AG, Peter JC, Peacock WJ, Vaughan CL. Functional status of patients with cerebral palsy according to the international classification of functioning, disability and health model: a 20-year follow-up study after selective dorsal rhizotomy. Arch Phys Med Rehabil. 2009;90(6):994–1003.

38. Hurvitz EA, Marciniak CM, Daunter AK, Haapala HJ, Stibb SM, McCormick SF, et al. Functional outcomes of childhood dorsal rhizotomy in adults and adolescents with cerebral palsy. J Neurosurg Pediatr. 2013;11(4):380–8.
39. Daunter AK, Kratz AL, Hurvitz EA. Long-term impact of childhood selective dorsal rhizotomy on pain, fatigue, and function: a case-control study. Dev Med Child Neurol. 2017;59(10):1089–95.
40. Rosenbaum P, Paneth N, Leviton A, Goldstein M, Bax M, Damiano D, et al. A report: the definition and classification of cerebral palsy April 2006. Dev Med Child Neurol Suppl. 2007;109(Suppl 109):8–14.
41. Bolster EA, van Schie PE, Becher JG, van Ouwerkerk WJ, Strijers RL, Vermeulen RJ. Long-term effect of selective dorsal rhizotomy on gross motor function in ambulant children with spastic bilateral cerebral palsy, compared with reference centiles. Dev Med Child Neurol. 2013;55(7):610–6.
42. Langerak NG, Hillier SL, Verkoeijen PP, Peter JC, Fieggen AG, Vaughan CL. Level of activity and participation in adults with spastic diplegia 17-26 years after selective dorsal rhizotomy. J Rehabil Med. 2011;43(4):330–7.
43. Morgan P, McGinley J. Gait function and decline in adults with cerebral palsy: a systematic review. Disabil Rehabil. 2014;36(1):1–9.
44. Maanum G, Jahnsen R, Froslie KF, Larsen KL, Keller A. Walking ability and predictors of performance on the 6-minute walk test in adults with spastic cerebral palsy. Dev Med Child Neurol. 2010;52(6):e126–32.
45. Smith KJ, Peterson MD, O'Connell NE, Victor C, Liverani S, Anokye N, et al. Risk of depression and anxiety in adults with cerebral palsy. JAMA Neurol. 2019;76(3):294–300.
46. van Der Slot WM, Nieuwenhuijsen C, Van Den Berg-Emons RJ, Bergen MP, Hilberink SR, Stam HJ, et al. Chronic pain, fatigue, and depressive symptoms in adults with spastic bilateral cerebral palsy. Dev Med Child Neurol. 2012;54(9):836–42.
47. van der Slot WM, Nieuwenhuijsen C, van den Berg-Emons RJ, Wensink-Boonstra AE, Stam HJ, Roebroeck ME, et al. Participation and health-related quality of life in adults with spastic bilateral cerebral palsy and the role of self-efficacy. J Rehabil Med. 2010;42(6):528–35.
48. Roebroeck ME, Jahnsen R, Carona C, Kent RM, Chamberlain MA. Adult outcomes and lifespan issues for people with childhood-onset physical disability. Dev Med Child Neurol. 2009;51(8):670–8.
49. Steinbok P, Schrag C. Complications after selective posterior rhizotomy for spasticity in children with cerebral palsy. Pediatr Neurosurg. 1998;28(6):300–13.
50. Kim DS, Choi JU, Yang KH, Park CI, Park ES. Selective posterior rhizotomy for lower extremity spasticity: how much and which of the posterior rootlets should be cut? Surg Neurol. 2002;57(2):87–93.
51. Ontario HQ. Lumbosacral dorsal Rhizotomy for spastic cerebral palsy: a health technology assessment. Ontario Health Technology Assessment Series. 2017;17(10):1.
52. Steinbok P, Hicdonmez T, Sawatzky B, Beauchamp R, Wickenheiser D. Spinal deformities after selective dorsal rhizotomy for spastic cerebral palsy. J Neurosurg. 2005;102(4 Suppl):363–73.
53. Silva S, Nowicki P, Caird MS, Hurvitz EA, Ayyangar RN, Farley FA, et al. A comparison of hip dislocation rates and hip containment procedures after selective dorsal rhizotomy versus intrathecal baclofen pump insertion in nonambulatory cerebral palsy patients. J Pediatr Orthop. 2012;32(8):853–6.
54. Mishra D, Barik S, Raj V, Kandwal P. A systematic review of complications following selective dorsal rhizotomy in cerebral palsy. Neuro-Chirurgie. 2023;69(3):101425.
55. Tu A, Steinbok P. Long term outcome of selective dorsal Rhizotomy for the management of childhood spasticity-functional improvement and complications. Childs Nerv Syst. 2020;36(9):1985–94.

Part V
Future Perspectives

Chapter 16
Patient Selection in Selective Dorsal Rhizotomy (SDR)

Benjamin J. Hall, Conor S. Gillespie, Christine Sneade, Alder Hey Children's Hospital Physiotherapy Group, Deborah Quirk, Dawn Hennigan, and Benedetta Pettorini

Abbreviations

SDR	Selective dorsal rhizotomy
MDT	Multidisciplinary team
PT	Physiotherapist
GMFCS	Gross Motor Function Classification System
CP	Cerebral palsy
CCP	Clinical Commissioning Policy
CPQoL	Cerebral Palsy Quality of Life Questionnaire
PEDI	Paediatric Evaluation of Disability Inventory
MAS	Modified Ashworth Scale
TUG	Timed Up and Go

B. J. Hall (✉)
Department of Neurosurgery, Alder Hey Children's Hospital NHS Foundation Trust, Liverpool, UK

Department of Neurosurgery, The Walton Centre NHS Foundation Trust, Liverpool, UK
e-mail: benjaminhall@doctors.org.uk

C. S. Gillespie
Department of Clinical Neurosciences, University of Cambridge, Cambridge, UK
e-mail: conor.gillespie1@nhs.net

C. Sneade · Alder Hey Children's Hospital Physiotherapy Group · D. Quirk · D. Hennigan · B. Pettorini (✉)
Department of Neurosurgery, Alder Hey Children's Hospital NHS Foundation Trust, Liverpool, UK
e-mail: Christine.sneade@alderhey.nhs.uk; deborah.quirk@alderhey.nhs.uk; dawn.hennigan@alderhey.nhs.uk; benedetta.pettorini@alderhey.nhs.uk

N. Morota, P. Steinbok (eds.), *Dorsal Rhizotomy: Neurosurgery for Childhood Spasticity*, Advances and Technical Standards in Neurosurgery 51,
https://doi.org/10.1007/978-3-031-86441-4_16

PVL Periventricular leukomalacia
EMG Electromyography

16.1 Introduction

Appropriate patient selection is a key component of determining the likelihood of success of a surgical procedure and maximising safety for the patients involved. While this process is guided by a handful of variables consistent across surgery such as age and clinical performance status, there are a number of more procedure-specific variables to be considered. These considerations can be classified according to their position in relation to surgery, or broadly as preoperative and postoperative.

In the paediatric population wherein surgical procedures convey the greatest lifelong impact, even greater consideration must be applied to patient selection. In particular, there are few surgical interventions that have sparked such protracted discussion surrounding patient selection as selective dorsal rhizotomy (SDR). SDR is most frequently employed as a means of treating spasticity in children with cerebral palsy (CP), an extremely heterogenous patient cohort that present several challenges when deciding eligibility for surgery. Unlike many other surgical procedures, a particular caveat of patient selection in SDR is that 'selection' itself is not solely governed by anatomical or physiological parameters of the patient. Accurately interpreting patient goals, anticipating expectations of the caregiver, and assessing the likelihood of engagement with postoperative therapies: all are challenges faced by clinicians in the setting of SDR. One could argue that prescience is perhaps the most useful skill when identifying patients for SDR! In lieu of being able to predict the future, this chapter seeks to review contemporary approaches toward patient selection for SDR, as well as glance at potential advances to be made in this complex and controversial process.

16.2 Preoperative Considerations

16.2.1 Age

Age is frequently a determinant of patient suitability for surgery, though its role in patient selection for SDR is particularly controversial. While earlier intervention is generally preferred to optimise the potential for functional improvement and to capitalise on neuroplasticity during developmental years, the successful use of SDR in adult patients is evidence enough that benefit may be conveyed to patients of all ages. A recent review highlights the remarkable range of ages considered for SDR across the literature [1], with some series demonstrating narrow intervals of between

3 and 7 years and others with much broader inclusivity of between 3 and 21 years [2–6]. In the United Kingdom, the Clinical Commissioning Policy (CCP) for SDR currently supports children aged 3–9 years in undergoing the surgery [7], though there is evidence to suggest older patients may gain a similar degree of benefit.

In a comparison of patient groups aged between 3–9 years and 10–18 years, spasticity improved significantly for both groups after SDR, with older patients gaining a similar degree of benefit to their younger counterparts [8]. Variables that considered quality of life such as the Cerebral Palsy Quality of Life (CPQoL) questionnaire and Paediatric Evaluation of Disability Inventory (PEDI) self-care score also improved significantly after SDR in both groups. Interestingly, these assessments of quality of life demonstrated a significantly greater degree of improvement after SDR in the older patient cohort [8]. While this underlines the overall benefit that SDR can provide, it specifically highlights the potential it has for improving quality of life in patients outside of the current status quo for selection.

16.2.2 Aetiology and Comorbidities

The term 'cerebral palsy' (CP) encompasses a spectrum of neurological dysfunction affecting tone, movement, and posture arising from an acquired, nonprogressive brain injury during early childhood development. In most cases, this is as a result of intraventricular haemorrhage related to prematurity. CP remains a strictly clinical diagnosis, and while it is typically the most common aetiological indication for SDR, there has been evidence of successful application in several other causes of spasticity including hereditary spastic paraplegia (HSP), spinal cord insults [9, 10], and neurometabolic disorders [11].

Comorbidities are not uncommon in those being considered for SDR and may be a determining factor in whether to undertake the procedure. Epilepsy is frequently associated with CP [12] and in some cases has previously been included as an exclusion criterion for SDR [13]. Other chronic conditions often seen in CP include gastro-oesophageal reflux disease (GORD), excessive upper airway secretions, and neurogenic bladder and bowel dysfunction [14]. In severe spasticity with the resultant scoliosis, a reduction in thoracic volume can also significantly impair ventilatory function.

All of the above are factors that may increase risk of complications associated with a general anaesthetic and therefore must be weighed against the benefit of undergoing SDR through extensive discussion with anaesthetic colleagues. If such significant comorbidities exist that a general anaesthetic is accompanied by too great a risk to proceed, then SDR is invariably not an option. However, with increasingly accurate neurophysiology support and implementation of single-level surgery, progressively shorter operating times may permit SDR in patients that previously may have been ineligible.

16.2.3 Spasticity, Functional Limitations, and Physical Assessment

Historically, the severity of spasticity and its impact on functional ability has often been regarded as the critical determinant of patient selection in SDR. The Gross Motor Function Classification System (GMFCS) is used to classify the degree of motor function in patients preoperatively [15], with candidates for SDR usually having significant spasticity that impairs mobility, gait, and activities of daily living. The battery of preoperative assessment measures available to treating teams is ever increasing and can provide a wealth of insight into the functionality of each individual patient. Spasticity may be assessed grossly using the Modified Ashworth Scale (MAS) [16] or with a quantitative spasticity assessment through the use of an isokinetic dynamometer. The MAS measures resistance during muscle stretching and is used to gauge baseline function and effectiveness of treatment by assessing the lower limb adductors as well as the hip, knee, and ankle flexors. These are scored from normal tone to rigid tone in flexion and extension.

Of equal importance to the assessment of spasticity is the concurrently assessment of underlying muscle strength and range of movement. In subtle cases, it can be challenging to elicit evidence of spasticity in individual muscle functionality. For this reason, performing thorough gait analysis is critical in ambulatory children. The typical features of a spastic gait pattern consist of persistent flexion at the hips with an associated hyperlordosis, with inward rotation and adduction of the hip joints resulting in the classical 'scissoring' of the knees. Hamstring spasticity may result in a crouched deformity with shortening of the stride length, while at the ankles, there is elevation and outward rotation of the heel at foot strike. By assessing each patient's ability to stand from a sitting position through measures such as 'Timed Up and Go' (TUG), the strength of antigravity muscles is assessed [17]. Many children with spasticity who are able to mobilise independently or with use of a mobility aid rely on the structural support provided by their spasticity to do so. With this removed, the underlying muscle strength may not be sufficient to allow locomotion.

The irreversible nature of SDR may then in turn lead to a deterioration in mobility and function, if muscle strength is not suitably assessed preoperatively. Physical examination of muscle strength and range of motion may also be supported by electromyography (EMG) as part of the preoperative assessment process. The presence of underlying weakness often serves as the rationale for avoiding SDR in patients that achieve good function despite or, in some cases, because of their spasticity. However, the potential for improving mobility even in those of GMFCS level 1 has been recognised [8].

During this process, evidence of joint deformity or contractures may also come to light. Much like the deleterious effect that reducing spasticity can have in those with inadequate underlying muscle strength, removing it in those with contractures and severe fixed flexion deformity can also be detrimental. Loss of antagonistic muscle group contraction can ultimately worsen the deformity, resulting in reduction of functionality and quality of life.

An additional concept increasingly used in this aspect of the selection process is to 'simulate' the loss of spasticity observed in SDR, prior to committing to the procedure itself. This can be achieved through the use of intrathecal baclofen, either as a single 'test dose' delivered via lumbar puncture or as an infusion over 24–48 hours via lumbar catheter. This assessment process is undertaken as part of an inpatient admission, with younger patients often requiring sedation or general anaesthesia to undergo implantation of the lumbar catheter and administration of the baclofen. A comprehensive physiotherapy assessment is then undertaken to determine the impact of spasticity reduction on the patient's functional status. The results of the test often support clinical decision-making, guiding the multidisciplinary team (MDT) in determining whether implantation of an ITB pump or proceeding to SDR may be more suitable [18].

When presented with a list of some of the most common contraindications to SDR, it is clear that the procedure has not historically been intended for those of GMFCS level 4 or 5. 'Lack of antigravity muscle function' and 'absence of good motor control' are clearly absent in this group yet are frequently contraindications to surgery. If improving or indeed permitting independent mobility is the goal, then wheelchair-bound patients who are unlikely to achieve independence, with or without SDR, are rarely eligible for surgery. At the opposite end of the spectrum are those of GMFCS level 1 or 2, who also undergo SDR less frequently given that they do not necessarily rely on any adjuncts to aid in mobilisation at their baseline. The risk of surgery then often 'outweighs the benefit' of what is traditionally seen as a 'negligible improvement in function'. The resultant population selected to undergo SDR then consists predominantly of GMFCS level 3 patients, in whom the surgery may relieve them of needing mobility aids and indeed improve their stamina overall. While the impact of SDR may be most dramatic in this middle cohort, this traditional selection approach has led to clinicians potentially neglecting either pole of the GMFCS spectrum.

There is growing evidence, however, to indicate the beneficial impact of SDR is significant across GMFCS levels. A recent multicentre review identified that there was no difference in the degree of improvement observed in five out of eight outcome measures between GMFCS levels [8]. Rather, it was observed that some of the greatest change postoperatively was seen in the GMFCS level 4 group, in particular in relation to quality of life (CPQoL) and self-care (PEDI self-care score) [8]. The use of SDR in non-ambulant patients has also been specifically explored by the same group, observing an increase in gross motor function in 77.6%, reduction in pain in 60.7%, and improvement in bladder function in 30.9% of patients [19].

In another cohort of GMFCS level 4 and 5 patients, SDR not only resulted in a significant reduction in lower limb spasticity scores but also a significant reduction in upper limb spasticity scores, both of which were maintained at 8 and 14 months postoperatively [20]. The same study also reported rates of pre- and postoperative bladder dysfunction in this cohort, with urological assessment identifying preexisting bladder dysfunction in 70% and 90% of GMFCS 4 and 5 patients, respectively. Following SDR, improvement in urinary continence was observed in 71% of affected GMFCS 4 and 42.8% of GMFCS 5 patients [20].

GMFCS level 1 patients, while already independently mobile, have been identified as also gaining significant improvements in both self-care and mobility [8]. The assumption made about either end of the GMFCS spectrum is that the goals of each patient are the same as those in the middle, which is evidently false and must be considered when each new referral is received.

16.2.4 Dystonia

In between 7% and 14% of CP patients, there is coexistence of spasticity and dystonia [21, 22]. As in some cases whereby children ultimately rely on their spasticity to mobilise, spasticity can also conceal the severity of dystonia. In these instances, removal of spasticity even in part can result in a substantial deterioration in quality of life. As such, significant dystonia is often a criterion for exclusion when considering SDR given the irreversible nature of the procedure. Instead, intrathecal baclofen (ITB) pumps are often the preferred choice of management thanks to their titratable functionality and reversibility. However, recent evidence suggests that a mixed clinical picture of spasticity and dystonia may not be a definitive exclusion criterion from SDR as it once was. In six of eight outcome measures observed, there was no significant difference in the degree of improvement obtained between those with dystonia and those without [8]. In the two metrics where there was significant difference between the groups, PEDI mobility and TUG, those with a mixed picture of spasticity and dystonia gained a significantly greater improvement [8]. This, unlike the historical notion that dystonia is an absolute contraindication to SDR, suggests benefit may be conveyed even in the presence of some degree of dystonia. The severity of dystonia and at what point the impact of SDR becomes detrimental, however, require further delineation. Advances in electromyographic techniques may prove useful in better defining this threshold [23]. It is worth noting that children with spastic quadriplegia are more likely to present with concurrent dystonia, though as iterated elsewhere in this chapter the presence of quadriplegia should not be in and of itself a contraindication to SDR.

16.2.5 Imaging Studies and Investigations

Few preoperative surgical assessments are undertaken without the use of comprehensive imaging, which in the setting of SDR the majority of which is constituted by magnetic resonance imaging (MRI) of the brain and spine. While clinical history may often be obvious in the diagnosis of CP (in the presence of severe prematurity, intraventricular haemorrhage, and neonatal meningitis), underlying causes of spasticity are frequently multifactorial. Imaging modalities therefore enable a more thorough assessment of aetiology and may be performed to clarify the diagnosis where there may be uncertainty.

Periventricular leukomalacia (PVL) is frequently present on the MRI of those with classical spastic diplegia and usually takes the form of small, hyperintense lesions on T1-weighted sequences abutting the trigone, surrounded by a larger area of hyperintensity on T2. These lesions impede supratentorial communication with the spinal interneuron pool, resulting in disinhibition of spinal reflex arcs [24]. In larger lesions, those with substantial periventricular cyst formation and thinning of the corpus callosum, the deficit is typically more severe and may also be evident in the upper limbs resulting in a spastic quadriplegia.

MRI may also highlight findings that result in exclusion of patients from SDR. Significant lesions of the basal ganglia and thalamus or cerebellum may indicate eventual development of significant dystonia or ataxia, respectively, thus precluding many patients from undergoing SDR. Similarly, those with radiological evidence of injuries to the brainstem may also be ineligible from undergoing SDR given the degree of difficulty anticipated in postoperative recovery and rehabilitation.

MRI of the spine is also frequently undertaken to ensure no high spinal lesions are contributing to the spasticity observed but also to prepare the surgeon for any anatomical variation that may complicate the procedure. Additionally, any occult spinal dysraphism would exclude the patient from SDR. Neurogenic bladder dysfunction is also well recognised in CP, occurring in approximately 16% of patients [25]. As such, there is an increasing role for the use of urodynamic studies in the pre- and postoperative assessment of those reporting bladder dysfunction.

Historically, extra-neuraxial imaging has also played a role in the preoperative assessment of patients for SDR. The 'extrusion index', or Reimer's index (RI), describes the extent of bony coverage of the femoral head by the acetabulum observed on X-ray. Morphologically normal values typically lie between 17% and 27%, with values above that indicating hip dysplasia [26]. With less anatomical security of the femoral head within the acetabulum comes greater risk of hip subluxation, a risk that is exacerbated further with greater spasticity. The relevance of RI varies between centres, with some allowing RIs of up to 40% as part of their inclusion criteria for SDR, while others propose any degree of hip dysplasia as a contraindication [24].

16.3 Postoperative Considerations

Individualised care is rightly becoming the gold standard across all aspects of healthcare, though few procedures require the extent of bespoke planning as SDR. In order to determine suitability for SDR, the treating team must not only comprehensively review patients preoperatively but also be able to discern the likely postoperative course of two important variables: firstly, by gauging the patient and their family's expectations of what goals can be achieved with SDR, and secondly, their concordance with the team in trying to achieve those goals.

16.3.1 Establishing Achievable Goals

As the positive effects of SDR are more widely reported, perceptions of a 'miracle treatment' amongst many parents and caregivers can arise. The potentially life-changing reputation of the procedure however does in itself risk impacting patients negatively, if the outcomes they expect do not match those they encounter. Thus, it is critical that realistic goals are established as early as possible in the preoperative assessment process. As has been discussed previously, these goals may vary dramatically between patients.

While patients of all GMFCS levels may benefit from SDR, each must be considered uniquely. For example, in the case of GMFCS level 1 patients, patients and families but be adequately counselled to ensure they recognise that with every surgery there is a small risk not only of complication directly related to surgery but also of potential deterioration. In order to mitigate this risk, they must be willing to engage fully in the preoperative assessment process.

Regarding GMFCS level 4 and 5 patients, the same degree of counselling is mandatory. Patients and families must understand that the goal of SDR in many of these cases will be to improve ease of care, transfer, and comfort, rather than to enable independent mobility. It is critical that the entire SDR team are concordant in their interactions with patients and their families: ensuring that they have ample opportunity to reflect on their preoperative goals throughout rehabilitation and allowing them to objectively measure the progress they make.

16.3.2 Engaging with Therapy

While surgeons may lead in the technical component of SDR, it is the therapy team and their work with the patient both pre- and postoperatively that enable them to achieve the positive outcomes they hope for. Undergoing SDR necessitates that patients and their families assume responsibility for engaging with therapy teams both during preoperative assessment and during the postoperative recovery and ensuring that patients are aware of the importance of this is vital. Failure to adequately commit to their prescribed postoperative therapy and rehabilitation risks may not only prevent the patient from achieving their desired goals but may ultimately result in deterioration to a functional level beneath that of their baseline.

Early involvement of the therapy team in assessing and getting to know the patient is essential in ensuring they and their families feel supported in their decision to undergo SDR. This also reiterates to them the role their own efforts play in ensuring the shared goal of a positive outcome is met. If during the assessment process there are concerns that perhaps patient or family may not be able to provide the long-term commitment to rehabilitation required, they should have these concerns brought to them. If concerns remain despite discussion around the magnitude of the procedure and the commitment required, then this will likely exclude the patient from undergoing surgery. Importantly, being able to 'engage with therapy' encompasses a broad range of abilities. While in the past, cognitive deficits have been employed as an exclusion criterion for SDR, the authors support the notion that patients who are active and willing to play will often be able to engage suitably, regardless of their conscious effort to do so. As such, strictly excluding patients based on cognitive function may no longer be appropriate.

16.3.3 Orthopaedic Surgery: Before or After SDR

Orthopaedic surgeons play an important role in the multidisciplinary assessment and management of patients with spasticity, necessitating an ample understanding of their role by the neurosurgical team. A number of orthopaedic procedures are available to patients and, much like SDR, require substantial preoperative workup before implementation. The overarching goals of orthopaedic procedures in spasticity are to increase range of movement and correct deformity, thereby improving function, ease of care, and discomfort [27].

A staple in the armamentarium of orthopaedic procedures for spasticity, a tenotomy involves tendon sectioning and can be performed in both the upper and lower limbs to affect position and range of movement at almost every joint. In some circumstances, percutaneous tenotomy can also be performed without the need for general anaesthetic, thus remaining applicable to patients with comorbidities that would normally preclude them from surgery. However, with complete tendon detachment comes the risk of potential for loss of functional active movement. To combat this risk, tendon lengthening or transfer procedures may be applied to achieve a similar goal, and while some active function is expected to remain, the extent to which it does can be hard to predict. In more severe circumstances, particularly later in the development of the patient, bony and joint deformities can also be treated with orthopaedic procedures [27].

Of the many obstacles that face children with CP, however, spasticity is invariably the root of each. The contractures and deformity that result in impaired mobility, difficulty in self-care, and pain ultimately arise as a result of chronically increased muscle tone. This chronic hypertonic state then should be the primary treatment target of any surgical intervention for spasticity, followed or supported by deformity correction itself.

By first aiming to ameliorate a patient's spasticity through neurosurgical procedures such as SDR, the clinician reduces the likelihood of eventual contracture and therefore the need for orthopaedic surgery. By reversing the order and undertaking similarly irreversible orthopaedic procedures first, there remains a risk that post-SDR the patient may experience a dramatic loss of function, potentially debilitating them more than without surgery in the first place. Orthopaedic surgery therefore remains an important complementary adjunct to neurosurgery in the management of spasticity but should ideally be reserved for those who have already received maximal neurosurgical intervention. Although it is ideal that children undergo SDR prior to orthopaedic surgery, if the latter has already been performed, it is recommended that SDR by at least 6 months to allow muscle strength to recover. The role of MDT discussion is critical in these particular cases.

16.3.4 Absolute Contraindications

This chapter outlines the developments made toward expanding patient eligibility for SDR in recent years, though there remains some absolute contraindications to the procedure: primarily, any comorbidities that may preclude a patient from undergoing a general anaesthetic in the prone position. To determine whether these are present necessitates discussion with general paediatric and anaesthetic colleagues during the preoperative assessment process.

Secondly, while there is evidence to suggest that some degree of dystonia may not contraindicate SDR, severe dystonia is well recognised as resulting in a poor outcome. Thus, significant and measurable lower limb dystonia preoperatively would also exclude patients from undergoing SDR. Further advances in EMG techniques may one day define this threshold more precisely, but until then, comprehensive physiotherapy and neurosurgical review will continue to form the mainstay of diagnosis.

The final and arguably most important contraindication to SDR comes down to the patient and family themselves. The toll of the surgical procedure and intense postoperative rehabilitation cannot be underestimated, and both require enormous commitment from all involved. While a great number of patients may be referred to an SDR service, it is of the utmost importance that during the preoperative assessment the patient and their family are counselled on the importance of their engagement and willingness to see the entire process through to completion. Without this, there is substantial risk that the patient may ultimately lose function beyond that of their preoperative baseline, and as such, inability to fully engage with the team is also an absolute contraindication (Table 16.1).

16.4 Summary

The recent resurgence in popularity of SDR is testament to its efficacy in managing spasticity, after largely being abandoned during the middle of the twentieth century. While selection criteria for SDR vary between centres and individual surgeons, the renewed interest in use of the procedure continues to grow. As more neurosurgical units integrate SDR into their treatment paradigm for spasticity and access increases, so too will the volume of outcome data to analyse. With this, our approach to patient selection will also continue to develop: perhaps stratifying selection criteria

Table 16.1 Comparison of preoperative criteria and subsequent patient eligibility for SDR

Variable	Ideal candidate	MDT consideration	Controversial	Contraindication
Age	3–9 years	≥10 years	–	–
Aetiology of spasticity	Cerebral palsy	Hereditary spastic paraplegia (HSP), traumatic brain injury (TBI), multiple sclerosis (MS)	Spinal cord injury, neurometabolic disorder	Tumour-related spasticity
GMFCS	Level 2 or 3	Level 1, 4, or 5	–	–
Joint deformity	None	–	–	Contracture
Previous orthopaedic surgery	None	At least 6 month interval after orthopaedic procedure	–	–
Hip dysplasia (Reimer's index)	RI ≤27%	RI 28–40%	RI ≥40%	–
MRI brain	Injury concordant with CP (e.g. PVL)	Basal ganglia, thalamic, cerebellar lesions	Brainstem lesion	
Dystonia	None	Mild	Moderate	Severe (consider ITB trial)
Athetosis	None	–	–	Yes
Nonmedical	Engaged patient, supportive caregivers with appropriate goals	–	–	Patient disinterested; caregiver unable to support engagement

according to GMFCS level, rather than generalising to across all patients. In whichever direction these advances occur, the multidisciplinary team will remain central in determining patient eligibility for SDR.

Special Thanks to Alder Hey Children's Hospital Physiotherapy Group *Chris Sneade, Beata Migas, Colm MacEoin, Helen Gedrim, Nicola Idowu, Joe Ford, Jamie Loydon, and Ryan Hughes.*

References

1. Nicolini-Panisson RD, Tedesco AP, Folle MR, Donadio MVF. Rizotomia dorsal seletiva na paralisia cerebral: critérios de indicação e protocolos de reabilitação fisioterapêutica pós-operatória. Rev Paul Pediatr. 2018;36(1):100–8.
2. Graubert C, Song KM, McLaughlin JF, Bjornson KF. Changes in gait at 1 year post-selective dorsal rhizotomy: results of a prospective randomized study. J Pediatr Orthop. 2000;20(4):496–500.
3. Steinbok P, McLeod K. Comparison of motor outcomes after selective dorsal Rhizotomy with and without preoperative intensified physiotherapy in children with spastic Diplegic cerebral palsy. Pediatr Neurosurg. 2002;36(3):142–7.
4. Wright FV, Sheil EMH, Drake JM, Wedge JH, Naumann S. Evaluation of selective dorsal rhizotomy for the reduction of spasticity in cerebral palsy: a randomized controlled trial. Develop Med Child Neuro. 1998;40(4):239–47.
5. Josenby AL, Wagner P, Jarnlo G, Westbom L, Nordmark E. Motor function after selective dorsal rhizotomy: a 10-year practice-based follow-up study. Develop Med Child Neuro. 2012;54(5):429–35.
6. McLaughlin JF, Bjornson KF, Astley SJ, Graubert C, Hays RM, Roberts TS, et al. Selective dorsal rhizotomy: efficacy and safety in an investigator-masked randomized clinical trial. Develop Med Child Neuro. 1998;40(4):220–32.
7. NHS England Specialised Services Clinical Reference Group for Paediatric Neurosciences. Clinical commissioning policy: selective dorsal Rhizotomy (SDR) for the treatment of spasticity in cerebral palsy (children aged 3-9 years). England: NHS; 2019.
8. Gillespie CS, Hall B. Alder hey physiotherapy group, George AM, Toh S, Islim AI, et al. the effect of GMFCS level, age, sex, and dystonia on multi-dimensional outcomes after selective dorsal rhizotomy: prospective observational study. Childs Nerv Syst. 2021;37(5):1729–40.
9. Mazarakis NK, Ughratdar I, Vloeberghs MH. Excellent functional outcome following selective dorsal rhizotomy in a child with spasticity secondary to transverse myelitis. Childs Nerv Syst. 2015;31(11):2189–91.
10. Reynolds RM, Morton RP, Walker ML, Massagli TL, Browd SR. Role of dorsal rhizotomy in spinal cord injury–induced spasticity: report of 3 cases. PED. 2014 Sep;14(3):266–70.
11. Mazarakis NK, Vloeberghs MH. Spasticity secondary to Leigh syndrome managed with selective dorsal rhizotomy: a case report. Childs Nerv Syst. 2016;32(9):1745–8.
12. Pavone P, Gulizia C, Le Pira A, Greco F, Parisi P, Di Cara G, et al. Cerebral palsy and epilepsy in children: clinical perspectives on a common comorbidity. Children. 2020;8(1):16.
13. Cole GF, Farmer SE, Roberts A, Stewart C, Patrick JH. Selective dorsal rhizotomy for children with cerebral palsy: the Oswestry experience. Arch Dis Child. 2007;92(9):781–5.
14. Minocha P, Sitaraman S, Sachdeva P. Clinical spectrum, comorbidities, and risk factor profile of cerebral palsy children: a prospective study. J Pediatr Neurosci. 2017;12(1):15.
15. Morris C, Bartlett D. Gross motor function classification system: impact and utility. Dev Med Child Neurol [Internet]. 2004;46(01) [cited 2023 Dec 14]. Available from: http://doi.wiley.com/10.1017/S0012162204000118
16. Bohannon RW, Smith MB. Interrater reliability of a modified Ashworth scale of muscle spasticity. Phys Ther. 1987;67(2):206–7.
17. Carey H, Martin K, Combs-Miller S, Heathcock JC. Reliability and responsiveness of the timed up and go test in children with cerebral palsy. Pediatr Phys Ther. 2016;28(4):401–8.
18. Boster AL, Bennett SE, Bilsky GS, Gudesblatt M, Koelbel SF, McManus M, et al. Best practices for intrathecal baclofen therapy: screening test. Neuromodulation: Technol Neural Interface. 2016;19(6):616–22.
19. Gillespie CS, Hall BJ, George AM, Hennigan D, Sneade C, Cawker S, et al. Selective dorsal rhizotomy in non-ambulant children with cerebral palsy: a multi-center prospective study. Childs Nerv Syst [Internet]. 2023; [cited 2023 Dec 14]. Available from: https://link.springer.com/10.1007/s00381-023-06062-4

20. D'Aquino D, Moussa AA, Ammar A, Ingale H, Vloeberghs M. Selective dorsal rhizotomy for the treatment of severe spastic cerebral palsy: efficacy and therapeutic durability in GMFCS grade IV and V children. Acta Neurochir. 2018;160(4):811–21.
21. Evensen TL, Vik T, Andersen GL, Bjellmo S, Hollung SJ. Prevalence, birth, and clinical characteristics of dyskinetic cerebral palsy compared with spastic cerebral palsy subtypes: a Norwegian register-based study. Develop Med Child Neuro. 2023;65(11):1464–74.
22. Michael-Asalu A, Taylor G, Campbell H, Lelea LL, Kirby RS. Cerebral palsy. Adv Pediatr. 2019;66:189–208.
23. Beattie C, Gormley M, Wervey R, Wendorf H. An electromyographic protocol that distinguishes spasticity from dystonia. PRM. 2016;9(2):125–32.
24. Graham D, Aquilina K, Mankad K, Wimalasundera N. Selective dorsal rhizotomy: current state of practice and the role of imaging. Quant Imaging Med Surg. 2018;8(2):209–18.
25. Murphy KP, Boutin SA, Ide KR. Cerebral palsy, neurogenic bladder, and outcomes of lifetime care. Develop Med Child Neuro. 2012;54(10):945–50.
26. Tannast M, Hanke MS, Zheng G, Steppacher SD, Siebenrock KA. What are the radiographic reference values for acetabular under- and Overcoverage? Clin Orthop Relat Res. 2015;473(4):1234–46.
27. Sindou M, Duraffourg M, Georgoulis G. Neuro-orthopedic surgery for the correction of spastic disorders. In: Neurosurgery for spasticity [internet]. Cham: Springer; 2022. p. 285–300. [cited 2023 Dec 14]. Available from: https://link.springer.com/10.1007/978-3-030-92717-2_14.

Chapter 17
Start-Up of Rhizotomy Program in a Developing Country

Tufan Hiçdönmez

17.1 Background

The selective dorsal rhizotomy (SDR) procedure is an effective surgical treatment of spasticity in children with cerebral palsy (CP) and an important component of current pediatric neurosurgical practice [1, 2]. It reduces lower limb spasticity, increases the range of motion of extremities, and improves the patient's Gross Motor Function Classification System (GMFCS) levels [2]. Additionally, in children who underwent SDR for lower limb spasticity, some improvements in upper extremity spasticity were also noted [3, 4].

I had the opportunity to learn pediatric neurosurgery and also the philosophy of childhood spasticity and its surgical treatment by SDR in Canada between 2002 and 2003. I was the clinical fellow of Dr. Paul Steinbok at the British Columbia's Children's Hospital (BCCH) in Vancouver, British Columbia. Paul Steinbok, a leading pediatric neurosurgeon, was at that time the head of the Division of Pediatric Neurosurgery at the BCCH. Dr. Steinbok always had a particular interest in childhood spasticity. This made him not only one of the founders of today's modern SDR surgery but also made the BCCH one of the most experienced centers for spasticity.

Years later, while working as an attending pediatric neurosurgeon at Liv Hospital Vadi Istanbul, an affiliate center of Istinye University, the hospital administration informed me of the request of the Mongolian Ministry of Health to start the rhizotomy program in their country and asked me whether I could perform the SDR procedure in Mongolia.

I was aware of a recent trend among neurosurgeons from North America and Europe concerning efforts to engage in global neurosurgery partnerships and

T. Hiçdönmez (✉)
Pediatric Neurosurgery, Liv Hospital Vadi İstanbul, İstinye University Faculty of Medicine, İstanbul, Türkiye

N. Morota, P. Steinbok (eds.), *Dorsal Rhizotomy: Neurosurgery for Childhood Spasticity*, Advances and Technical Standards in Neurosurgery 51,
https://doi.org/10.1007/978-3-031-86441-4_17

sustainable programs, aiming to cooperate with neurosurgeons around the world for care everywhere and training needs worldwide, as reported in recent literature [5–7]. In this light, I found this opportunity exciting.

This short report is about the contribution of a Turkish pediatric neurosurgeon to the start-up of a rhizotomy program in Ulaanbaatar, Mongolia, in two visits in September 2022 and March 2023.

17.2 The First Visit to Ulaanbaatar, the Setting-Up of the Rhizotomy Team, and the First SDR Surgery

Before our departure, we were in online contact with ministry officials and the hospital administration of the Third State Central Hospital of Ulaanbaatar. We were informed that the surgical tools for a standard osteoplastic lumbar laminotomy including high-speed drill and cut system, the operating microscope, and neurosurgical microinstruments were all available. Also, local officials reported that the attending neurosurgeons would be able to assist us in surgery.

Additionally, anesthesiologists stated that total intravenous anesthesia (TIVA) could be performed during SDR surgery. We only had to bring with us our neuromonitoring tools, consisting of a portable personal computer and specific electrodes used in neuromonitoring.

After having completed the official paperwork with the Mongolian Ministry of Health, we were ready for departure with Mr. Uğur Özcan, the electrophysiology technician responsible for neuromonitoring, and Mrs. Zhannera Khayrdzhankyzy of Liv Hospital responsible for official local relationships and Russian language translation.

17.3 Selecting Patient Candidates for SDR

At the first visit, we evaluated many spastic children with CP who were candidates for SDR. All children were examined in the outpatient clinic together with pediatric neurologists, neurosurgeons, and physiotherapists (Fig. 17.1). Five patients were selected for SDR. Children with cerebral palsy associated with generalized dystonia were excluded as well as children with athetoid and choreiform CP.

The first patient was a 6-year-old boy with GMFCS level 2 spastic diplegia. His mental status and functions of the upper limbs were normal. He was walking on tiptoes. He had regular physiotherapy on a daily basis. Three patients were spastic diplegic children with GMFCS level 3. Lastly, a wheelchair-bound GMFCS level 4 8-year-old girl with excessive contractions, poor extremity, and head control but fairly good mental function was selected for SDR. Our aim in this last patient was basically to facilitate her care beside improvement in upper and lower limbs. This patient would be an example of a combined therapy of SDR with intensive physiotherapy, to reduce spasticity even in GMFCS levels 4 and 5 patients [8].

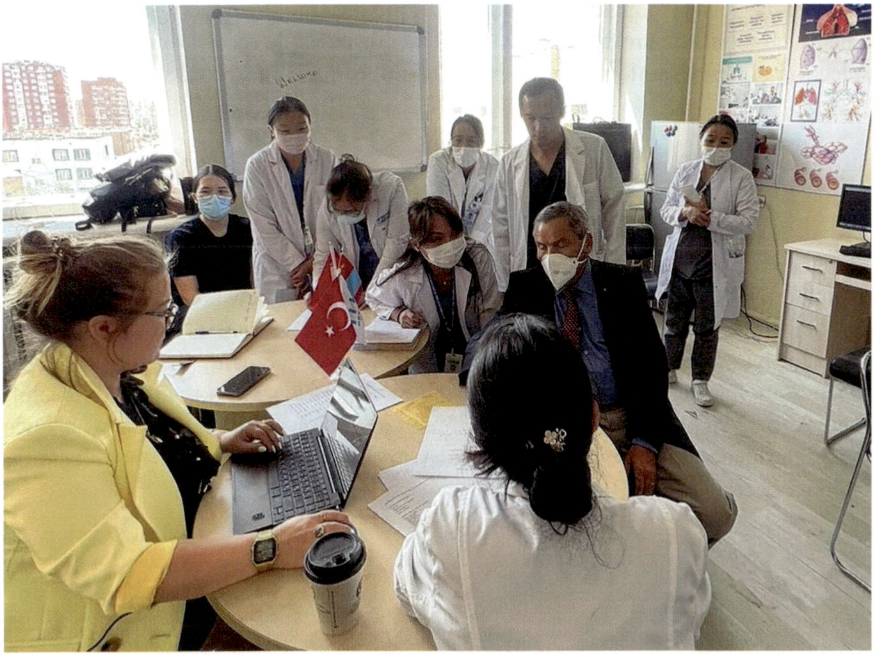

Fig. 17.1 Discussion about spastic children with Mongolian colleagues on the first visit to Ulaanbaatar

17.4 The SDR Technique We Used in Spastic Children, the SDR Team, and Surgery

In our practice, all children underwent surgery under general and total intravenous anesthesia (TIVA). In all patients, a rostrally reflected osteoplastic laminotomy between L2 to S1 levels is used. Under operating microscope, each dorsal nerve root is divided into several rootlets. The amount of rootlet cut varied according to the preoperatively determined Modified Ashworth Scale of each muscle group functions.

During the SDR, two local attending neurosurgeons assisted the surgery. They performed many rootlet cuttings under our guidance, and they learned how to perform rhizotomy by doing it practically.

The dorsal rhizotomy is a relatively simple surgery and may be easily performed in a standard neurosurgery operating room. However, selective dorsal rhizotomy needs an electrophysiology technician in the selection of nerve rootlets. The selection is based on intraoperative electrophysiologic data obtained with stimulation of each nerve rootlet.

Therefore, the electrophysiology technician's role in SDR surgery is essentially unique.

My experience is that the minimum SDR practice in the operating room requires a neurosurgeon, a neuromonitoring technician responsible for neuromonitoring and selection of nerve rootlets, and an anesthesiologist for TIVA procedure.

17.5 The Second Visit to Ulaanbaatar

Six months after the initial surgeries, we visited Ulaanbaatar again for the follow-up examination of operated children and for consultation of new children with spastic cerebral palsy (Fig. 17.2). We had the chance to see four patients who underwent SDR during our previous visit. We were already in contact with physiotherapy and rehabilitation specialists taking care of the SDR patients. On a regular basis, children were given physiotherapy with exercises in sessions using orthotics to enhance the performance of lower limbs relaxed with rhizotomy. Children made a fairly good recovery after SDR.

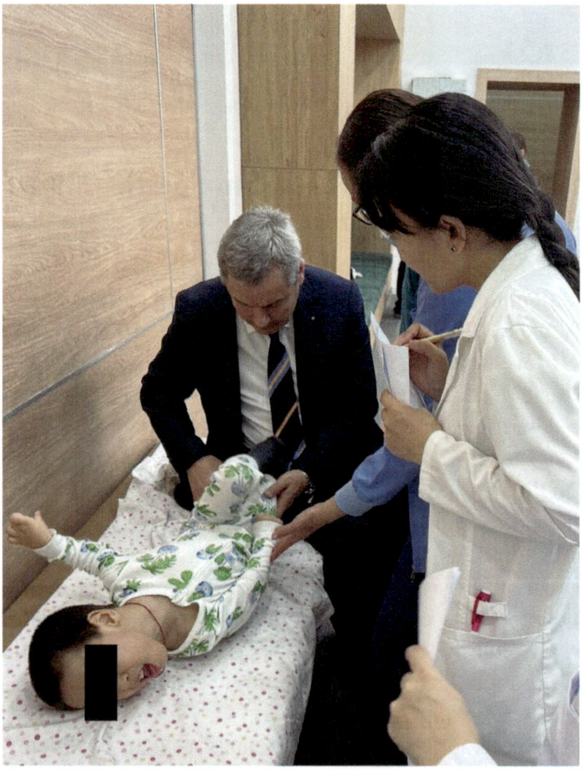

Fig. 17.2 Examination of a spastic child in the outpatient clinic on the second visit to Ulaanbaatar

17.6 Considerations and Factors for the Sustainable Rhizotomy Practice

The selection of rootlets to cut based on electrophysiologic findings is the crucial point of the SDR procedure. The role of the electrophysiology technician experienced in SDR surgery is vital.

In my practice of spasticity surgery, my personal motto is always: *Instead of rowing (physiotherapy) against the current (ongoing spasticity), row (more effective physiotherapy) with the current behind you (after rhizotomy).* The presence of sustainable physiotherapy and rehabilitation facilities and family support are mandatory. In spastic cerebral palsy, rehabilitation is a long process extending for years depending on the patient's clinical status. For a sustainable general rhizotomy program, easy access to physiotherapy and a rehabilitation facility is needed. Family support is essential for regularly doing muscle group exercises at home.

The limitation of this study is that we have only initiated SDR surgery and have the opportunity to see early results 6 months later. Administratively, more permanent and longer-term cooperation between institutions is expected. Although we have tried to initiate SDR surgeries in a foreign country, one cannot say that we have reached the desired level of sustainability. In order to overcome this inconvenience and make the SDR program more permanent and sustainable, much longer- and long-term visits, more surgeries, and the training of a qualified local SDR team are required.

In conclusion, based on our experience, I think that the minimum of a SDR surgery team for starting up rhizotomy surgery in a foreign country is a pediatric neurosurgeon experienced with SDR surgery, an electrophysiology technician responsible for selection of nerve rootlets, an anesthesiologist, and a physiotherapist responsible for patient selection and rehabilitation follow-up, with accessible physiotherapy and rehabilitation facilities and continuous family support.

Acknowledgements I wish to thank Mr. Uğur Özcan for his electrophysiologic support in all SDR surgeries; Mrs. Zhannera Khayrdzhankyzy, Liv Hospital, for organization; Dr. Abay Siyez, attending neurosurgeon, Third State Central Hospital of Ulaanbaatar; Dr. Byambatsend Dorjsuren, attending pediatric neurosurgeon, National Center for Maternal and Child Health; Dr. Munhdelger Suren from Ministry of Health, Mongolia, for her help in Ulaanbaatar; Dr. Ozan Başkurt for editorial assistance; and Dr. Sinan Hiçdönmez for revising the manuscript.

Declaration of Interest There is no conflict of interest. The author declares that the study is conducted in the absence of any commercial or financial relationships and did not receive any specific grant from funding agencies in the public, commercial, or not-for-profit sectors.

Compliance with Ethical Standards None.

References

1. Albright AL. Spasticity and movement disorders in cerebral palsy. Child's Nerv Syst ChNS Off J Int Soc Pediatr Neurosurg. 2023;39(10):2877–86. https://doi.org/10.1007/s00381-023-06045-5.
2. Steinbok P. Outcomes after selective dorsal rhizotomy for spastic cerebral palsy. Child's Nerv Syst ChNS Off J Int Soc Pediatr Neurosurg. 2001;17(1–2):1–18. https://doi.org/10.1007/pl00013722.
3. Mortenson P, Sadashiva N, Tamber MS, Steinbok P. Long-term upper extremity performance in children with cerebral palsy following selective dorsal rhizotomy. Child's Nerv Syst ChNS Off J Int Soc Pediatr Neurosurg. 2021;37(6):1983–9. https://doi.org/10.1007/s00381-020-05018-2.
4. Tu A, Steinbok P. Long term outcome of selective dorsal Rhizotomy for the management of childhood spasticity-functional improvement and complications. Child's Nerv Syst ChNS Off J Int Soc Pediatr Neurosurg. 2020;36(9):1985–94. https://doi.org/10.1007/s00381-020-04747-8.
5. Mediratta S, Lippa L, Venturini S, Demetriades AK, El-Ouahabi A, Gandía-González ML, et al. Current state of global neurosurgery activity amongst European neurosurgeons. J Neurosurg Sci. 2022;68:371–8. https://doi.org/10.23736/S0390-5616.21.05447-3.
6. Dewan MC, Baticulon RE, Rattani A, Johnston JM, Warf BC, Harkness W. Pediatric neurosurgical workforce, access to care, equipment and training needs worldwide. Neurosurg Focus. 2018;45(4):E13. https://doi.org/10.3171/2018.7.FOCUS18272.
7. Davis MC, Rocque BG, Singhal A, Ridder T, Pattisapu JV, Johnston JMJ. State of global pediatric neurosurgery outreach: survey by the international education subcommittee. J Neurosurg Pediatr. 2017;20(2):204–10. https://doi.org/10.3171/2017.3.PEDS16433.
8. D'Aquino D, Moussa AA, Ammar A, Ingale H, Vloeberghs M. Selective dorsal rhizotomy for the treatment of severe spastic cerebral palsy: efficacy and therapeutic durability in GMFCS grade IV and V children. Acta Neurochir. 2018;160(4):811–21. https://doi.org/10.1007/s00701-017-3349-z.

Chapter 18
New Developments in the Surgery for Spasticity

J. M. N. Enslin

18.1 Introduction

Management of spasticity in the twenty-first century is still based mainly on two tiers: lesioning procedures on the one hand—selective dorsal rhizotomy (SDR), selective peripheral neurotomy (SPN), and dorsal root entry zone lesioning (DREZotomy)—and medical treatment with oral and intrathecal Baclofen (ITB) on the other. Botulinum toxin, in its various formulations, is used to affect the injected abnormal muscle tone temporarily. The lesioning techniques have been in use since the late 1800s [1], while ITB was first used in 1991 [2] and approved for use in treating spasticity in children in 1996 [3]. Figure 18.1 shows the timeline of significant developments in managing spasticity.

Unfortunately, we are only treating the symptoms with these methods. We are still not able to cure cerebral palsy nor prevent it, and we are not able to reverse the causes of spasticity.

A common criticism against using lesioning techniques for spasticity treatment is that "this will disqualify the patient from future, better treatments and possible cures." The concern is, however, that we have had more than 200 years since Sherrington's physiological description, which formed our early understanding of spasticity [4]. Nevertheless, we are not much closer to treating the cause nor are we

J. M. N. Enslin (✉)
Division of Neurosurgery, Groote Schuur Hospital, University of Cape Town, Observatory, Cape Town, South Africa

Red Cross War Memorial Children's Hospital, Rondebosch, Cape Town, South Africa

Neuroscience Institute, University of Cape Town, Observatory, Cape Town, South Africa
e-mail: johannes.enslin@uct.ac.za

N. Morota, P. Steinbok (eds.), *Dorsal Rhizotomy: Neurosurgery for Childhood Spasticity*, Advances and Technical Standards in Neurosurgery 51,
https://doi.org/10.1007/978-3-031-86441-4_18

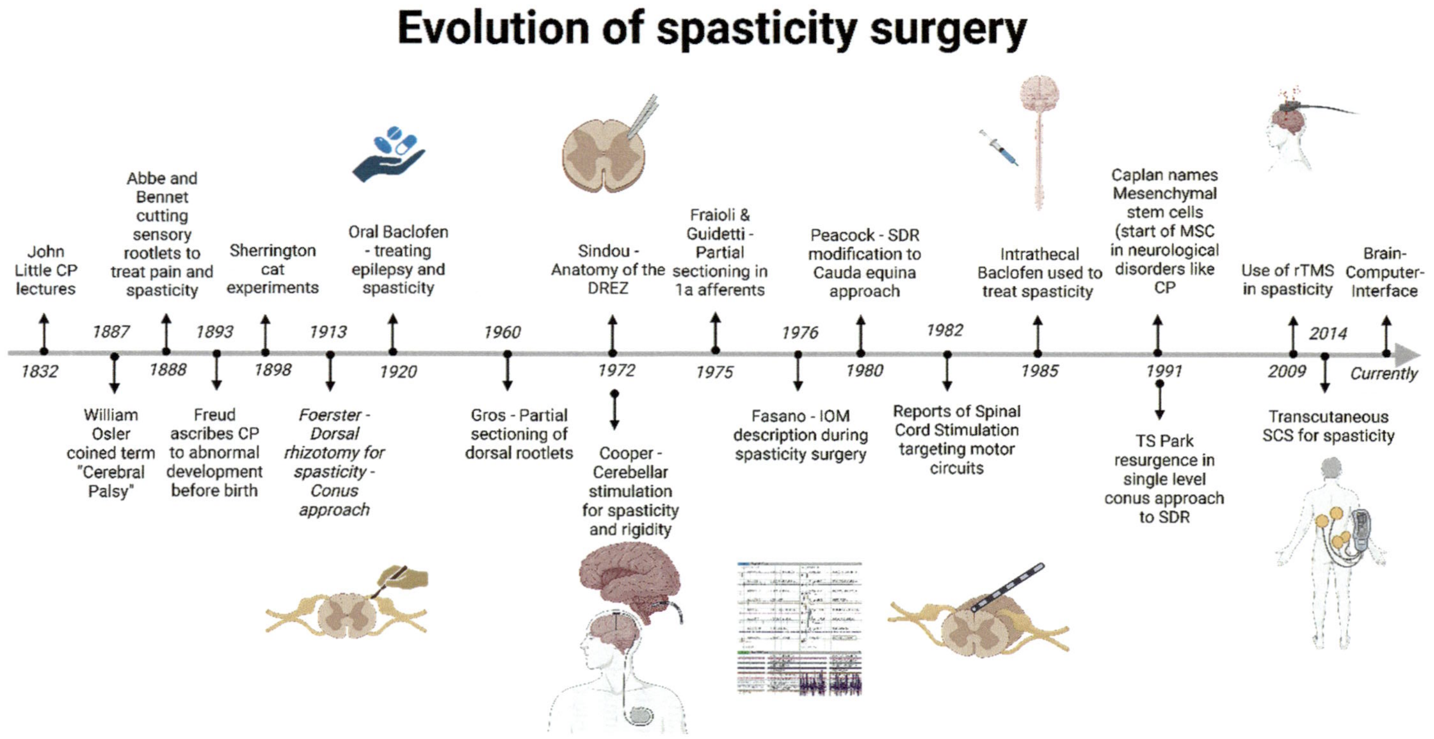

Fig. 18.1 Timeline on the evolution of spasticity management. (Created with BioRender.com) [1–12]

very good at selectively modifying the biomechanical impairments of the individual with difficulty performing activities of daily living and walking. Until such a time, we must continue searching for the best treatment strategy.

18.2 Improvements in Intraoperative Neuromonitoring (IONM) for Surgery

Over the past two decades, we have made many intraoperative neuromonitoring (IONM) advances. Fasano further refined the original principles espoused by Foerster and later Gros, and we still use these principles, as recommended by Fasano, in our current SDR techniques [5–12]. Various groups have published their unique findings and intraoperative monitoring principles during SDR [13–18], and there is constant improvement in our search for selectivity that will allow better preservation of proprioceptive and postural function and, hopefully, isolate and impact the nerve fascicles that contribute to spasticity. This area will continue progressing in the years to come and will allow us to identify the fascicles to section and, more importantly, which to leave alone, all helping to improve function in patients with spasticity.

18.3 Advances in Surgical Approaches to SDR

Our approach to SDR is becoming more refined, with fewer complications, better wound healing, and less postoperative pain being the goal. Many different surgical approaches and access to the spinal cord have been described and summarized by Warsi et al. [19]. Most surgeons try to follow a minimal exposure technique, while others [20] also modify the cauda equina exposure technique.

18.4 Neuromodulation Techniques

The significant advances are probably going to lie in neuromodulation techniques [21, 22]. These techniques are advertised as less invasive and cause no permanent changes. From the data on deep brain stimulation for movement disorders, we know this is not entirely true, as all neuromodulation leads to neural plasticity changes [23]. The less destructive approach does, however, lead to more families being open to considering these techniques for managing spasticity in their children. The author will briefly discuss spinal cord stimulation and deep brain stimulation as two forms of neuromodulation.

18.5 Spinal Cord Stimulation

The first report on spinal cord stimulation used for refractory pain in a patient with multiple sclerosis was published by Cook and Weinstein in 1973 [24]. Their patient also had good improvement in spasticity [24]. Many groups are currently evaluating the role of spinal cord stimulation in managing spasticity, with promising results [25]. Patients with spinal cord injury have additional benefits in improving their bladder capacity and pain, as well as autonomic functions [25, 26].

Noninvasive spinal cord stimulation has also been shown to improve lower limb spasticity in patients after spinal cord injury, specifically in a meta-analysis by Massey et al. [27]. Jocelyne Bloch and colleagues in Switzerland are doing fantastic work combining epidural spinal cord stimulation with brain control via electrocorticography and motor cortex activation in patients with spinal cord injury and spasticity [28]. This seems to be a promising development in spasticity surgery.

18.6 Deep Brain Stimulation

Cooper started implanting cerebellar stimulation electrodes on the surface of the cerebellum in the 1970s already [29]. Current advances in deep brain stimulation and better imaging and targeting techniques have led to neurosurgeons performing deep brain stimulation of the dentate nuclei [30] and other nuclei [31] in patients with cerebral palsy and other causes of spasticity.

Chronic cerebellar stimulation to the superomedial cortex of the cerebellum has been shown to reduce spasticity and athetoid movements [32]. In a double-blind study, Davis showed a 60% improvement in motor function and joint range of motion in patients with chronic cerebellar stimulation [32]. These results also seem to be effective over the long term, with their patients showing improvement for up to 17 years [32].

In most studies looking at deep brain stimulation, there seems to be some benefit in patients' spasticity, associated movement disorders, and overall functioning, with up to 40% improvement in some dystonia scales, mainly [30]. With advances in closed-loop technology, our improved ability to visualize targets, and different stimulation parameters, this may be a therapy to watch in the future.

18.7 Extracorporeal Shockwave Therapy

With extracorporeal shock wave therapy (ESW), a sequence of acoustic impulses is applied to the spastic limb of a patient with spasticity. Some preliminary studies show sound effects, but further research is still needed. A meta-analysis done recently was inconclusive, although promising [33].

18.8 Transcranial Magnetic Stimulation

Transcranial magnetic stimulation (TMS) is a form of neuromodulation whereby an electrical current, which passes through a coil on the head, will generate a magnetic field [34]. This magnetic field creates a membrane depolarization in a predictable focal area of the brain. Repetitive transcranial magnetic stimulation (rTMS) is the clinical application of this technique, whereby action potentials are created within the cerebral cortex. In a systematic review, where 19 publications were reviewed [34], the authors showed a reduction in spasticity when TMS is combined with a comprehensive rehabilitation strategy, including regular physiotherapy and medication.

The beneficial effects are only significant in spasticity secondary to spinal cord injury [34]. The authors found no evidence for the use of TMS in stroke patients [34]. There also seems to be a significant variance in the effects of TMS on spasticity related to the type of stimulation protocol applied [34]. Mori and colleagues have demonstrated a clear benefit of the H-reflex, as a measure of stretch reflex, after TMS to the leg motor cortex, with a reduction in spasticity [35]. There may, therefore, be room for further advances in this area, primarily related to treating spasticity in spinal cord injured patients and those with spinal cord pathology.

18.9 Transcranial Direct Current Stimulation (tDCS)

Transcranial direct current stimulation is another noninvasive tool that differs from the other forms of cortical stimulation, such as TMS, in that it is seen as a neuromodulation technique. tDCS does not induce neuronal action potentials, as does TMS [36]. The stimulated cortex is polarized, and neuronal excitability is modified by low current density and tonic stimulation [36].

In patients with multiple sclerosis (MS), the group of El Habashy has shown that there is some improvement in spasticity compared to the sham group [37]. This protocol requires transcortical stimulation over the primary motor cortex, on the same side as the MS lesion, for 20 minutes for 5 days [37]. These same benefits could not be achieved in patients after stroke, however [38]. There is no benefit shown in cerebral palsy, either [39].

18.10 Transcutaneous Electrical Nerve Stimulation and Transcutaneous Spinal Cord Stimulation

Transcutaneous electrical nerve stimulation (TENS) is a form of electrical stimulation whereby biphasic and asymmetric square waves treat pain [39]. This modality can also be delivered at low frequencies of 1–2 Hz, leading to sensory stimulation only and reduced hyperexcitability. Some studies show that, combined with a comprehensive physiotherapy exercise program, there may be some minor benefit to spasticity in patients if used regularly [39]. When stimulating the muscles that are affected by spasticity directly (neuromuscular stimulation), especially as part of a planned motor activation strategy—called functional electrical stimulation (FES)—the rehabilitation process is augmented with active-assisted functional limb movements, for example, dorsiflexion during gait training [27, 39]. This also shows minor improvements in tone in patients [39].

In studies that looked at transcutaneous spinal cord stimulation, there were also good results with reduced spasticity and improved function for up to 2 h after a 30-min transcutaneous (noninvasive) spinal cord stimulation in patients with spasticity after spinal cord injury [40, 41]. This makes home-based therapy an option for patients.

It is still early to evaluate the effectiveness of spinal cord stimulation on chronic spasticity, but it does seem promising in the future.

18.11 Whole-Body Vibration Therapy

Whole-body vibration therapy reduces whole-body spasticity for a period after the therapy. Researchers postulate that the vibration stimulates the alpha motor neurons and muscle spindles, thereby reducing spasticity [39]. This short-term treatment may be helpful in combination with other treatments and rehabilitation [39].

18.12 Gene Therapy

Many recent studies demonstrate that more than 10% of children with cerebral palsy have a genetic cause [42–46]. One study reported that up to one in four children with cerebral palsy may have a genetic component to their spasticity [47]. With the advances in genetic diagnostic processes and the identification of single-gene therapies, many new genetic treatment strategies may be available for patients with congenital and hereditary spasticity. The best current example is hereditary spastic paraparesis (HSP), where gene therapies are already being used [48, 49]. These strategies are not aimed at spasticity but, rather, the cause of the spasticity and may even be able to prevent spasticity in the future.

18.13 Stem Cell Therapy

Treatment or reversal of the underlying cause of the spasticity—albeit cerebral palsy, cerebral infarction, trauma, and demyelination—remains the holy grail of caring for patients with spasticity. The therapies mentioned above, except gene therapy, are all symptomatic treatments at best. We still cannot cure the conditions and reverse the associated spasticity. Stem cell therapy offers a glimmer of hope that somewhere in the future, we may be able to treat the cause and have ways of completely reversing or preventing spasticity.

There have been many trials, and many are still in process, on using stem cells in treating stroke and cerebral palsy patients [50]. The studies that have concluded thus far show no clear benefit in the spasticity component [51, 52]. Hopefully, a breakthrough will happen soon, and we can all stop lesioning or performing neuromodulation for most patients with spasticity.

18.14 Conclusion

With significant advances in our understanding of the human nervous system, better imaging, and ongoing gene discoveries, we may be on the threshold of understanding and curing spasticity and the conditions that cause it. The work on gene therapies and brain–spine–computer interfaces are all very promising. In the meantime, many patients with function-impairing spasticity require our help today. It is unlikely that all cases will be curable in the future, and we should continue researching and teaching the lesioning and neuromodulation techniques so that future generations can also aid patients with spasticity using these techniques.

References

1. Enslin JMN, Langerak NG, Fieggen AG. The evolution of selective dorsal rhizotomy for the management of spasticity. Neurotherapeutics. 2019;15(16):3–8.
2. Winter G, Beni-Adani L, Ben-Pazi H. Intrathecal baclofen therapy—practical approach: clinical benefits and complication management. J Child Neurol. 2018;33(11):734–41. https://doi.org/10.1177/0883073818785074.
3. Turner MS. Early use of intrathecal baclofen in brain injury in pediatric patients. Acta Neurochir Suppl. 2003;87:81–3. https://doi.org/10.1007/978-3-7091-6081-7_17.
4. Sherrington CS. On reciprocal innervation of antagonistic muscles. In: Third note, Proceedings of the Royal Society of London, vol. 60; 1897. p. 414–7. https://doi.org/10.1098/rspl.1896.0062.
5. Foerster P. Resection of the posterior spinal nerve-roots in the treatment of gastric crises and spastic paralysis. SAGE Publications; 1911.
6. Privat J, Benezech J, Frerebeau P, Gros C. Sectorial posterior rhizotomy, a new technique of surgical treatment for spasticity. Acta Neurochir. 1976;35:181–95.
7. Foerster O. On the indications and results of the excision of posterior spinal nerve roots in men. Surg Gynecol Obstet. 1913;16:463–75.
8. Gros C, Ouaknine G, Vlahovitch B, Frerebeau P. La radicotomie sélective postérieure dans le traitement neuro-chirurgical de lhypertonie pyramidale. Neurochirurgie. 1967;13:505−+.
9. Smyth MD, Peacock WJ. The surgical treatment of spasticity. Muscle Nerve: Official J American Assoc Electrodiagnostic Med. 2000;23:153–63.

10. Gros C. Spasticity—clinical classification and surgical treatment, advances and technical standards in neurosurgery. Springer; 1979. p. 55–97.
11. Fasano V, Broggi G, Barolat-Romana G, Sguazzi A. Surgical treatment of spasticity in cerebral palsy. Pediatr Neurosurg. 1978;4:289–305.
12. Fasano VA, Barolat-Romana G, Zeme S, Sguazzi A. Electrophysiological assessment of spinal circuits in spasticity by direct dorsal root stimulation. Neurosurgery. 1979;4:146–51.
13. Jiang W, Zhan Q, Wang J, Mei R, Xiao B. Intraoperative neurophysiological monitoring in selective dorsal rhizotomy (SDR). Brain Sci Adv. 2020;6(1):56–67. https://doi.org/10.26599/BSA.2020.9050009.
14. Nishida T, Storrs BB. Electrophysiological monitoring in selective posterior rhizotomy for spasticity: principles, techniques and interpretation of responses. In: Sindou MP, Abbott IR, Keravel Y, editors. Neurosurgery for spasticity. Vienna: Springer; 1991. https://doi.org/10.1007/978-3-7091-6708-3_23.
15. De Vloo P, Huttunen TJ, Forte D, Jankovic I, Lee A, Hair M, Cawker S, Chugh D, Carr L, Crowe BH, Pitt M. Intraoperative electrophysiology during single-level selective dorsal rhizotomy: technique, stimulation threshold, and response data in a series of 145 patients. J Neurosurg Pediatr. 2020;25(6):597–606.
16. Georgoulis G, Sindou M. Muscle responses to radicular stimulation during lumbo-sacral dorsal rhizotomy for spastic diplegia: insights to myotome innervation. Clin Neurophysiol. 2020;131(5):1075–86.
17. Georgoulis G, Brînzeu A, Sindou M. Dorsal rhizotomy for children with spastic diplegia of cerebral palsy origin: usefulness of intraoperative monitoring. J Neurosurg Pediatr. 2018;22(1):89–101.
18. Sindou M, Georgoulis G, Joud A, Neromyliotis E, Dinopoulos A. Excitability of the radiculomedullary circuitry in spastic cerebral palsy: an intraoperative neurophysiological study in children undergoing selective dorsal rhizotomy. Dev Med Child Neurol. 2023;65(1):78–85.
19. Warsi NM, Tailor J, Coulter IC, Shakil H, Workewych A, Haldenby R, Breitbart S, Strantzas S, Vandenberk M, Dewan MC, Ibrahim GM. Selective dorsal rhizotomy: an illustrated review of operative techniques. J Neurosurg Pediatr. 2020;7:1–8. https://doi.org/10.3171/2019.12.PEDS19629. Epub ahead of print
20. Sindou M, Georgoulis G. Keyhole interlaminar dorsal rhizotomy for spastic diplegia in cerebral palsy. Acta Neurochir. 2015;157(7):1187–96. https://doi.org/10.1007/s00701-015-2453-1. Epub 2015 May 24
21. Damián Carrillo-Ruíz J, Quetzalcoatl Beltran J, Rodrigo Carrillo-Márquez J, Luis Navarro-Olvera J, García L, Villegas-López F, et al. Neurosurgical spasticity treatment: from lesion to Neuromodulation procedures [internet]. Frontiers Clinical Neurosurgery IntechOpen. 2021; Available from: https://doi.org/10.5772/intechopen.960
22. Hodge JO, Brandmeir CL, Brandmeir NJ. Neuromodulation therapies for spasticity control: now and beyond. Neurol India. 2020;68(8):241.
23. van Hartevelt TJ, Cabral J, Deco G, Møller A, Green AL, Aziz TZ, Kringelbach ML. Neural plasticity in human brain connectivity: the effects of long term deep brain stimulation of the subthalamic nucleus in Parkinson's disease. PLoS One. 2014;9(1):e86496. https://doi.org/10.1371/journal.pone.0086496. PMID: 24466120; PMCID: PMC3899266.
24. Cook AW, Weinstein SP. Chronic dorsal column stimulation in multiple sclerosis. Preliminary report. N Y State J Med. 1973;73(24):2868–72.
25. Huang XL, Chen YC, Kuo CC, Tsai ST. Potential benefits of spinal cord stimulation treatment on quality of life for paralyzed patients with spinal cord injury. Tzu Chi Med J. 2022;35(2):131–6. https://doi.org/10.4103/tcmj.tcmj_102_22. PMID: 37261296; PMCID: PMC10227680
26. Rowald A, Komi S, Demesmaeker R, et al. Activity-dependent spinal cord neuromodulation rapidly restores trunk and leg motor functions after complete paralysis. Nat Med. 2022;28:260–71. https://doi.org/10.1038/s41591-021-01663-5.

27. Massey S, Vanhoestenberghe A, Duffell L. Neurophysiological and clinical outcome measures of the impact of electrical stimulation on spasticity in spinal cord injury: systematic review and meta-analysis. Front Rehabil Sci. 2022;16(3):1058663.
28. Bloch J, et al. Study in progress: ClinicalTrials.gov Identifier: NCT05665998.
29. Cooper IS, Riklan M, Amin I, Waltz JM, Cullinan T. Chronic cerebellar stimulation in cerebral palsy. Neurology. 1976;26(8):744–53.
30. Cajigas I, Morrison MA, San Luciano M, Starr P. Cerebellar deep brain stimulation in cerebral palsy: promising early results and a look forward to a larger clinical trial. World Neurosurg. 2023;174:223.
31. Elias GJ, Namasivayam AA, Lozano AM. Deep brain stimulation for stroke: current uses and future directions. Brain Stimul. 2018;11(1):3–28.
32. Davis R. Cerebellar stimulation for cerebral palsy spasticity, function, and seizures. Arch Med Res. 2000;31(3):290–9. https://doi.org/10.1016/s0188-4409(00)00065-5.
33. Zhang H-L, Jin R-J, Guan L, Zhong D-L, Li Y-X, Liu X-B, Xiao Q-W, Xiao X-L, Li J. Extracorporeal shock wave therapy on spasticity after upper motor neuron injury: a systematic review and meta-analysis. Am J Phys Med Rehabil. 2022;101(7):615–23. https://doi.org/10.1097/PHM.0000000000001977.
34. Korzhova J, Sinitsyn D, Chervyakov A, Poydasheva A, Zakharova M, Suponeva N, Chernikova L, Piradov M. Transcranial and spinal cord magnetic stimulation in treatment of spasticity: a literature review and meta-analysis. Eur J Phys Rehabil Med. 2018;54(1):75–84.
35. Mori F, Koch G, Foti C, Bernardi G, Centonze D. The use of repetitive transcranial magnetic stimulation (rTMS) for the treatment of spasticity. Prog Brain Res. 2009;175:429–39.
36. Nitsche MA, Cohen LG, Wassermann EM, Priori A, Lang N, Antal A, Paulus W, Hummel F, Boggio PS, Fregni F, Pascual-Leone A. Transcranial direct current stimulation: state of the art 2008. Brain Stimul. 2008;1(3):206–23.
37. El Habashy HR, El Sawy N, Al Menabbawy S, Dahshan A. Transcranial direct current stimulation for spasticity in patients with multiple sclerosis: exploring novel routes. Mult Scler Relat Disord. 2022;1(67):104191.
38. Elsner B, Kugler J, Pohl M, et al. Transcranial direct current stimulation for improving spasticity after stroke: a systematic review with meta-analysis. J Rehabil Med. 2016;48(7):565–70.
39. Naro A, Leo A, Russo M, Casella C, Buda A, Crespantini A, Porcari B, Carioti L, Billeri L, Bramanti A, Bramanti P. Breakthroughs in the spasticity management: are non-pharmacological treatments the future? J Clin Neurosci. 2017;39:16–27.
40. Alashram AR, Padua E, Raju M, Romagnoli C, Annino G. Transcutaneous spinal cord stimulation effects on spasticity in patients with spinal cord injury: a systematic review. J Spinal Cord Med. 2023;46(4):582–9.
41. Hofstoetter US, Freundl B, Danner SM, Krenn MJ, Mayr W, Binder H, Minassian K. Transcutaneous spinal cord stimulation induces temporary attenuation of spasticity in individuals with spinal cord injury. J Neurotrauma. 2020;37(3):481–93.
42. Jin SC, Lewis SA, Bakhtiari S, Zeng X, Sierant MC, Shetty S, Nordlie SM, Elie A, Corbett MA, Norton BY, van Eyk CL. Mutations disrupting neuritogenesis genes confer risk for cerebral palsy. Nat Genet. 2020;52(10):1046–56.
43. Lewis SA, Shetty S, Wilson BA, Huang AJ, Jin SC, Smithers-Sheedy H, Fahey MC, Kruer MC. Insights from genetic studies of cerebral palsy. Front Neurol. 2021;11:625428.
44. Li N, Zhou P, Tang H, He L, Fang X, Zhao J, Wang X, Qi Y, Sun C, Lin Y, Qin F. In-depth analysis reveals complex molecular aetiology in a cohort of idiopathic cerebral palsy. Brain. 2022;145(1):119–41.
45. Gonzalez-Mantilla PJ, Hu Y, Myers SM, Finucane BM, Ledbetter DH, Martin CL, Moreno-De-Luca A. Diagnostic yield of exome sequencing in cerebral palsy and implications for genetic testing guidelines: a systematic review and meta-analysis. JAMA Pediatr. 2023;177:472.
46. Friedman JM, van Essen P, van Karnebeek CD. Cerebral palsy and related neuromotor disorders: overview of genetic and genomic studies. Mol Genet Metab. 2022;137(4):399–419.

47. Chopra M, Gable DL, Love-Nichols J, Tsao A, Rockowitz S, Sliz P, Barkoudah E, Bastianelli L, Coulter D, Davidson E, DeGusmao C, Fogelman D, Huth K, Marshall P, Nimec D, Sanders JS, Shore BJ, Snyder B, Stone SSD, Ubeda A, Watkins C, Berde C, Bolton J, Brownstein C, Costigan M, Ebrahimi-Fakhari D, Lai A, O'Donnell-Luria A, Paciorkowski AR, Pinto A, Pugh J, Rodan L, Roe E, Swanson L, Zhang B, Kruer MC, Sahin M, Poduri A, Srivastava S. Mendelian etiologies identified with whole exome sequencing in cerebral palsy. Ann Clin Transl Neurol. 2022;9:193–205. https://doi.org/10.1002/acn3.51506.
48. Brent JR, Deng HX. Paving a way to treat spastic paraplegia 50. J Clin Invest. 2023;133(10):e170226.
49. Mohan N, Qiang L, Morfini G, Baas PW. Therapeutic strategies for mutant SPAST-based hereditary spastic paraplegia. Brain Sci. 2021;11(8):1081.
50. Jensen A. Cerebral palsy–brain repair with stem cells. J Perinat Med. 2023;51(6):737–51.
51. Vaquero J, Zurita M, Rico MA, Aguayo C, Bonilla C, Marin E, et al. Intrathecal administration of autologous mesenchymal stromal cells for spinal cord injury: safety and efficacy of the 100/3 guideline. Cytotherapy. 2018;20(6):806–19.
52. Levi AD, Anderson KD, Okonkwo DO, Park P, Bryce TN, Kurpad SN, et al. Clinical outcomes from a multi-center study of human neural stem cell transplantation in chronic cervical spinal cord injury. J Neurotrauma. 2019;36(6):891–902.

GPSR Compliance

The European Union's (EU) General Product Safety Regulation (GPSR) is a set of rules that requires consumer products to be safe and our obligations to ensure this.

If you have any concerns about our products, you can contact us on ProductSafety@springernature.com

In case Publisher is established outside the EU, the EU authorized representative is:

Springer Nature Customer Service Center GmbH
Europaplatz 3
69115 Heidelberg, Germany

Batch number: 10726060

Printed by Printforce, the Netherlands